AMERICAN ACADEMY
OF OPHTHALMOLOGY®
Protecting Sight. Empowering Lives.

MW01701988

13 | Refractive Surgery

Last major revision 2021–2022

2022–2023

BCSC

Basic and Clinical Science Course™

EB

Published after collaborative review with the European Board of Ophthalmology subcommittee

The American Academy of Ophthalmology is accredited by the Accreditation Council for Continuing Medical Education (ACCME) to provide continuing medical education for physicians.

The American Academy of Ophthalmology designates this enduring material for a maximum of 10 *AMA PRA Category 1 Credits*™. Physicians should claim only the credit commensurate with the extent of their participation in the activity.

CME expiration date: June 1, 2024. *AMA PRA Category 1 Credits*™ may be claimed only once between June 1, 2021, and the expiration date.

BCSC® volumes are designed to increase the physician's ophthalmic knowledge through study and review. Users of this activity are encouraged to read the text and then answer the study questions provided at the back of the book.

To claim *AMA PRA Category 1 Credits*™ upon completion of this activity, learners must demonstrate appropriate knowledge and participation in the activity by taking the posttest for Section 13 and achieving a score of 80% or higher. For further details, please see the instructions for requesting CME credit at the back of the book.

The Academy provides this material for educational purposes only. It is not intended to represent the only or best method or procedure in every case, nor to replace a physician's own judgment or give specific advice for case management. Including all indications, contraindications, side effects, and alternative agents for each drug or treatment is beyond the scope of this material. All information and recommendations should be verified, prior to use, with current information included in the manufacturers' package inserts or other independent sources, and considered in light of the patient's condition and history. Reference to certain drugs, instruments, and other products in this course is made for illustrative purposes only and is not intended to constitute an endorsement of such. Some material may include information on applications that are not considered community standard, that reflect indications not included in approved FDA labeling, or that are approved for use only in restricted research settings. **The FDA has stated that it is the responsibility of the physician to determine the FDA status of each drug or device he or she wishes to use, and to use them with appropriate, informed patient consent in compliance with applicable law.** The Academy specifically disclaims any and all liability for injury or other damages of any kind, from negligence or otherwise, for any and all claims that may arise from the use of any recommendations or other information contained herein.

Cover image: From BCSC Section 12, *Retina and Vitreous.* Confocal scanning laser ophthalmoscopy multicolor fundus image (30° field of view) of a healthy eye. *(Courtesy of Lucia Sobrin, MD.)*

FSC
www.fsc.org
MIX
Paper from responsible sources
FSC® C001701

Printed in China.

Basic and Clinical Science Course

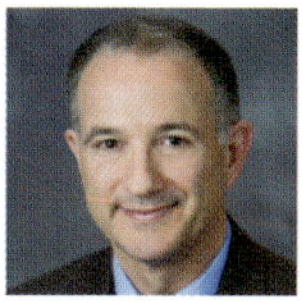

Christopher J. Rapuano, MD, Philadelphia, Pennsylvania
Senior Secretary for Clinical Education

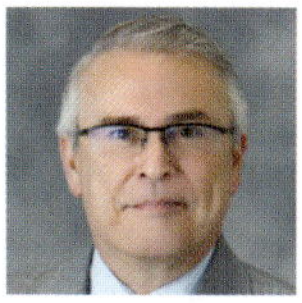

J. Timothy Stout, MD, PhD, MBA, Houston, Texas
Secretary for Lifelong Learning and Assessment

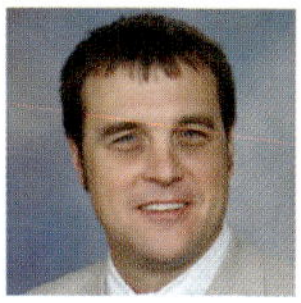

Colin A. McCannel, MD, Los Angeles, California
BCSC Course Chair

Section 13

Faculty for the Major Revision

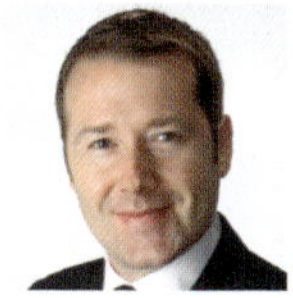

George O. Waring IV, MD
Chair
Charleston, South Carolina

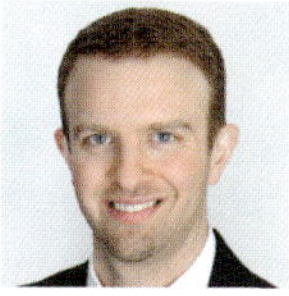

Sherman W. Reeves, MD, MPH
Minnetonka, Minnesota

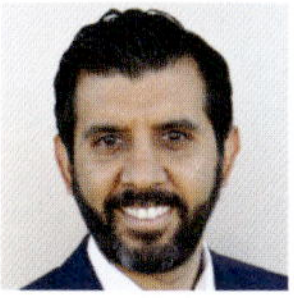

Sumit (Sam) Garg, MD
Irvine, California

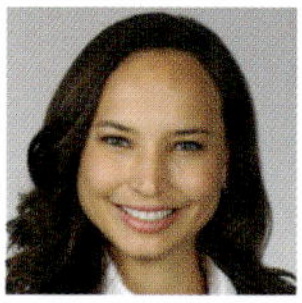

Karolinne Maia Rocha, MD, PhD
Charleston, South Carolina

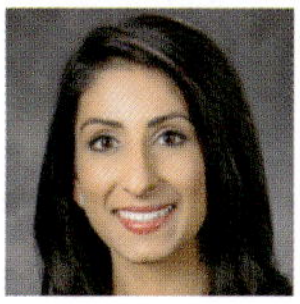

Preeya K. Gupta, MD
Durham, North Carolina

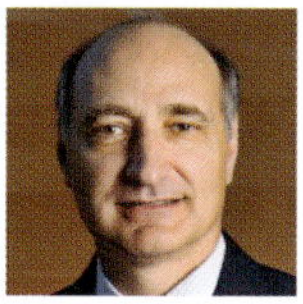

Michael J. Taravella, MD
Aurora, Colorado

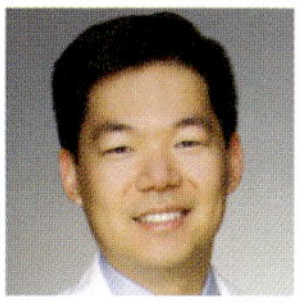

Bryan S. Lee, MD, JD
Los Altos, California

The Academy acknowledges the following committees for review of the major revision:

Committee on Aging: Ronald Luke Rebenitsch, MD, Oklahoma City, Oklahoma

Vision Rehabilitation Committee: Anne Riddering, PhD, Detroit, Michigan

BCSC Resident/Fellow Reviewers: Sharon L. Jick, MD, *Chair,* St Louis, Missouri; Shawn Lin, MD; Grace L. Paley, MD; Duo (David) Xu, MD

Practicing Ophthalmologists Advisory Committee for Education: Michelle S. Ying, MD, *Primary Reviewer,* Ladson, South Carolina; Bradley D. Fouraker, MD, *Chair,* Tampa, Florida; Cynthia S. Chiu, MD, Oakland, California; George S. Ellis Jr, MD, New Orleans, Louisiana; Stephen R. Klapper, MD, Carmel, Indiana; Gaurav K. Shah, MD, Town and Country, Missouri; Rosa A. Tang, MD, MPH, MBA, Houston, Texas; Troy M. Tanji, MD, Waipahu, Hawaii

In addition, the Academy acknowledges the following committee for assistance in developing Study Questions and Answers for this BCSC Section:

Resident Self-Assessment Committee: Evan L. Waxman, MD, PhD, *Chair,* Pittsburgh, Pennsylvania; Robert A. Beaulieu, MD, Royal Oak, Michigan; Benjamin W. Botsford, MD, New York, New York; Olga M. Ceron, MD, Grafton, Massachusetts; Eva DeVience, MD, Windsor Mill, Maryland; Kevin Halenda, MD, Cleveland, Ohio; Amanda D. Henderson, MD, Baltimore, Maryland; Andrew M. Hendrick, MD, Atlanta, Georgia; Joshua Hendrix, MD, Dalton, Georgia; Matthew B. Kaufman, MD, Portland, Oregon; Zachary A. Koretz, MD, MPH, Pittsburgh, Pennsylvania; Kevin E. Lai, MD, Indianapolis, Indiana; Kenneth C. Lao, MD, Temple, Texas; Yasha S. Modi, MD, New York, New York; Mark E. Robinson, MD, MPH, Columbia, South Carolina; Jamie B. Rosenberg, MD, New York, New York; Tahira Scholle, MD, Houston, Texas; Syed Mahmood Shah, MD, Pittsburgh, Pennsylvania; Ann Shue, MD, Sunnyvale, California; Jeong-Hyeon Sohn, MD, Shavano Park, Texas; Misha F. Syed, MD, League City, Texas; Parisa Taravati, MD, Seattle, Washington; Tanu O. Thomas, MD, El Paso, Texas; Sarah Van Tassel, MD, New York, New York; Matthew S. Wieder, MD, Scarsdale, New York; Jules A. Winokur, MD, Great Neck, New York

EB

European Board of Ophthalmology: Jesper Hjortdal, MD, PhD, *Chair,* Aarhus, Denmark; Marie-José Tassignon, MD, PhD, FEBO, *Liaison,* Edegem, Belgium; Roberto Bellucci, MD, Salò, Italy; Daniel Epstein, MD, PhD, Zurich, Switzerland; José L. Güell, MD, FEBO, Barcelona, Spain; Markus Kohlhaas, MD, Dortmund, Germany; Rudy M.M.A. Nuijts, MD, PhD, Maastricht, Netherlands

Financial Disclosures

Academy staff members who contributed to the development of this product state that within the 24 months prior to their contributions to this CME activity and for the duration of development, they have had no financial interest in or other relationship with any entity that produces, markets, resells, or distributes health care goods or services consumed by or used in patients, or with any competing commercial product or service.

The authors and reviewers state that within the 24 months prior to their contributions to this CME activity and for the duration of development, they have had the following financial relationships:*

Dr Bellucci: Alcon Laboratories (C), Bausch + Lomb Surgical (C)

Dr Fouraker: Addition Technology (C, L), AJL Ophthalmic, SA (C, L), Alcon (C, L), OASIS Medical (C, L)

Dr Garg: Abbott (C, L), Aerie Pharmaceuticals (C), Alcon (C), Allergan (C), Avedro (C), Dompé (C), EyePoint Pharmaceuticals (C), Eyevance Pharmaceuticals (C), Glaukos (C), Johnson & Johnson Vision (C), Kala Pharmaceuticals (C), LensGen (C, O), New World Medical (C), Novartis (C), Ocutrx (O), RPS (O), RxSight (C), RySurg (C), Shire/Takeda (C, L), SightLife Surgical (C), Sight Sciences (C), Tarsus Pharmaceuticals (C), Verana Health (C), VisionCare (C), ZEISS (C)

Dr Güell: Alcon Laboratories (C), Calhoun Vision (O), OPHTEC, BV (C), ZEISS (C)

Dr Gupta: Alcon (C), Allergan (C), Aurea Medical (C), Bio-Tissue (C), Johnson & Johnson Vision (C), Kala Pharmaceuticals (C), New World Medical (C), NovaBay Pharmaceuticals (C), Novartis (C), Ocular Science (C), ReGenTree (C), Shire/Takeda (C), Sight Sciences (C), Sun Pharma (C), TearLab Corporation (C), TearScience (C), ZEISS (C, L)

Dr Hjortdal: Carl Zeiss Meditec (L)

Dr Klapper: AdOM Advanced Optical Technologies (O)

Dr Lee: AcuFocus (S), Aerie Pharmaceuticals (C), Allergan (C), Carl Zeiss Meditec (S), Katena Products (C), New World Medical (C)

Dr Modi: Alimera Sciences (C), Allergan (C), Genentech (C), Théa (C), ZEISS (C)

Dr Nuijts: Alcon Laboratories (L, S), ASICO (P), Bausch + Lomb (C)

Dr Rebenitsch: AcuFocus (L), Carl Zeiss Meditec (C), FDA Ophthalmic Devices Committee (C), STAAR Surgical (L), Zeimer USA (L)

Dr Reeves: Abbott Medical Optics (C), Avedro (C, O), Johnson & Johnson Vision (L), Unifeye Vision Partners (O)

Dr Robinson: Horizon Therapeutics (O)

Dr Rocha: Alcon (C), Allergan (C), Bausch + Lomb (C), Dompé (C), Johnson & Johnson Vision (C), LaserACE (C)

Dr Tang: EMD Serono (L), Horizon Therapeutics (C, S), Immunovant (S), Novartis (S), Quark Pharmaceuticals, (C, S), Regenera Pharma (S), Sanofi (L), ZEISS (L)

Dr Taravella: Abbott Medical Optics (C), Coronet Medical Technologies (C), Eyevance (C), Ocular Therapeutix (C)

Dr Tassignon: Morcher GmbH (P)

* C = consultant fee, paid advisory boards, or fees for attending a meeting; E = employed by or received a W2 from a commercial company; L = lecture fees or honoraria, travel fees or reimbursements when speaking at the invitation of a commercial company; O = equity ownership/stock options in publicly or privately traded firms, excluding mutual funds; P = patents and/or royalties for intellectual property; S = grant support or other financial support to the investigator from all sources, including research support from government agencies, foundations, device manufacturers, and/or pharmaceutical companies

Dr Van Tassel: Aerie Pharmaceuticals (C), Allergan (C), Equinox (C), New World Medical (C)

Dr Waring: Abbott Medical Optics (C, L), ACE Vision Group (C), AcuFocus (C, L), Alcon (C, L), Allergan (C, L), Allotex (C), Avedro (C, L), Bausch + Lomb (C, L), Centricity Vision (C), Gerson Lehrman Group (C), GlassesOff (C), Glaukos (C, L), Ivantis (C), Johnson & Johnson Vision (C, L), Minosys (C), Novartis (C), OASIS Medical (C, L), OCULUS (C, L), Omega Ophthalmics (C), Omeros (C), Optoquest (C), Perfect Lens (C), Refocus Group (C), Reichert (C), Shire/Takeda (C), Sight Sciences (C), SRD Vision (C), Visiometrics (C, O)

The other authors and reviewers state that within the 24 months prior to their contributions to this CME activity and for the duration of development, they have had no financial interest in or other relationship with any entity that produces, markets, resells, or distributes health care goods or services consumed by or used in patients, or with any competing commercial product or service.

Recent Past Faculty

Renato Ambrósio Jr, MD, PhD
Gregg J. Berdy, MD
Richard S. Davidson, MD
M. Bowes Hamill, MD
Parag A. Majmudar, MD
Neda Shamie, MD

In addition, the Academy gratefully acknowledges the contributions of numerous past faculty and advisory committee members who have played an important role in the development of previous editions of the Basic and Clinical Science Course.

American Academy of Ophthalmology Staff

Dale E. Fajardo, EdD, MBA, *Vice President, Education*
Beth Wilson, *Director, Continuing Professional Development*
Denise Evenson, *Director, Brand & Creative*
Susan Malloy, *Acquisitions and Development Manager*
Stephanie Tanaka, *Publications Manager*
Rayna Ungersma, *Manager, Curriculum Development*
Jasmine Chen, *Manager, E-Learning*
Sarah Page, *Online Education and Licensing Manager*
Lana Ip, *Senior Designer*
Beth Collins, *Medical Editor*
Eric Gerdes, *Interactive Designer*
Lynda Hanwella, *Publications Specialist*
Debra Marchi, *Permissions Assistant*

American Academy of Ophthalmology
655 Beach Street
Box 7424
San Francisco, CA 94120-7424

Contents

Introduction to the BCSC

The Basic and Clinical Science Course (BCSC) is designed to meet the needs of residents and practitioners for a comprehensive yet concise curriculum of the field of ophthalmology. The BCSC has developed from its original brief outline format, which relied heavily on outside readings, to a more convenient and educationally useful self-contained text. The Academy updates and revises the course annually, with the goals of integrating the basic science and clinical practice of ophthalmology and of keeping ophthalmologists current with new developments in the various subspecialties.

The BCSC incorporates the effort and expertise of more than 100 ophthalmologists, organized into 13 Section faculties, working with Academy editorial staff. In addition, the course continues to benefit from many lasting contributions made by the faculties of previous editions. Members of the Academy Practicing Ophthalmologists Advisory Committee for Education, Committee on Aging, and Vision Rehabilitation Committee review every volume before major revisions, as does a group of select residents and fellows. Members of the European Board of Ophthalmology, organized into Section faculties, also review volumes before major revisions, focusing primarily on differences between American and European ophthalmology practice.

Organization of the Course

The Basic and Clinical Science Course comprises 13 volumes, incorporating fundamental ophthalmic knowledge, subspecialty areas, and special topics:

1. Update on General Medicine
2. Fundamentals and Principles of Ophthalmology
3. Clinical Optics and Vision Rehabilitation
4. Ophthalmic Pathology and Intraocular Tumors
5. Neuro-Ophthalmology
6. Pediatric Ophthalmology and Strabismus
7. Oculofacial Plastic and Orbital Surgery
8. External Disease and Cornea
9. Uveitis and Ocular Inflammation
10. Glaucoma
11. Lens and Cataract
12. Retina and Vitreous
13. Refractive Surgery

References

Readers who wish to explore specific topics in greater detail may consult the references cited within each chapter and listed in the Additional Materials and Resources section at the back of the book. These references are intended to be selective rather than exhaustive, chosen by the BCSC faculty as being important, current, and readily available to residents and practitioners.

Multimedia

This edition of Section 13, *Refractive Surgery*, includes videos related to topics covered in the book. Selected by members of the BCSC faculty, the videos are available to readers of the print and electronic versions of Section 13 (www.aao.org/bcscvideo_section13). Mobile-device users can scan the QR code below (a QR-code reader may need to be installed on the device) to access the video content.

Self-Assessment and CME Credit

Each volume of the BCSC is designed as an independent study activity for ophthalmology residents and practitioners. The learning objectives for this volume are given on page 1. The text, illustrations, and references provide the information necessary to achieve the objectives; the study questions allow readers to test their understanding of the material and their mastery of the objectives. Physicians who wish to claim CME credit for this educational activity may do so by following the instructions given at the end of the book.*

Conclusion

The Basic and Clinical Science Course has expanded greatly over the years, with the addition of much new text, numerous illustrations, and video content. Recent editions have sought to place a greater emphasis on clinical applicability while maintaining a solid foundation in basic science. As with any educational program, it reflects the experience of its authors. As its faculties change and medicine progresses, new viewpoints emerge on controversial subjects and techniques. Not all alternate approaches can be included in this series; as with any educational endeavor, the learner should seek additional sources, including Academy Preferred Practice Pattern Guidelines.

The BCSC faculty and staff continually strive to improve the educational usefulness of the course; you, the reader, can contribute to this ongoing process. If you have any suggestions or questions about the series, please do not hesitate to contact the faculty or the editors.

The authors, editors, and reviewers hope that your study of the BCSC will be of lasting value and that each Section will serve as a practical resource for quality patient care.

* This activity meets the Self-Assessment CME requirements defined by the American Board of Ophthalmology (ABO). Please be advised that the ABO is not an accrediting body for purposes of any CME program. ABO does not sponsor this or any outside activity, and ABO does not endorse any particular CME activity. Complete information regarding the ABO Self-Assessment CME Maintenance of Certification requirements is available at https://abop.org/maintain-certification/cme-self-assessment/.

Objectives

Upon completion of BCSC Section 13, *Refractive Surgery,* the reader should be able to

- state the contributions of the cornea's shape and tissue layers to the optics of the eye and how these components are affected biomechanically by different types of keratorefractive procedures
- describe the basic concepts of wavefront analysis and its relationship to different types of optical aberrations
- identify the general types of lasers used in refractive surgeries
- explain the steps—including medical and social history, ocular examination, and ancillary testing—in evaluating whether a patient is an appropriate candidate for refractive surgery
- for incisional keratorefractive surgery (radial keratotomy, transverse keratotomy, arcuate keratotomy, and limbal relaxing incisions), describe the history, patient selection, surgical techniques, outcomes, and complications
- for surface ablation procedures, describe patient selection, epithelial removal, refractive outcomes, and complications
- for laser in situ keratomileusis (LASIK), describe patient selection, surgical techniques, outcomes, and complications
- describe the different methods for creating a LASIK flap with a microkeratome or a femtosecond laser, as well as the instrumentation and possible complications associated with each
- state considerations for, and possible contraindications to, refractive surgery in patients with preexisting ocular or systemic disease
- list some of the effects of prior refractive procedures on later intraocular lens (IOL) calculations, contact lens wear, and ocular surgery

- explain recent developments in the application of wavefront technology to surface ablation and LASIK
- describe how intraocular surgical procedures, including refractive lens exchange or implantation of a phakic IOL, can be used in refractive correction, with or without corneal intervention
- describe the different types of IOLs used for refractive correction
- explain the leading theories of accommodation and how they relate to potential treatment of presbyopia
- describe nonaccommodative and accommodative approaches to the treatment of presbyopia

Introduction to Section 13

Of all the subspecialties within ophthalmology, refractive surgery may be evolving the most rapidly. Accordingly, the current edition features a number of updates, including a greater emphasis on femtosecond lasers and advances in intraocular lens technology. The terminology for recording visual acuity is also changing, and the BCSC Section 13 Committee now uses the following conventions throughout the text: uncorrected distance visual acuity (UDVA) and corrected distance visual acuity (CDVA), which replaces best-corrected visual acuity (BCVA).

Considerations in the evaluation of new refractive surgical procedures are broadly predicated upon safety, efficacy, applicability, and endurance. Consensus standard reporting measures for outcomes in refractive surgery have been proposed, and we recommend that readers familiarize themselves with these standards when critically reviewing new technologies in the literature.

Refractive surgeons, like all medical specialists, also use numerous abbreviations and acronyms in discussing and describing their field. The following list of frequently used terms is included as an aid to readers of this text as well as of the refractive surgery literature in general.

Reinstein DZ, Waring GO 3rd. Graphic reporting of outcomes of refractive surgery. *J Refract Surg.* 2009;25(11):975–978.

Reinstein DZ, Archer TJ, Srinivasan S, et al. Standard for reporting refractive outcomes of intraocular lens-based refractive surgery. *J Cataract Refract Surg.* 2017;43(4):435–439.

Common Abbreviations and Acronyms in Refractive Surgery

ACS anterior ciliary sclerotomy

AHWP Asian Harmonization Working Party (for device regulation)

AK arcuate keratotomy

ArF argon-fluoride (laser)

ASA advanced surface ablation (synonym for *photorefractive keratectomy, PRK*)

BCVA best-corrected visual acuity (preferred term is *corrected distance visual acuity, CDVA*)

CCD charge-coupled device

CCL corneal crosslinking (also CXL)

CDVA corrected distance visual acuity (formerly called *best-corrected visual acuity, BCVA*)

CE mark Conformité Européenne mark (product approval used in European countries, similar to US Food and Drug Administration approval)

CK conductive keratoplasty

CXL corneal crosslinking (also CCL)

D diopter

DALK deep anterior lamellar keratoplasty

DLK diffuse lamellar keratitis

DMEK Descemet membrane endothelial keratoplasty

DSEK Descemet stripping endothelial keratoplasty

EDOF extended depth of focus (intraocular lens)

Epi-LASIK epipolis laser in situ keratomileusis

Femto-LASIK femtosecond laser–assisted laser in situ keratomileusis

FLEx femtosecond lenticule extraction

GAT Goldmann applanation tonometry

GHTF Global Harmonization Task Force (international medical device regulation)

HDE Humanitarian Device Exemption

Hex K hexagonal keratotomy

HOA higher-order aberration

Ho:YAG holmium:yttrium-aluminum-garnet (laser)

ICL implantable collamer lens

ICRS intrastromal corneal ring segment

IOL intraocular lens

IOP intraocular pressure

I–S inferior–superior (value)

KC keratoconus

LAL Light Adjustable Lens

LASEK laser subepithelial keratomileusis

LASIK laser in situ keratomileusis

logMAR base-10 logarithm of the minimum angle of resolution

LRI limbal relaxing incision

LTK laser thermokeratoplasty

LVC laser vision correction

MFIOL multifocal intraocular lens

MRSE manifest refraction spherical equivalent

Nd:YAG neodymium:yttrium-aluminum-garnet (laser)

OBL opaque bubble layer

OCT optical coherence tomography

OSC ocular surface disease

OSDI Ocular Surface Disease Index

PCO posterior capsule opacification

PERK Prospective Evaluation of Radial Keratotomy (study)

PIOL phakic intraocular lens

PISK pressure-induced stromal keratopathy

PKP penetrating keratoplasty

PMD pellucid marginal degeneration

PMMA polymethyl methacrylate

PRK photorefractive keratectomy

PROWL Patient-Reported Outcomes With Laser In Situ Keratomileusis (studies)

PTA percent of tissue altered

PTK phototherapeutic keratectomy

ReLEx refractive lenticule extraction

RGP rigid gas-permeable (contact lenses)

RK radial keratotomy

RLE refractive lens exchange

RMS root mean square

RSB residual stromal bed

SA spherical aberration

SIM K corneal power (K) simulation measurements

SMILE small-incision lenticule extraction

UCVA uncorrected visual acuity (preferred term is *uncorrected distance visual acuity, UDVA*)

UDVA uncorrected distance visual acuity (also called *uncorrected visual acuity, UCVA*)

WAMR wavefront-adjusted manifest refraction

CHAPTER 1

The Science of Refractive Surgery

This chapter includes a related video. Go to www.aao.org/bcscvideo_section13 or scan the QR code in the text to access this content.

Highlights

- A wide variety of refractive surgical techniques and technologies are available to reduce dependence on contact lenses or glasses.
- Wavefront analysis of higher-order aberrations is useful in calculating custom ablations to enhance vision correction and in explaining patients' visual symptoms.
- Corneal topography and tomography are key technologies in both preoperative screening and postoperative evaluation of patients with unexpected results.
- Three different types of laser–tissue interactions are used in keratorefractive surgery: photoablative, photodisruptive, and photothermal.

Introduction

The goal of refractive surgery is to reduce dependence on contact lenses or glasses for use in routine daily activities. A wide variety of surgical techniques and technologies are available to accomplish this goal. To ensure optimal refractive outcomes, surgeons must conduct careful preoperative evaluations using appropriate diagnostic tools to determine patient candidacy.

Refractive surgical procedures can be categorized broadly as corneal, scleral, or intraocular (Tables 1-1, 1-2). *Keratorefractive (corneal)* procedures include incisional, laser ablation, refractive lenticule extraction (ReLEx, FLEx, SMILE), corneal inlays and onlays, corneal collagen shrinkage, and corneal crosslinking techniques. *Scleral* procedures involve either scleral implants or laser excision of the anterior ciliary sclera. *Intraocular* refractive procedures include phakic intraocular lens (PIOL) implantation and cataract surgery or refractive lens exchange (RLE) with implantation of a monofocal, toric, multifocal, accommodative, or extended depth of focus intraocular lens. Each technique has advantages and disadvantages and should be specifically matched to the patient.

This chapter, focusing on keratorefractive procedures, provides an overview of relevant fundamental corneal properties, imaging for refractive surgery, and the effects of such surgery on the cornea. It includes review of the optical principles discussed in BCSC

Table 1-1 Overview of Keratorefractive Procedures

Location	Type of Procedure	Specific Procedures	Common Abbreviations	Refractive Error Treated
Cornea	Incisional	Radial keratotomy	RK	Myopia (historical)
		Astigmatic keratotomy	AK	Astigmatism
		Arcuate keratotomy		
		Femtosecond laser–assisted arcuate keratotomy	FLAAK	Astigmatism
		Limbal relaxing incisions	LRI	Astigmatism
	Excimer laser	Photorefractive keratectomy	PRK	Myopia, hyperopia, astigmatism
		Laser in situ keratomileusis	LASIK	Myopia, hyperopia, astigmatism
		Laser subepithelial keratomileusis	LASEK	Myopia, hyperopia, astigmatism
		Epipolis laser in situ keratomileusis	Epi-LASIK	Myopia, hyperopia, astigmatism
	Excimer and femtosecond lasers	Femtosecond laser–assisted laser in situ keratomileusis	Femto-LASIK	Myopia, hyperopia, astigmatism
	Femtosecond laser	Refractive lenticule extraction	ReLEx, FLEx, SMILE	Myopia, astigmatism
		Refractive indexing		Investigational
	Inlays/onlays	Corneal inlays/onlays		Presbyopia
	Nonlaser lamellar	Epikeratophakia, epikeratoplasty		Myopia, hyperopia, astigmatism (historical)
		Intrastromal corneal ring segments	ICRS	Myopia, keratoconus
	Collagen shrinkage	Laser thermokeratoplasty	LTK	Hyperopia, astigmatism (historical)
		Conductive keratoplasty	CK	Hyperopia, astigmatism
	Corneal crosslinking		CXL	Keratoconus, myopia (investigational)

Section 3, *Clinical Optics and Vision Rehabilitation;* refractive errors (both lower- and higher-order aberrations); corneal biomechanics; corneal topography and tomography; wavefront analysis; laser biophysics and laser–tissue interactions; and corneal wound healing.

Corneal Optics

The majority of the optical power of the eye derives from the combined effect of the air–tear interface and the corneal curvature. The normal tear film has minimal deleterious effect on vision. However, an abnormal tear film—such as excessive tear film (eg, epiphora) or altered tear film (eg, dry eye or blepharitis)—can dramatically decrease the quality of vision. The anterior corneal curvature contributes approximately two-thirds of the eye's

Table 1-2 Overview of Scleral and Intraocular Refractive Procedures

Location	Type of Procedure	Specific Procedures	Refractive Error Treated
Scleral		Scleral laser anterior ciliary excision	Presbyopia (investigational)
		PMMA microinserts placed in scleral tunnels	Presbyopia (investigational)
Intraocular	Phakic	Anterior chamber (angle-supported) phakic IOL implantation	Myopia (investigational)
		Iris-fixated phakic IOL implantation	Myopia, astigmatism
		Posterior chamber phakic IOL implantation	Myopia, astigmatism
	Pseudophakic	Refractive lens exchange (multifocal/ accommodating/ extended depth of focus IOLs)	Myopia, hyperopia, presbyopia, astigmatism

IOL = intraocular lens; PMMA = polymethyl methacrylate.

refractive power, about +48.00 diopters (D). However, the overall corneal power is approximately +42.00 D as a result of the negative power (approximately −6.00 D) of the posterior corneal surface.

Standard keratometers and Placido-based corneal topography instruments measure the anterior corneal radius of curvature and *estimate* total corneal power from the front-surface measurements. These instruments extrapolate the central corneal power *(K)* by measuring the rate of change in curvature from the paracentral 3–4-mm zone; this factor takes on crucial importance in the determination of IOL power after keratorefractive surgery (see Chapter 9). The normal cornea flattens from the center to the periphery by up to 4.00 D and is flatter nasally than temporally; this shape is described as *prolate* (Fig 1-1).

The majority of keratorefractive surgical procedures change the refractive state of the eye by altering corneal curvature. The tolerances involved in this process are relatively small. For example, achieving a refractive change of 2.00 D may require altering the cornea's thickness by less than 30 µm. Thus, attaining predictable results is sometimes problematic because minuscule changes in the shape of the cornea may produce large changes in refraction.

Refractive Error: Optical Principles and Wavefront Analysis

One of the major applications of the wave theory of light is in wavefront analysis (see also BCSC Section 3, *Clinical Optics and Vision Rehabilitation*). Currently, wavefront analysis can

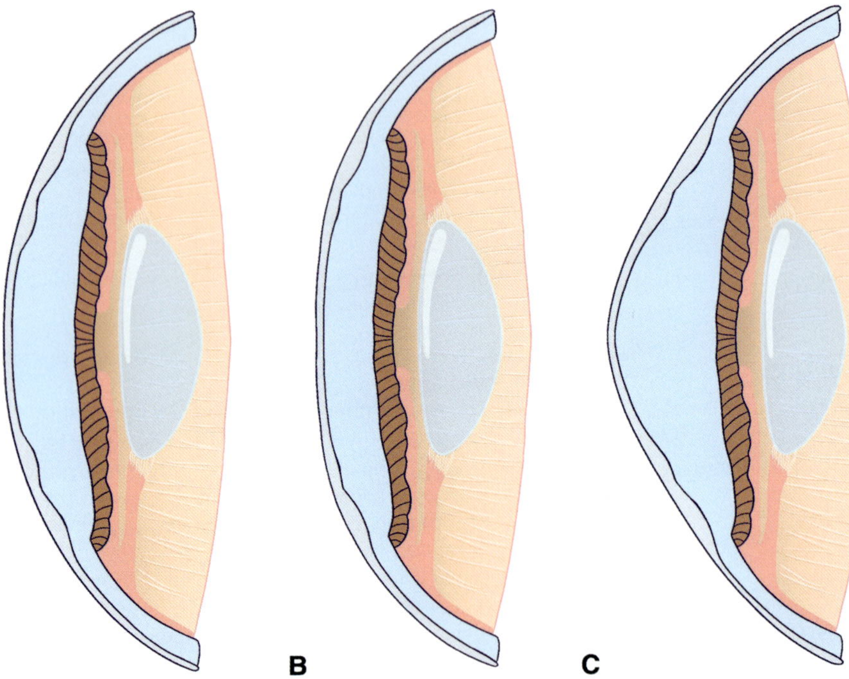

Figure 1-1 Examples of corneal profiles. **A,** Prolate cornea (the normal corneal shape), steeper centrally and flatter in the periphery. **B,** Oblate cornea (eg, after myopic ablation), flatter centrally and steeper in the periphery. **C,** Hyperprolate cornea (eg, after hyperopic ablation). *(Courtesy of Raquel Gouvea and Larissa Gouvea, MD.)*

be performed clinically by 4 methods: Hartmann-Shack, Tscherning, thin-beam single-ray tracing, and optical path difference. Each method generates a detailed report of *lower-order aberrations* (eg, sphere and cylinder) and *higher-order aberrations* (eg, spherical aberration, coma, and trefoil). This information is useful both in calculating custom ablations to enhance vision or to correct optical problems and in explaining patients' visual symptoms.

Measurement of Wavefront Aberrations and Graphical Representations

Of the several techniques for measuring wavefront aberrations, the most popular in clinical practice is based on the *Hartmann-Shack wavefront sensor.* With this device, a low-power laser beam is focused on the retina. A point on the retina acts as a point source, and the reflected light is then propagated back (anteriorly) through the optical elements of the eye to a detector. In an aberration-free eye, all the rays would emerge in parallel, and the reflected wavefront would be a flat plane. In reality, the reflected wavefront is not flat. To determine its shape, an array of lenses samples parts of the wavefront and focuses light on a detector (Fig 1-2; see also BCSC Section 3, *Clinical Optics and Vision Rehabilitation*). The extent of the divergence of the lenslet images from their expected focal points determines the wavefront error (see Figure 1-2B). Optical aberrations measured by an aberrometer can be resolved into a variety of basic shapes whose combination represents the total aberration of the patient's ocular system. This compares to the conventional refractive error, which is a combination of sphere and cylinder (Fig 1-3).

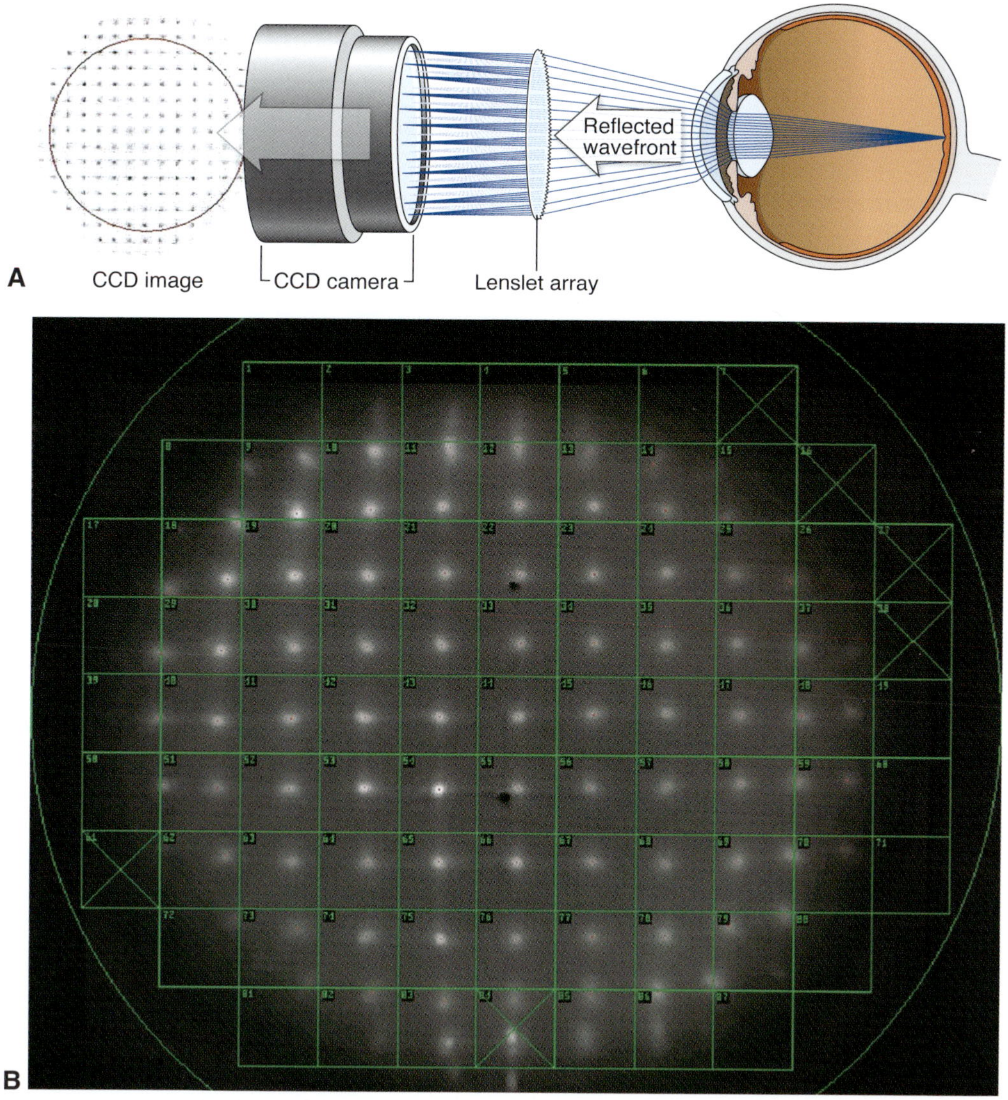

Figure 1-2 Schematic of a Hartmann-Shack wavefront sensor. **A,** The reflected wavefront passes through a grid of small lenses (the *lenslet array*), and the images formed are focused onto a charge-coupled device (CCD) chip. The degree of deviation of the focused images from the expected focal points determines the aberration and thus the wavefront error. **B,** Example of the images formed after the wavefront passes through the lenslet array. The green overlay lattice is registered to correspond to each lenslet in the array. *(Part A illustration by Mark Miller.)*

Currently, wavefront aberrations are most commonly specified by *Zernike polynomials,* which are the mathematical formulas used to describe the surfaces shown in Figures 1-4 through 1-8. Each aberration may be positive or negative in value and induces predictable alterations in the image quality. The magnitude of these aberrations is expressed as a root mean square (RMS) error, which is the deviation of the wavefront

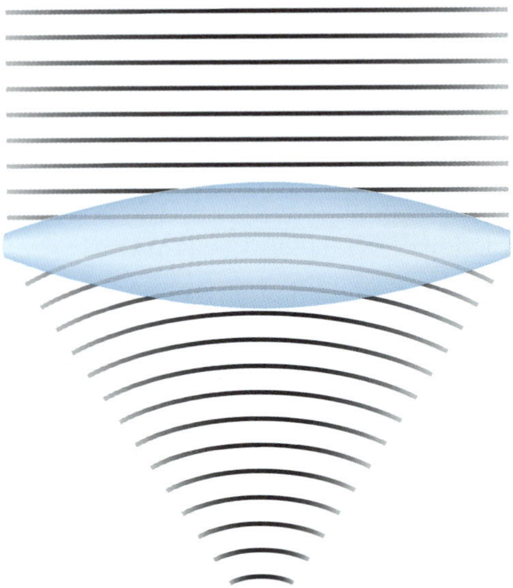

Figure 1-3 Wavefronts change shape after going through a lens. *(Redrawn by Cyndie C. H. Wooley from a schematic image from https://en.wikipedia.org/wiki/Wavefront.)*

averaged over the entire wavefront. The higher the RMS value, the greater is the overall aberration of a given eye. The majority of patients have total RMS values less than 0.3 μm for a 6-mm pupil. Most higher-order Zernike coefficients have mean values close to 0. The most important Zernike coefficients affecting visual quality are defocus, spherical aberration, coma, and secondary astigmatism.

Fourier analysis is an alternative method for evaluating the output from an aberrometer. This method involves a sine wave–derived transformation of a complex shape. Compared with shapes derived from Zernike polynomial analysis, those derived from Fourier analysis are more detailed, theoretically allowing for the measurement and treatment of more highly aberrated corneas.

Klyce SD, Karon MD, Smolek MK. Advantages and disadvantages of the Zernike expansion for representing wave aberration of the normal and aberrated eye. *J Refract Surg.* 2004;20(5):S537–S541.

Salmon TO, van de Pol C. Normal-eye Zernike coefficients and root-mean-square wavefront errors. *J Cataract Refract Surg.* 2006;32(12):2064–2074.

Lower-Order Aberrations

Myopia, hyperopia, and regular astigmatism are all lower-order, *or second-order,* aberrations. Myopia produces *positive defocus* (see Figure 1-4), whereas hyperopia produces *negative defocus.* Regular (cylindrical) astigmatism produces a wavefront aberration that has orthogonal (ie, facing at right angles) and oblique components (see Figure 1-5). Other lower-order aberrations are non–visually significant aberrations known as *first-order aberrations* such as vertical and horizontal prisms and zero-order aberrations such as piston, which has no impact on wavefront shape.

Higher-Order Aberrations

Wavefront aberration is strongly affected by pupil size, with higher-order aberrations becoming more apparent as the pupil dilates. Higher-order aberrations also increase with age, although the clinical effect is thought to be balanced by the increasing miosis of the pupil with age. Although lower-order aberrations decrease after laser vision correction, higher-order aberrations, particularly spherical aberration and coma, may increase after conventional surface ablation, laser in situ keratomileusis (LASIK), or radial keratotomy (RK) for myopia. (See the section "Effect of excimer laser ablation on higher-order aberrations.")

Spherical aberration

When peripheral light rays passing through a lens or the cornea focus in front of more central rays, the effect is called *spherical aberration* (see Figure 1-6 in this volume and also BCSC Section 3, *Clinical Optics and Vision Rehabilitation*). Clinically, this radially symmetric

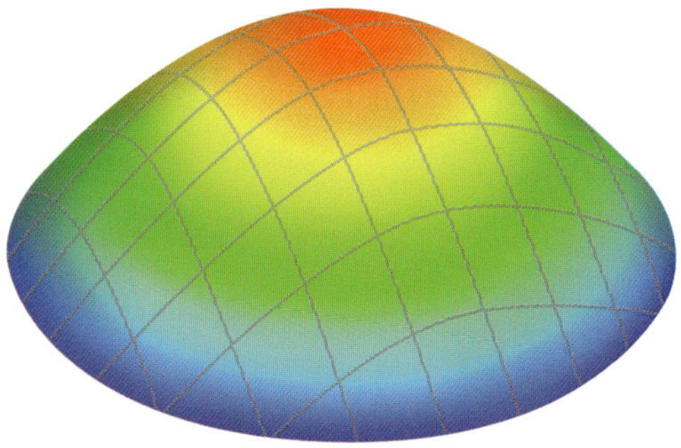

Figure 1-4 Zernike polynomial representation of defocus. *(Redrawn by Cyndie C. H. Wooley. Original image courtesy of Roger F. Steinert, MD.)*

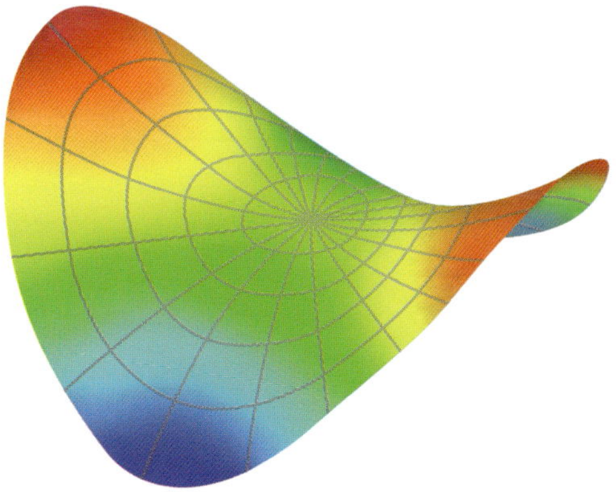

Figure 1-5 Zernike polynomial representation of astigmatism. *(Redrawn by Cyndie C. H. Wooley. Original image courtesy of Roger F. Steinert, MD.)*

fourth-order aberration is the cause of night myopia and is commonly increased after RK and myopic LASIK and surface ablation. It results in halos around point images. Spherical aberration is the most significant higher-order aberration. Although it may increase depth of field, it decreases contrast sensitivity.

Coma and trefoil

With *coma,* a third-order aberration, light rays at one edge of the pupil come into focus before those at the opposite edge do. The rays entering the system do not focus on a plane; rather, one edge of the incoming beam focuses either in front of or behind the opposite edge of the beam (see Figure 1-7). The image generated by an incoming light beam passing through an optical system with a coma aberration would appear "smeared," looking somewhat like a comet, with a zone of sharp focus at one edge tailing off to a fuzzy focus at the opposite edge of the beam. Coma is common in patients with decentered corneal grafts, keratoconus, and decentered laser ablations.

Trefoil, also a third-order aberration, can occur after refractive surgery. Trefoil produces less degradation in image quality than does coma of similar RMS magnitude (see Figure 1-8).

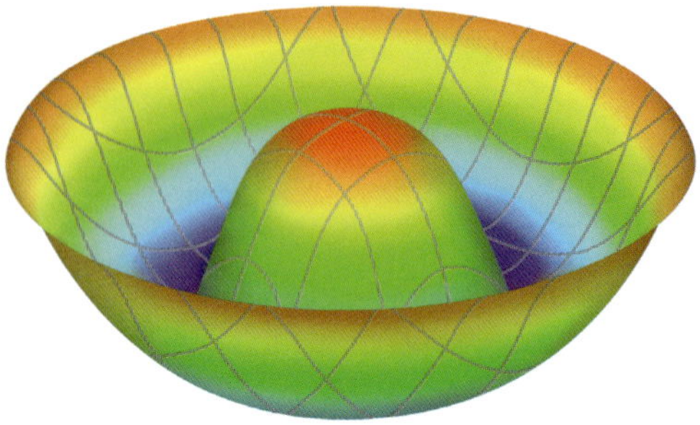

Figure 1-6 Zernike polynomial representation of spherical aberration. *(Redrawn by Cyndie C. H. Wooley. Original image courtesy of Roger F. Steinert, MD.)*

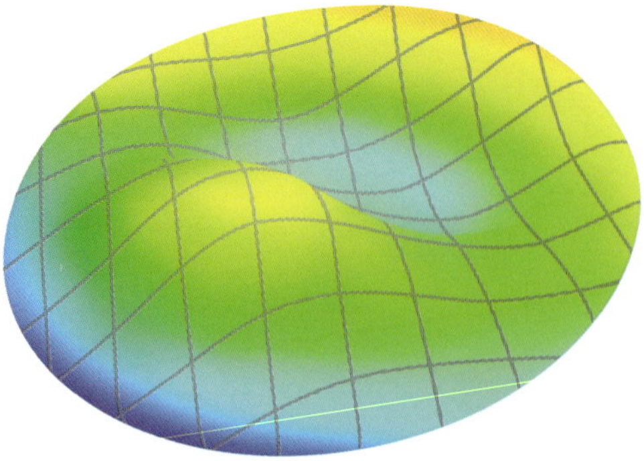

Figure 1-7 Zernike polynomial representation of coma. *(Redrawn by Cyndie C. H. Wooley. Original image courtesy of Roger F. Steinert, MD.)*

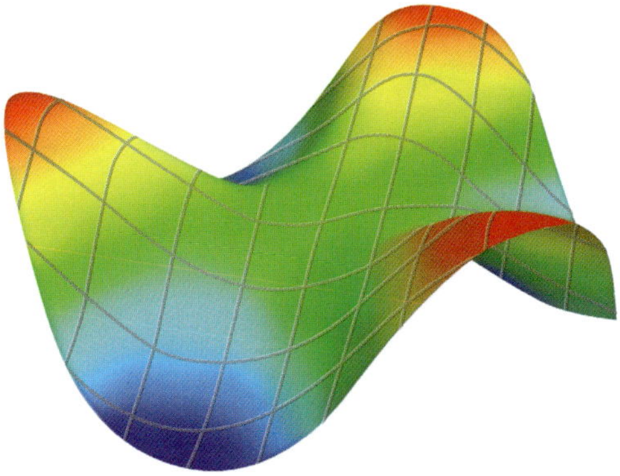

Figure 1-8 Zernike polynomial representation of trefoil. *(Redrawn by Cyndie C. H. Wooley. Original image courtesy of Roger F. Steinert, MD.)*

Other higher-order aberrations

Although there are numerous other higher-order aberrations, only a few are of clinical interest. As knowledge of surgically induced aberration increases, more types of aberrations may become clinically relevant.

Effect of excimer laser ablation on higher-order aberrations

The use of conventional excimer laser ablation typically increases higher-order aberrations, and the effect is correlated with the degree of preoperative refractive error. After standard myopic laser vision correction, the cornea assumes an oblate shape, inducing positive spherical aberration. In hyperopic ablation, treatment is applied to the midperipheral cornea relative to the central cornea, increasing the central curvature of the cornea, resulting in a hyperprolate cornea that generates greater amounts of negative spherical aberration (see the section Corneal Imaging for Keratorefractive Surgery and Figure 1-1).

Compared with conventional laser treatment, wavefront-optimized, wavefront-guided, and topography-guided ablations may decrease the number of induced higher-order aberrations and, in principle, may be able to reduce preexisting higher-order aberrations and provide better-quality vision, particularly in mesopic conditions.

Holland S, Lin DT, Tan JC. Topography-guided laser refractive surgery. *Curr Opin Ophthalmol.* 2013;24(4):302–309.

Corneal Imaging for Keratorefractive Surgery

Corneal shape, curvature, and thickness profiles can be generated from a variety of technologies such as Placido disk–based systems and elevation-based systems (including scanning-slit systems and Scheimpflug imaging). Each technology conveys different information about corneal curvature, anatomy, and biomechanical function. Computerized topographic and tomographic systems may also display other data, including pupil size and location, indices for estimating regular and irregular astigmatism, estimates of the probability of keratoconus, simulated keratometry, and corneal asphericity. Other topographic systems may integrate wavefront aberrometry data with topographic data. Although such additional information can be useful in preoperative surgical evaluations, no automated screening system can supplant clinical experience in evaluating corneal imaging.

The degree of asphericity of the cornea can be quantified by determining the Q value, with $Q = 0$ for *spherical* corneas, $Q < 0$ for *prolate* corneas (relatively flatter periphery), and $Q > 0$ for *oblate* corneas (relatively steeper periphery). A normal cornea is prolate, with an asphericity Q value of approximately −0.26. Prolate corneas minimize spherical aberrations by virtue of their relatively flat peripheral curve. Conversely, oblate corneal contours, in which the peripheral cornea is steeper than the center, increase the probability of induced positive spherical aberrations (see Figure 1-1).

Corneal Topography

Corneal topography provides highly detailed information about corneal curvature. Topography is evaluated using keratoscopic images, which are captured from Placido disk patterns *(mires)* that are reflected from the tear film overlying the corneal surface and then converted to computerized color scales (Fig 1-9). Because the image is generated from the anterior surface of the tear film, irregularities in tear composition or volume can have a major impact on the quality and results of a Placido disk–based system. Given this effect, it is very important to review the Placido image (image of the mires) before interpreting the maps and subsequent numerical data. Also, Placido disk–based systems are referenced from the line that the instrument makes to the corneal surface (called the *vertex normal*). This line is not necessarily the patient's line of sight or the visual axis, which may lead to confusion in interpreting topographic maps. For further discussion of computerized corneal topography, see BCSC Section 3, *Clinical Optics and Vision Rehabilitation.*

Corneal topography maps provide color scales to represent curvature data. Two types of scales are commonly used: absolute (or standard) scale and normalized (or relative) scale. These color scales appear on the left margin of the map; the top of the scale represents the steepest curvature, and the bottom of the scale represents the flattest curvature. Areas of steeper curvature are represented by warmer colors, such as red and orange, and areas of flatter curvature by cooler colors, such as green and blue. The *absolute scale* displays a fixed color-coding map, with each color representing a 1.5-D interval between 35 and 50 D. The same color always represents the same power, allowing easy comparisons between different maps. In contrast, the *normalized scale* spans the eye's total dioptric power, thus providing more detailed topographic information. It is important to note the diopter change between colors when using the normalized scale. Too large a difference between colors can mask significant abnormalities, while too little difference can "smooth" over significant abnormalities.

Axial power and curvature

Axial power representation derives from the assumption that the cornea is a sphere and that the angle of incidence of the instrument is normal to the cornea. *Axial power* is based on the concept of "axial distance" (Fig 1-10). As shown in the illustration, axial power underestimates steeper curvatures and overestimates flatter curvatures. This representation is also extremely dependent on the reference axis employed: optical or visual. Maps of the same cornea generated by these 2 reference axes will look very different from each another. Axial power representations actually average the corneal powers and thereby

A

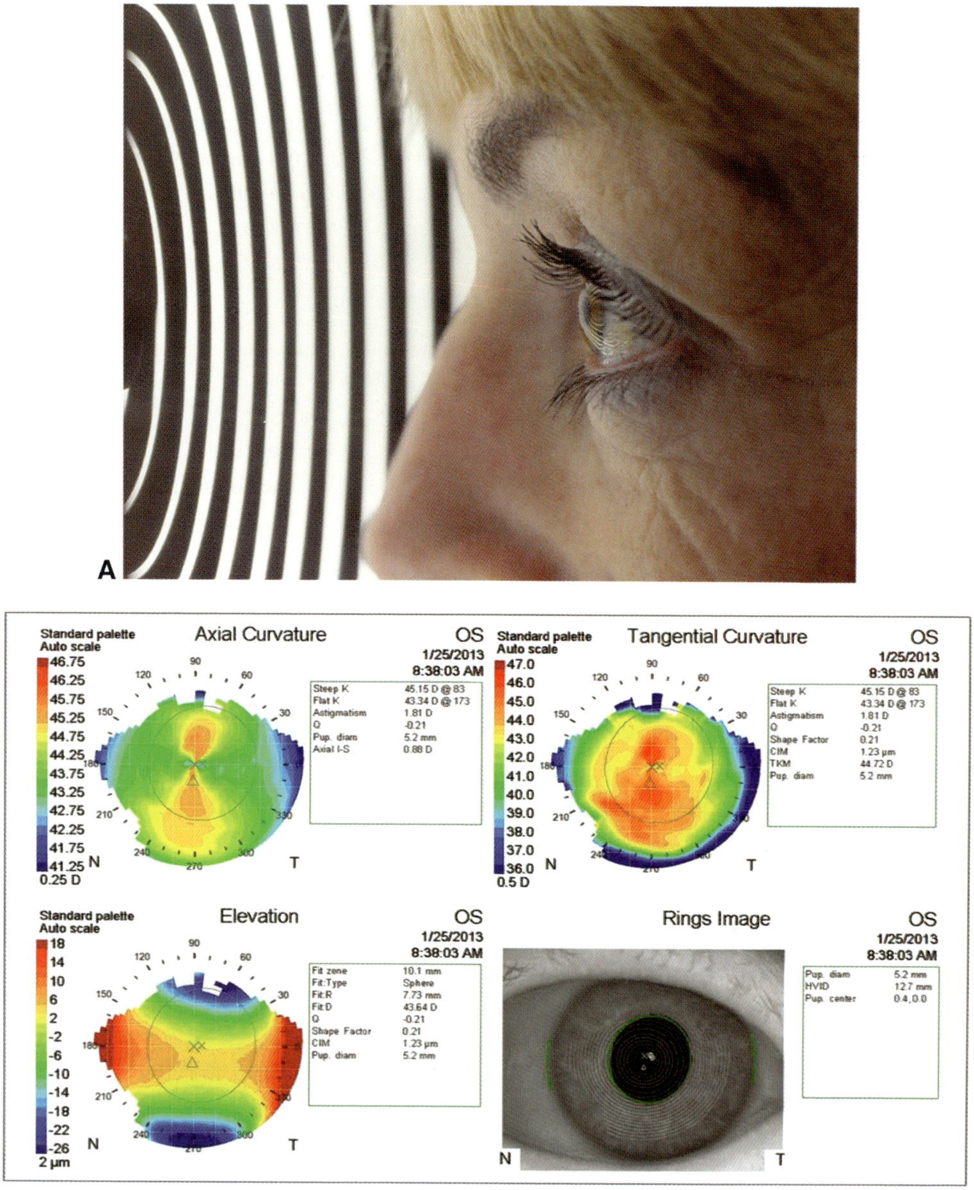

B

Figure 1-9 Placido imaging of the cornea. **A,** The reflected mires from the Placido device can be seen on this patient's cornea. This image is then captured and analyzed. **B,** The captured Placido image is seen in the lower right-hand corner, and the different types of color maps derived from it appear in the other corners. *(Courtesy of M. Bowes Hamill, MD.)*

provide a "smoother" depiction of corneal curvature than does the tangential, or instantaneous, method. Although the curvature and power of the central 1–2 mm of the cornea are generally not well imaged by Placido disk techniques, they can be closely approximated by the axial power and curvature indices (formerly called *sagittal curvature*); however, the central measurements are extrapolated and, thus, potentially inaccurate. These indices

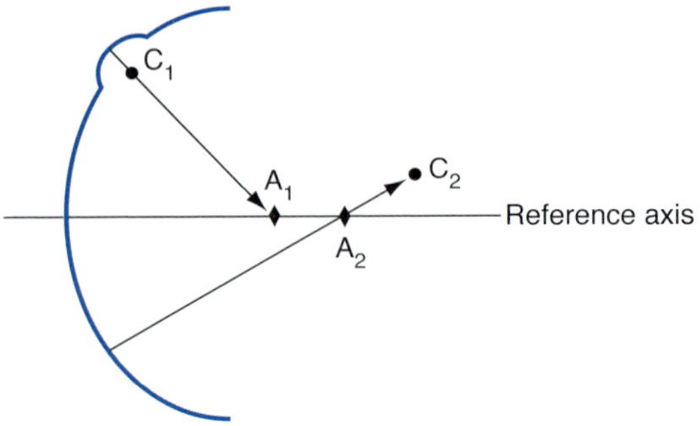

Figure 1-10 Schematic representation of the difference between axial distance (axial curvature) and radius of curvature for 2 points on a curved surface. Points C_1 and C_2 represent the centers of curvature of their respective surface points. Points A_1 and A_2 represent the endpoints of the axial distances for the given axis. Steeper, localized areas of curvature are underestimated, while flatter areas are overestimated. *(Adapted from Roberts C. Corneal topography: a review of terms and concepts.* J Cataract Refract Surg. *1996;22(5):624–629.)*

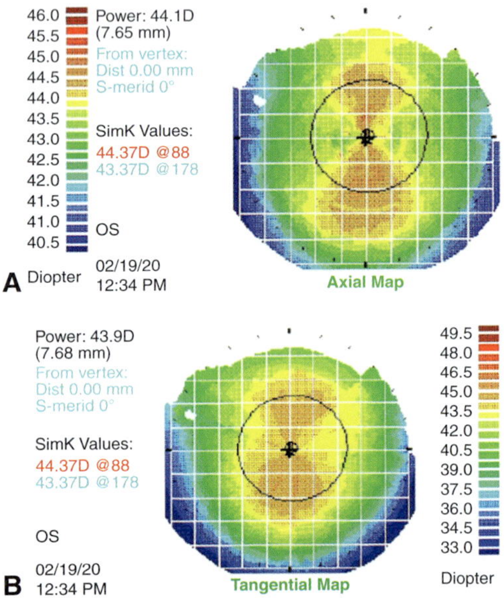

Figure 1-11 Examples of Placido-based curvature maps. **A,** Axial (sagittal); **B,** instantaneous (tangential). *(Courtesy of Karolinne Maia Rocha, MD, PhD.)*

also fail to describe the true shape and power of the peripheral cornea. Topographic maps displaying axial power and curvature provide an intuitive sense of the physiologic flattening of the cornea but do not represent the true refractive power or the true curvature of peripheral regions of the cornea (Figs 1-11A, 1-12).

Instantaneous power and curvature

A second method of describing the corneal curvature on Placido disk–based topography is the *instantaneous radius of curvature* (also called *meridional* or *tangential power*). The instantaneous radius of curvature is determined by taking a perpendicular path through the point in question from a plane that intersects the point and the visual axis, while allowing

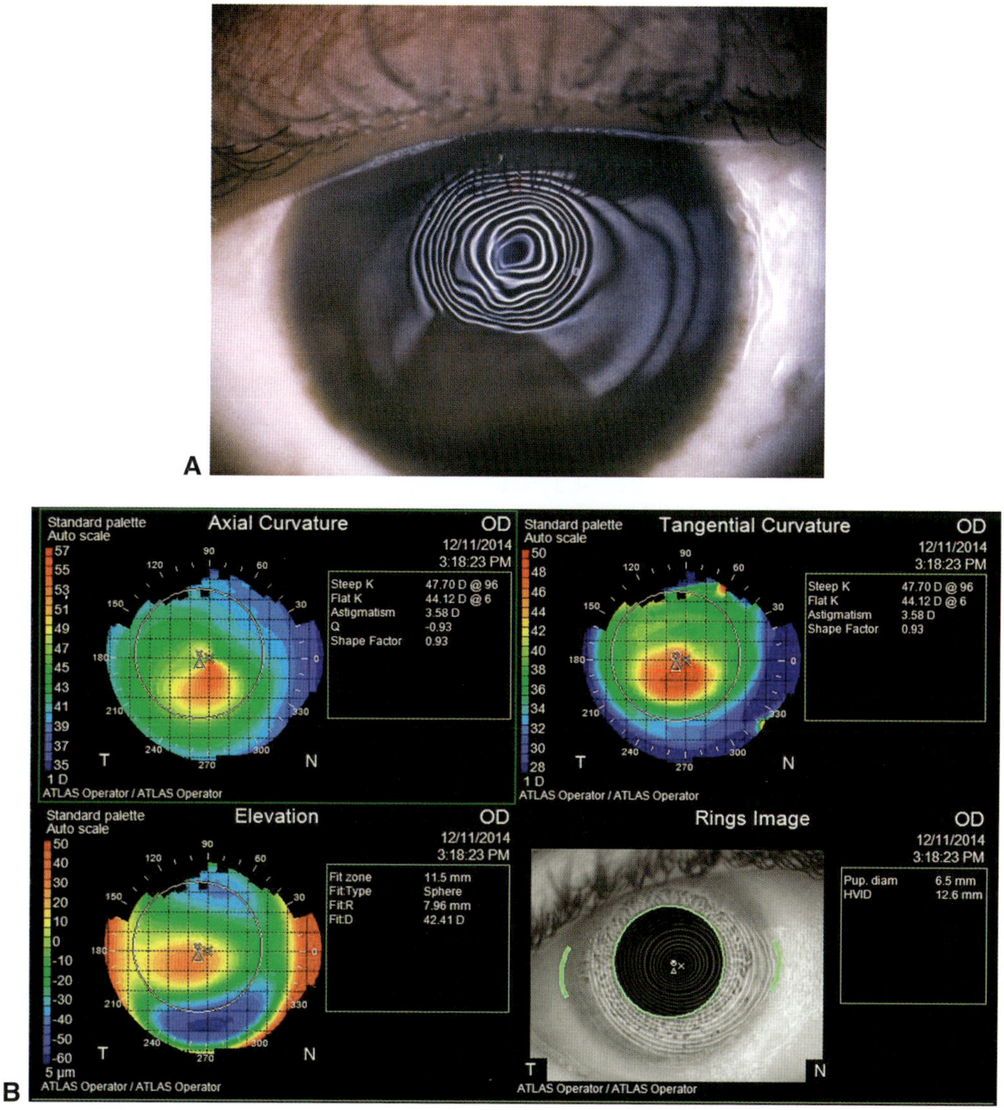

Figure 1-12 Corneal topography in keratoconus. **A,** Placido imaging showing distorted corneal mires. **B,** Axial, tangential, and elevation topography maps of the same cornea. *(Courtesy of M. Bowes Hamill, MD.)*

the radius to be the length necessary to correspond to a sphere with the same curvature at that point. The curvature, which is expressed in diopters, is estimated by the difference between the corneal index of refraction and 1.000, divided by this tangentially determined radius. A tangential map typically shows better sensitivity to peripheral changes, with less smoothing of the curvature than seen on an axial map (see Figures 1-11B and 1-12B). In these maps, diopters are relative units of curvature and are not the equivalent of diopters of corneal power. The potential benefit of this method's greater sensitivity is balanced by its tendency to document excessive detail ("noise"), which may not be clinically relevant.

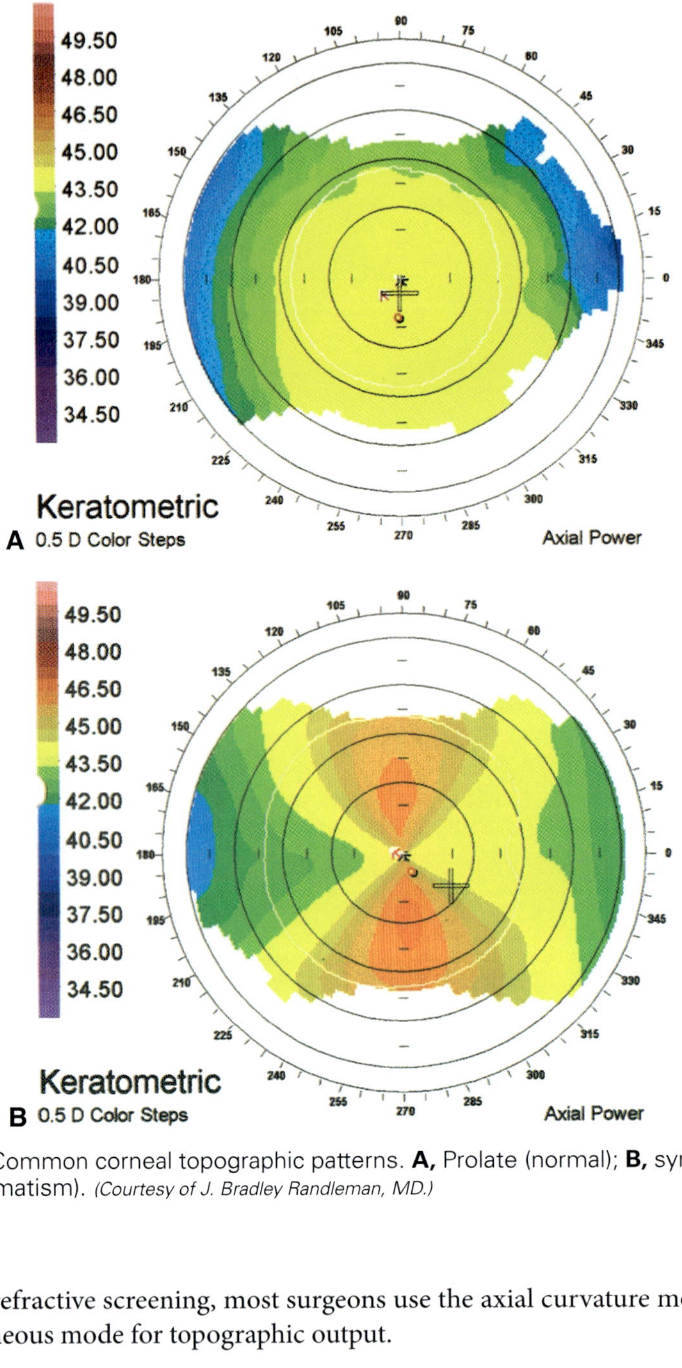

Figure 1-13 Common corneal topographic patterns. **A,** Prolate (normal); **B,** symmetric bow tie (regular astigmatism). *(Courtesy of J. Bradley Randleman, MD.)*

For routine refractive screening, most surgeons use the axial curvature mode rather than the instantaneous mode for topographic output.

Corneal topography and astigmatism

A topographic image of a normal cornea without astigmatism demonstrates a relatively uniform color pattern centrally with a natural flattening in the periphery (Fig 1-13A). *Regular astigmatism* is uniform steepening along a single corneal meridian that can be fully corrected with a cylindrical lens. Topographic imaging of regular astigmatism demonstrates a symmetric "bow-tie" pattern along a single meridian with a straight axis on both sides of center (Fig 1-13B). The bow-tie pattern on topographic maps is an artifact of Placido-based imaging; that is, because the Placido image cannot detect curvature at the central measurement point, the corneal meridional steepening seems to disappear centrally and become enhanced farther from center.

Irregular astigmatism is nonuniform corneal steepening from a variety of causes that cannot be corrected by cylindrical lenses. Irregular astigmatism decreases corrected distance visual acuity (CDVA) and may also reduce contrast sensitivity and increase visual aberrations, depending on the magnitude of irregularity. Rigid gas-permeable contact lenses can correct visual acuity reductions resulting from corneal irregular astigmatism by bridging the irregular corneal surface and the contact lens with the tear film. For more information on irregular astigmatism, see BCSC Section 3, *Clinical Optics and Vision Rehabilitation.*

Corneal topography is very helpful in evaluating eyes with irregular astigmatism. Topographic changes include nonorthogonal steep and flat meridians (ie, not 90° apart; Fig 1-14). Asymmetry between the superior and inferior or nasal and temporal halves of the cornea may also be revealed by corneal topography, although these patterns are not necessarily indicative of corneal pathology. In contrast, wavefront analysis can demonstrate higher-order aberrations such as coma, trefoil, quadrafoil, or secondary astigmatism. The ability to differentiate regular from irregular astigmatism has clinical significance in keratorefractive surgery. Traditional excimer laser ablation can correct spherocylindrical errors but does not effectively treat irregular astigmatism. Topography-guided ablation may be useful in treating irregular astigmatism not caused by early corneal ectatic disorders.

Ghoreishi M, Naderi Beni A, Naderi Beni Z. Visual outcomes of topography-guided excimer laser surgery for treatment of patients with irregular astigmatism. *Lasers Med Sci.* 2014;29(1):105–111.

Lin DT, Holland S, Tan JC, Moloney G. Clinical results of topography-based customized ablations in highly aberrated eyes and keratoconus/ectasia with cross-linking. *J Refract Surg.* 2012;28(11 Suppl):S841–S848.

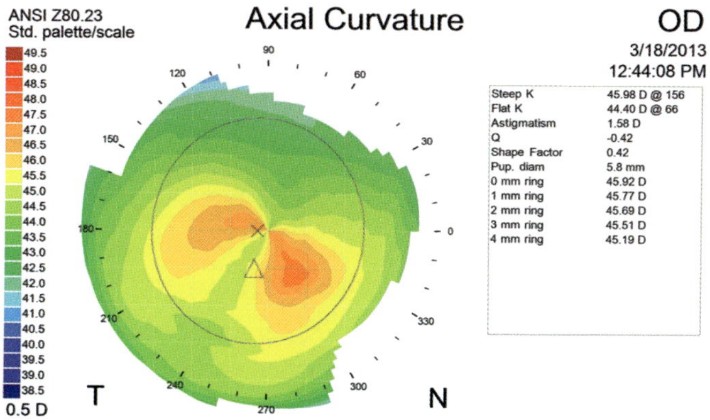

Figure 1-14 A curvature map showing nonorthogonal axes, which may indicate pathology that would contraindicate refractive surgery. *(Courtesy of Gregg J. Berdy, MD.)*

Limitations of corneal topography

In addition to the limitations of specific algorithms and the variations in terminology among manufacturers, the accuracy of corneal topography may be affected by other potential problems:

- tear film irregularities
- misalignment (misaligned corneal topography may give a false impression of corneal apex decentration suggestive of keratoconus)
- instability (test-to-test variation)
- insensitivity to focus errors
- limited area of coverage (central and limbal)
- decreased accuracy of corneal power simulation measurements (SIM K) after refractive surgical procedures
- decreased accuracy of posterior surface elevation values (with scanning-slit technology) in the presence of corneal opacities or, often, after refractive surgery

Roberts C. Corneal topography: a review of terms and concepts. *J Cataract Refract Surg.* 1996;22(5):624–629.

Corneal Tomography

Whereas surface corneal curvature (power) is best expressed by Placido-based topography, overall corneal shape, including spatial thickness profiles, is best expressed by tomography. Various imaging systems are available that take multiple slit images and reconstruct them into a corneal shape profile, including anterior and posterior corneal elevation data (Fig 1-15). Among the methods used are scanning-slit technology, Scheimpflug-based imaging systems, and anterior segment optical coherence tomography (OCT) that can provide epithelial mapping for refractive surgery. To represent shape directly, color maps may be used to display a *z-height* from an arbitrary plane such as the iris plane; however, in order to be clinically useful, corneal surface maps are plotted to show differences from best-fit spheres or other objects that closely mimic the normal corneal shape (Fig 1-16). In general, each device calculates the best-fit sphere individually for each map. For this reason, elevation maps cannot be compared precisely because they often have different referenced best-fit sphere characteristics.

Elevation-based tomography is especially helpful in refractive surgery for depicting the anterior and posterior surface shapes of the cornea and lens. With such information, alterations to the shape of the ocular structures, especially postoperative changes, can be determined with greater accuracy.

Indications for Corneal Imaging in Refractive Surgery

Corneal topography is an essential part of the preoperative evaluation of refractive surgery candidates. About two-thirds of patients with normal corneas have a symmetric astigmatism pattern that is round, oval, or bow-tie shaped (see Figure 1-13). Asymmetric patterns include asymmetric bow-tie patterns, inferior steepening, superior steepening, skewed radial axes, or other nonspecific irregularities.

Corneal topography detects irregular astigmatism, which may result from abnormal tear film, contact lens warpage, keratoconus and other corneal ectatic disorders, corneal surgery, trauma, scarring, and postinflammatory or degenerative conditions. Repeated topographic examinations may be helpful when the underlying etiology is in question, especially in cases of suspicious steepening patterns in patients who wear contact lenses or who have an abnormal tear film. It is often helpful to have contact lens users discontinue their lens wear for an extended period before preoperative planning; this allows the corneal map and refraction to stabilize. Patients with keratoconus or other ectatic disorders are not routinely considered for ablative keratorefractive surgery because the abnormal cornea may exhibit an unpredictable response or progressive ectasia. *Forme fruste,* or *subclinical, keratoconus* typically is considered a contraindication to ablative refractive surgery. Studies are under way to determine the suitability of some keratorefractive procedures in combination with corneal crosslinking as alternative therapeutic modalities for these patients (see also BCSC Section 8, *External Disease and Cornea*).

Corneal topography and tomography can also be used to demonstrate the effects of keratorefractive procedures. Preoperative and postoperative maps may be compared to determine the refractive effect achieved (*difference map;* Fig 1-17). Corneal mapping can also help explain unexpected results, including undercorrection and overcorrection; induced astigmatism; and induced aberrations from small optical zones, decentered ablations, or central islands (Fig 1-18).

Ambrósio R Jr, Alonso RS, Luz A, Coca Velarde LG. Corneal-thickness spatial profile and corneal-volume distribution: tomographic indices to detect keratoconus. *J Cataract Refract Surg.* 2006;32(11):1851–1859.

De Paiva CS, Harris LD, Pflugfelder SC. Keratoconus-like topographic changes in keratoconjunctivitis sicca. *Cornea.* 2003;22(1):22–24.

Rabinowitz YS, Yang H, Brickman Y, et al. Videokeratography database of normal human corneas. *Br J Ophthalmol.* 1996;80(7):610–616.

Corneal Biomechanics

Characteristics of the Stroma

The *corneal stroma* is the dominant structural component of the cornea and consists of collagen fibrils arranged in approximately 200 lamellar sheets. This network of collagen is largely responsible for the mechanical strength of the cornea. Lamellae are oriented parallel to the corneal surface at alternating angles to the adjacent lamellae, and the predominant fiber orientations in the posterior two-thirds of the stroma are vertical and horizontal. The fibrils demonstrate more branching and interweaving in the anterior third of the stroma, which confers greater biomechanical strength to the anterior stroma. In keratoconus, branching fibers are sparse in the area of the cone, which may cause local weakness. Structural differences between the anterior and posterior stroma are relevant in assessing the relative impact of procedures such as LASIK, PRK, and SMILE.

The type and distribution of glycosaminoglycans differ between the anterior and posterior stroma, and the more hydrophilic proteins in the posterior stroma influence

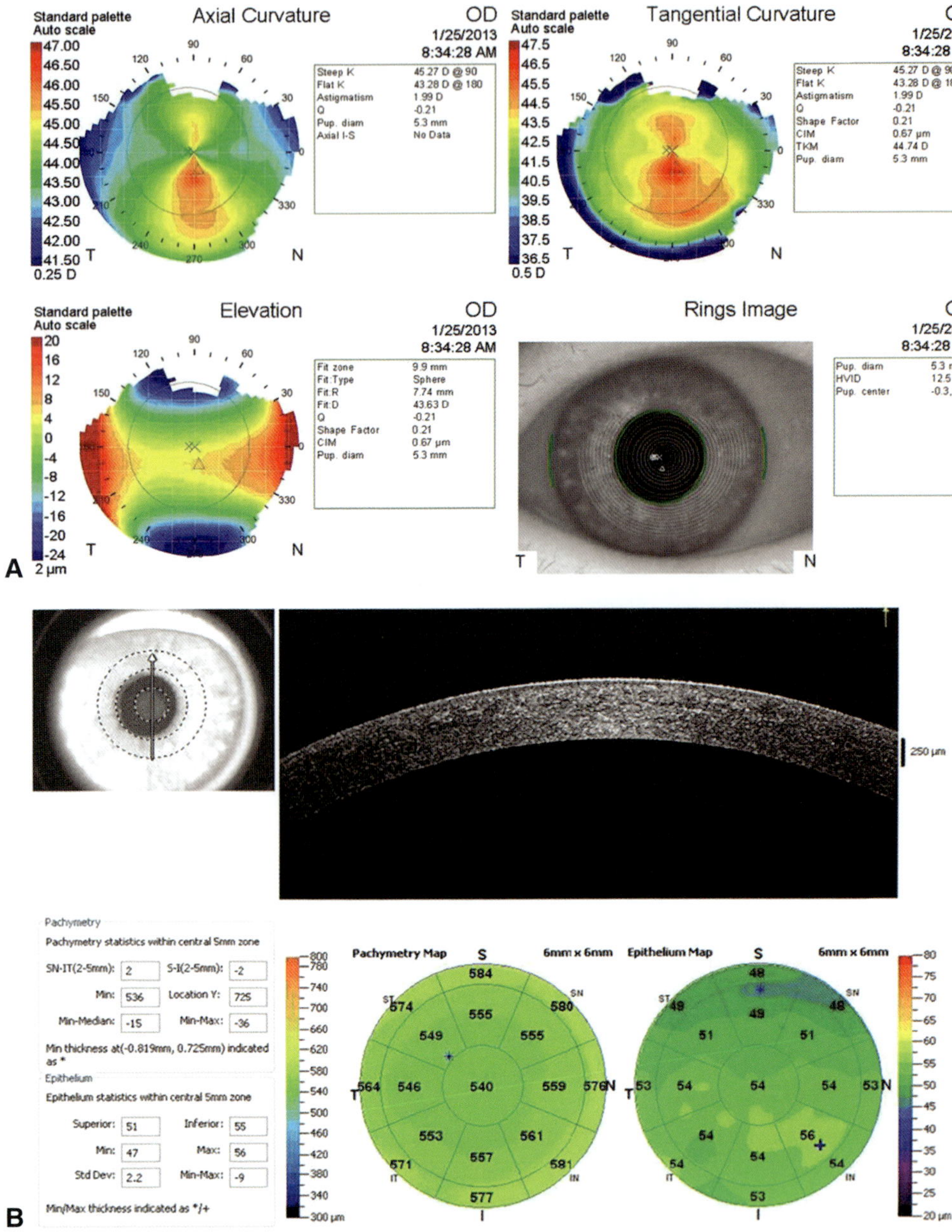

Figure 1-15 Different options for corneal imaging. All images are of the same patient taken at the same visit. **A,** Placido disk–based corneal curvature map showing axial and tangential curvature maps as well as the elevation map and the Placido mires. This mapping technology analyzes *only* the surface characteristics of the cornea. **B,** Optical coherence tomography image. Note that the corneal thickness profile (of the stroma as well as the epithelium) is well demonstrated, but the overall surface curvature is not.

(Continued)

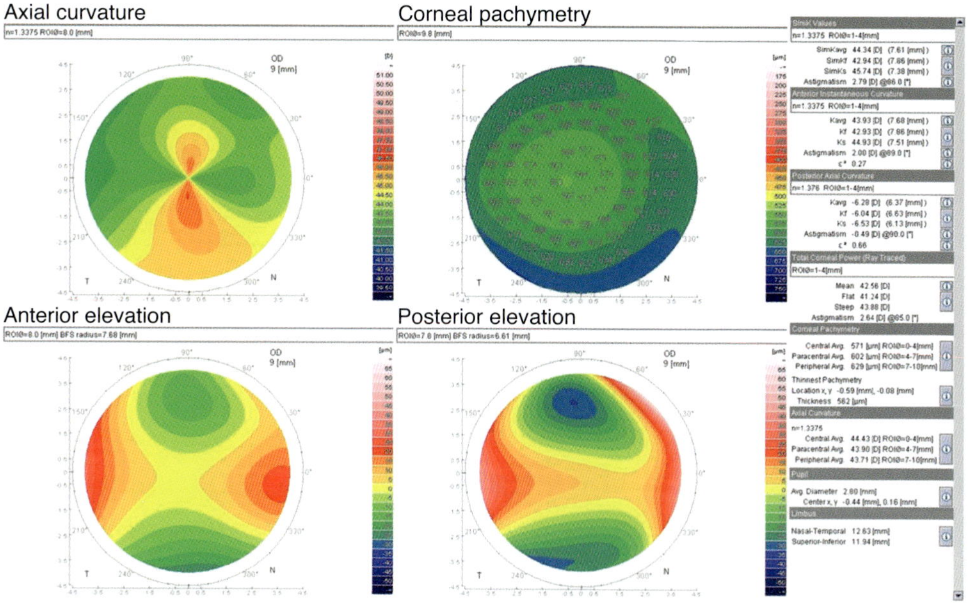

C

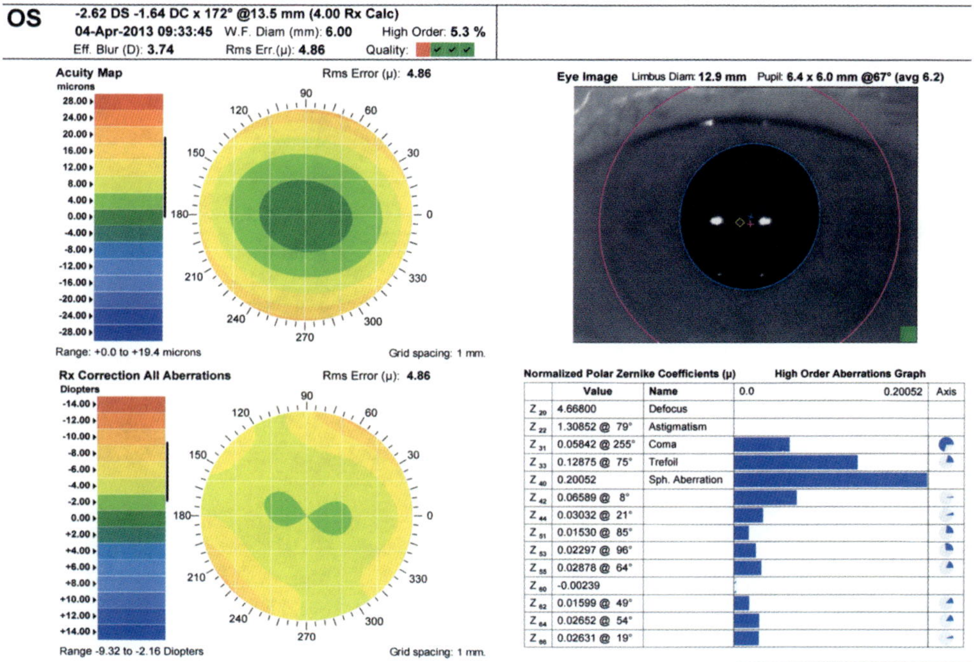

D

Figure 1-15 *(continued)* **C,** Corneal tomography image using dual Scheimpflug/Placido–based technology. The surface curvature, pachymetry, and anterior and posterior elevation mappings are shown. Numerical values appear along the right side. **D,** Wavescan image from a device like that illustrated in Fig 1-2A, taken of the fellow eye of the one seen in parts **A, B,** and **C.** Note that this map does not show corneal surface contours or features but rather provides information about the optics of the entire ocular system. As such, it can provide information on the refractive error and aberrations of the entire eye. *(Courtesy of M. Bowes Hamill, MD.)*

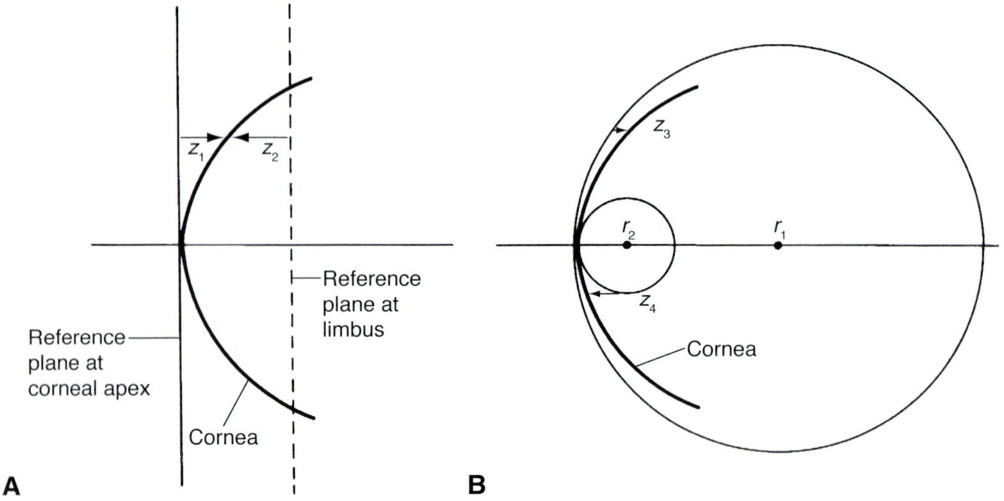

Figure 1-16 Height maps (typically in µm). **A,** Height relative to plane surface; z_1 is below the surface parallel to the corneal apex, and z_2 is above the surface parallel to the corneal limbus. **B,** Height relative to reference sphere; z_3 is below a flat sphere of radius r_1, and z_4 is above a steep sphere of radius r_2. *(Illustration by Christine Gralapp.)*

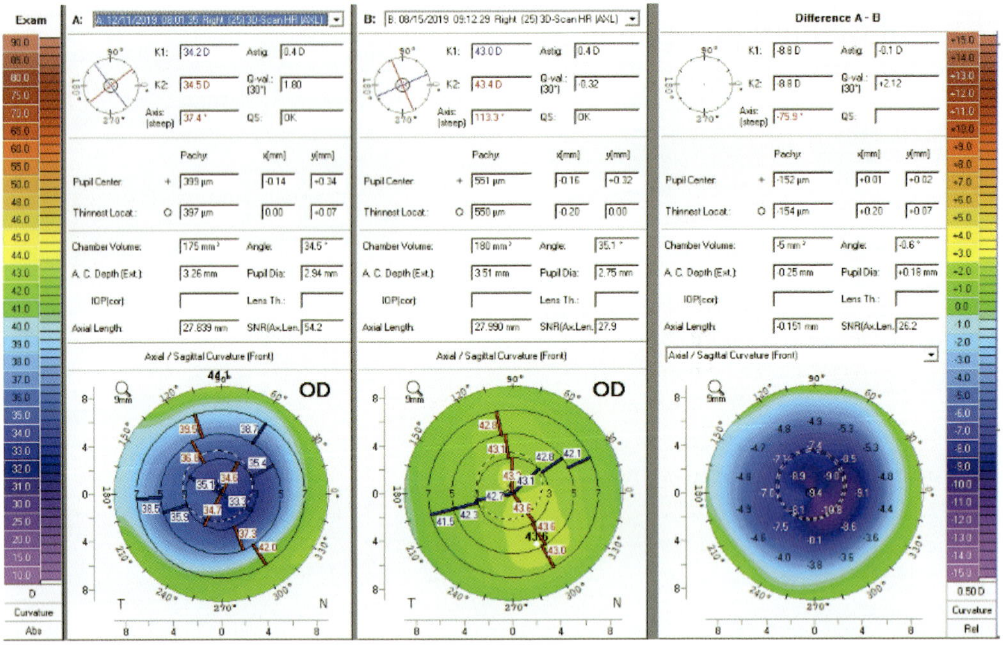

Figure 1-17 Scheimpflug tomography difference maps demonstrating corneal power change before and after myopic LASIK. *(Courtesy of Karolinne Maia Rocha, MD, PhD.)*

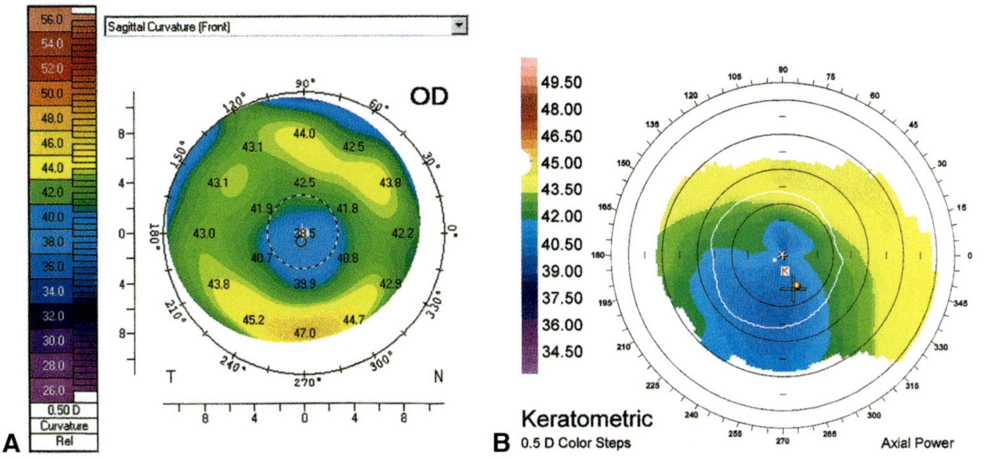

Figure 1-18 Postablation topographic maps. **A,** Small optical zone after excimer laser ablation; **B,** decentered ablation. *(Courtesy of J. Bradley Randleman, MD.)*

the stroma's swelling and load-bearing properties. When the cornea is in a normally hydrated state, stress is distributed relatively evenly across the corneal depth. In the presence of corneal edema, the anterior lamellae take up most of the stress and the posterior fibers become lax, which can be visualized as stromal folds that propagate to the Descemet membrane.

Evaluation Methods

Diagnostic techniques that directly evaluate biomechanics before refractive surgery, ideally to help differentiate between healthy and abnormal corneas, are available and in development. Devices currently available rely on bidirectional applanation tonometry or corneal deformation measurement with Scheimpflug imaging.

With *noncontact bidirectional applanation,* a focused air jet is used to indent the cornea and record 2 pressure measurements: the pressure at which the cornea moves inward, reaching the first applanation, and the pressure at which the cornea recovers from a slight concavity as the air pump decreases pressure at an inverse rate (the second applanation). The pressure at the second applanation is lower than that at the first; this difference is called *corneal hysteresis (CH),* which represents the viscous (time-dependent) dissipation of energy in the cornea (Fig 1-19, left). Low CH has been associated with keratoconus (Fig 1-19, right) and identified as an independent risk factor for progressive visual field loss in glaucoma. The mean of these 2 pressures is the *Goldmann-correlated IOP (IOPg).* The *corneal-compensated IOP (IOPcc)* is a pressure measurement that takes into account the biomechanical properties and is independent of the central corneal thickness. The *corneal resistance factor (CRF)* is an indicator of the overall resistance to the air puff that is weighted more toward the instantaneous (elastic) properties of the cornea.

The *corneal deformation method* uses an ultra-high-speed Scheimpflug camera to monitor the deformation of the cornea from a noncontact tonometer air-puff indentation.

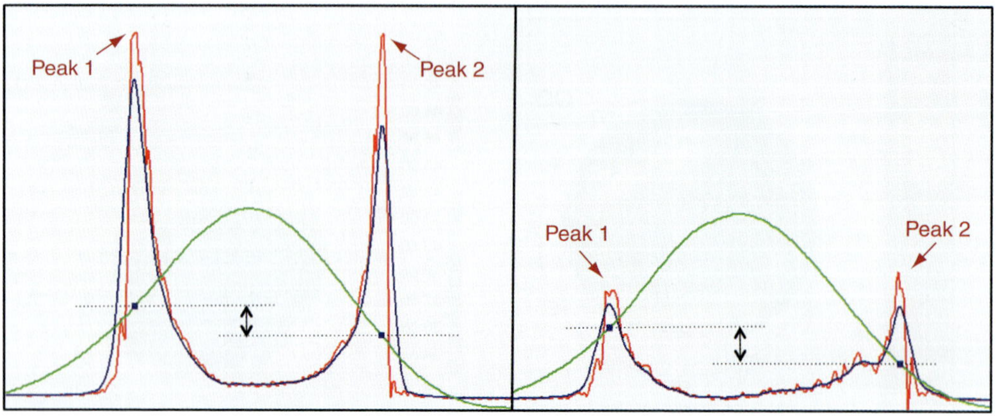

Figure 1-19 Noncontact bidirectional applanation. The device delivers a collimated stream of air onto the corneal apex *(green curve);* the optical signal *(red curve)* represents the dynamic motion of the cornea during the rapid in/out deformation. The filtered applanation signals are plotted in blue *(blue line).* The difference between the inward and outward pressure values defines corneal hysteresis. *(Left)* Repeatable high-amplitude peaks with minimal signal noise are seen in normal corneas. *(Right)* Low-amplitude peaks and signal noise are observed in keratoconus patients. *(Courtesy of Karolinne Maia Rocha, MD, PhD.)*

This method provides detailed information about the biomechanical characteristics of the cornea by determining velocity, length, and time lapse during different phases of applanation.

Abahussin M, Hayes S, Knox Cartwright NE, et al. 3D collagen orientation study of the human cornea using x-ray diffraction and femtosecond laser technology. *Invest Ophthalmol Vis Sci.* 2009;50(11):5159–5164.

Blackburn BJ, Jenkins MW, Rollins AM, Dupps WJ. A review of structural and biomechanical changes in the cornea in aging, disease, and photochemical crosslinking. *Front Bioeng Biotechnol.* 2019;7:66.

Damgaard IB, Reffat M, Hjortdal J. Review of corneal biomechanical properties following LASIK and SMILE for myopia and myopic astigmatism. *Open Ophthalmol J.* 2018;12:164–174.

Dupps WJ Jr, Wilson SE. Biomechanics and wound healing in the cornea. *Exp Eye Res.* 2006;83(4):709–720.

Garcia-Porta N, Fernandes P, Queiros A, Salgado-Borges J, Parafita-Mato M, González-Méijome JM. Corneal biomechanical properties in different ocular conditions and new measurement techniques. *ISRN Ophthalmol.* 2014;2014:724546.

Glass DH, Roberts CJ, Litsky AS, Weber PA. A viscoelastic biomechanical model of the cornea describing the effect of viscosity and elasticity on hysteresis. *Invest Ophthalmol Vis Sci.* 2008;49(9):3919–3926.

Changes in Corneal Biomechanics After Refractive Procedures

Corneal biomechanical properties are of major importance in keratorefractive surgeries. The various procedures differ in the biomechanical response they produce, depending on the biomechanical load of the ablated or dissected cornea. In LASIK, a corneal flap is created with a microkeratome or femtosecond laser, followed by thinning of the stromal bed with excimer laser ablation. In photorefractive keratectomy (PRK), the laser is applied directly to the anterior corneal stroma without creating a flap. In small-incision lenticule extraction (SMILE), a femtosecond laser is used to create a 3-dimensional lenticule, which is then extracted through a small corneal incision ranging from 2 to 5 mm. Because no flap is created and the most anterior stromal lamellae remain intact (except in the region of the small incision), this procedure may provide better biomechanical stability. Some studies have demonstrated better CH and CRF measurements following SMILE compared with LASIK or laser subepithelial keratomileusis (LASEK), possibly because the stiffer anterior stroma is preserved. However, ectasia has been reported after SMILE, as well.

Chen M, Yu M, Dai J. Comparison of biomechanical effects of small incision lenticule extraction and laser-assisted subepithelial keratomileusis. *Acta Ophthalmol.* 2016;94(7): e586–e591.

Dou R, Wang Y, Xu L, Wu D, Wu W, Li X. Comparison of corneal biomechanical characteristics after surface ablation refractive surgery and novel lamellar refractive surgery. *Cornea.* 2015;34(11):1441–1446.

Ganesh S, Brar S, Arra RR. Refractive lenticule extraction small incision lenticule extraction: a new refractive surgery paradigm. *Indian J Ophthalmol.* 2018;66(1):10–19.

Sachdev G, Sachdev MS, Sachdev R, Gupta H. Unilateral corneal ectasia following small-incision lenticule extraction. *J Cataract Refract Surg.* 2015;41(9):2014–2018.

Wang D, Liu M, Chen Y, et al. Differences in the corneal biomechanical changes after SMILE and LASIK. *J Refract Surg.* 2014;30(10):702–707.

Wu D, Wang Y, Zhang L, Wei S, Tang X. Corneal biomechanical effects: small-incision lenticule extraction versus femtosecond laser-assisted laser in situ keratomileusis. *J Cataract Refract Surg.* 2014;40(6):954–962.

Corneal Effects of Keratorefractive Surgery

All keratorefractive procedures induce refractive changes by altering corneal curvature; however, the method by which the alteration is accomplished varies by the procedure and the refractive error. Treatment of myopia requires a *flattening,* or decrease, in central corneal curvature, whereas treatment of hyperopia requires a *steepening,* or increase, in central corneal curvature. Keratorefractive surgery can be performed using a variety of techniques, including incisional, tissue addition or subtraction, alloplastic material addition, and laser ablation (see the section Laser Biophysics for discussion of laser ablation).

Overall patient satisfaction after the surgery depends largely on the successful correction of refractive error and creation of a corneal shape that maximizes visual quality. As discussed previously, the normal prolate corneal shape produces an aspheric optical system, while oblate corneas increase sphere aberration and visual symptoms such as glare, halos, and reduced contrast sensitivity. (See the section "Effect of excimer laser ablation on higher-order aberrations.")

Incisional Techniques

Incisions perpendicular to the corneal surface alter its shape, depending on the direction, depth, location, length, and number of incisions (see Chapter 3). All incisions cause a local flattening of the cornea. *Radial incisions* lead to flattening in both the meridian of the incision and the one 90° away. *Tangential (arcuate* or *linear) incisions* lead to flattening in the meridian of the incision and steepening in the meridian 90° away that may be equal to or less than the magnitude of the decrease in the primary meridian (Fig 1-20); this phenomenon is known as *coupling* (see Chapter 3, Fig 3-3). Reducing the optical zone of radial incisions increases their effect; similarly, placing tangential incisions closer to the visual axis increases the effect, as does increasing the length of a tangential incision, up to 3 clock-hours.

For optimum effect, an incision should be 85%–90% deep to retain an intact posterior lamella and maximum anterior bowing of the other lamellae. Nomograms for the number of incisions and optical zone size can be calculated using finite element analysis, but surgical nomograms are typically generated empirically (eg, see Chapter 3, Table 3-1). The important variables for radial and astigmatic surgery include patient age and the number, depth, and length of incisions. The same incision has greater effect in older patients than it does in younger patients. IOP and preoperative corneal curvature are not significant predictors of effect.

Technological developments have led to the use of femtosecond lasers for making arcuate incisions. Advanced imaging capabilities allow creation of femtosecond laser–assisted astigmatic or arcuate keratotomy (AK) with precise arc length, depth, and location (Video 1-1). Incorporation of iris registration technology allows cyclotorsion compensation and facilitates accurate placement of AK incisions on the intended meridian. Femtosecond laser–assisted AKs have been documented to yield good outcomes with low risks of wound dehiscence or corneal perforation.

VIDEO 1-1 Femtosecond laser astigmatic keratotomy post–penetrating keratoplasty.
Courtesy of Karolinne Maia Rocha, MD, PhD.

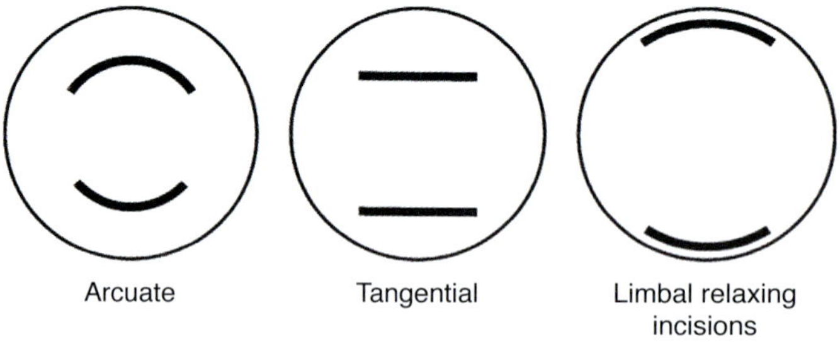

Figure 1-20 Schematic diagrams of incisions used in astigmatic keratotomy. Flattening is induced in the axis of the incisions (at 90° in this case), and steepening is induced 90° away from the incisions (at 180° in this case). *(Illustrations by Cyndie C. H. Wooley.)*

Chan TC, Cheng GP, Wang Z, Tham CC, Woo VC, Jhanji V. Vector analysis of corneal astigmatism after combined femtosecond-assisted phacoemulsification and arcuate keratotomy. *Am J Ophthalmol.* 2015;160(2):250–255.e252.
Chang JSM. Femtosecond laser-assisted astigmatic keratotomy: a review. *Eye Vis (Lond).* 2018;5:6.
Rowsey JJ. Ten caveats in keratorefractive surgery. *Ophthalmology.* 1983;90(2):148–155.
Visco DM, Bedi R, Packer M. Femtosecond laser-assisted arcuate keratotomy at the time of cataract surgery for the management of preexisting astigmatism [published correction appears in *J Cataract Refract Surg.* 2020;46(4):658]. *J Cataract Refract Surg.* 2019;45(12):1762–1769.

Tissue Addition or Subtraction Techniques

With the exception of laser ablation techniques (discussed in the section Laser Biophysics), lamellar procedures that alter corneal shape through tissue addition or subtraction are primarily of historical interest. *Keratomileusis* for myopia was originated by Barraquer as "carving" of the anterior surface of the cornea. It is defined as a method to modify the spherical or meridional surface of a healthy cornea by tissue subtraction. *Epikeratoplasty* (sometimes called *epikeratophakia*) adds a precision-lathed lenticule of donor tissue to the corneal surface to induce hyperopic or myopic changes. *Keratophakia* requires the addition of a tissue lenticule or synthetic inlay intrastromally.

However, there is renewed interest in tissue subtraction as a way to treat refractive error without excimer laser ablation. These current procedures—called *refractive lenticule extraction (ReLEx), femtosecond lenticule extraction (FLEx),* and *small-incision lenticule extraction (SMILE)*—use a femtosecond laser to excise an intrastromal lenticule and thus alter the corneal curvature.

Alloplastic Material Addition Techniques

The shape of the cornea can be altered by adding alloplastic material such as hydrogel on the surface or in the corneal stroma to modify the anterior shape or refractive index of the cornea. For example, the 2 arc segments of an intrastromal corneal ring can be placed in 2 pockets of the stroma to directly reshape the surface contour according to the profile and location of the individual segments (Fig 1-21; see also BCSC Section 8, *External Disease and Cornea*).

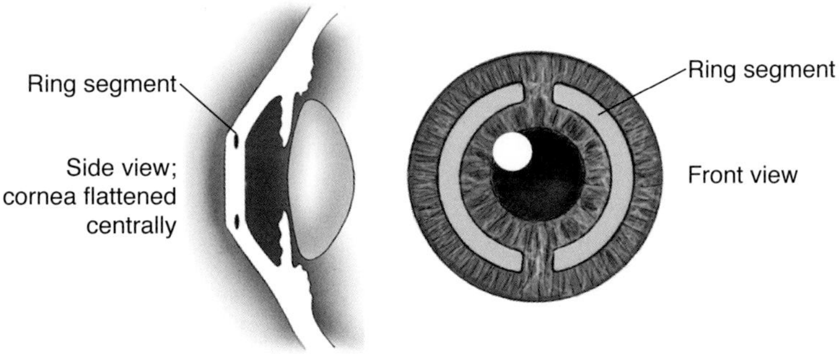

Figure 1-21 Schematic illustrations showing placement of intrastromal corneal ring segments. *(Illustrations by Jeanne Koelling.)*

A different type of inlay, which alters optical function by means of a small-aperture effect, was approved for treatment of presbyopia in 2015. Although other styles of corneal inlays and onlays have been investigated for presbyopia, studies were halted; in one case, an approved product was withdrawn from the market because of high rates of corneal haze. For further discussion, see Chapter 10.

Collagen Shrinkage Techniques

Alteration in corneal biomechanics can also be achieved by collagen shrinkage. Heating collagen to a critical temperature of 58°–76°C causes it to shrink, inducing changes in the corneal curvature. *Thermokeratoplasty* treatments such as *conductive keratoplasty (CK)* are generally avoided in the central cornea because of scarring but can be used in the mid-periphery to cause local collagen contraction with concurrent central corneal steepening (see Chapter 10, Figure 10-3).

Laser Biophysics

Laser–Tissue Interactions

Three different types of laser–tissue interactions are used in keratorefractive surgery: photoablative, photodisruptive, and photothermal. *Photoablation,* the most important laser–tissue interaction in refractive surgery, breaks chemical bonds by using excimer (from "*exci*ted di*mer*") lasers or other lasers of the appropriate wavelength. Laser energy of 4 eV per photon or greater is sufficient to break carbon–nitrogen or carbon–carbon tissue bonds.

Photoablative effects

Argon-fluoride lasers are excimer lasers that use electrical energy to stimulate argon to form dimers with fluorine gas. They generate a wavelength of 193 nm with 6.4 eV per photon. The 193-nm light is in the ultraviolet C (high ultraviolet) range, approaching the wavelength of x-rays. In addition to having high energy per photon, light at this end of the electromagnetic spectrum has very low tissue penetrance and thus is suitable for operating on the surface of a tissue. This laser energy is capable of great precision, with little thermal spread in tissue; moreover, its lack of penetrance or lethality to cells makes the 193-nm laser nonmutagenic, enhancing its safety. (DNA mutagenicity occurs in the range of 250 nm.) *Solid-state lasers* have been designed to generate wavelengths of light near 193 nm without the need for toxic gas, but the technical difficulties in manufacturing these lasers have limited their clinical use.

Photodisruptive effects

The *femtosecond laser* is approved by the US Food and Drug Administration (FDA) for creating corneal flaps for LASIK and for the SMILE procedure. It may also be used to create channels for intrastromal ring segments and for lamellar or penetrating keratoplasty. It uses a 1053-nm infrared beam that causes *photodisruption,* in which tissue is transformed into plasma, and the subsequent high pressure and temperature generated by this process lead to rapid tissue expansion and the formation of microscopic cavitation bubbles within the corneal stroma. Contiguous laser pulses allow creation of the corneal flap, lenticule of tissue, channel, or keratoplasty incision.

Photothermal effects

Photothermal effects are achieved by focusing a holmium:YAG laser with a wavelength of 2.13 μm into the anterior stroma. The beam's energy is absorbed by water in the cornea, and the resulting heat causes local collagen shrinkage and subsequent steepening of the cornea. This technique is FDA approved for low hyperopia but is not commonly used because of regression of effect.

Fundamentals of Excimer Laser Photoablation

All photoablative procedures result in the removal of corneal tissue. The amount of tissue removed centrally for myopic treatments using a broad-beam laser is estimated by the *Munnerlyn formula:*

$$\text{Ablation Depth } (\mu\text{m}) \approx \frac{\text{Degree of Myopia (D)} \times \text{Optical Zone Diameter [OZ (mm)]}^2}{3}$$

Clinical experience has confirmed that the effective change is independent of the initial curvature of the cornea. The Munnerlyn formula highlights some of the problems and limitations of laser vision correction. The amount of ablation increases by the square of the optical zone, but the complications of glare, halos, and regression increase when the optical zone decreases. To reduce these adverse effects, the optical zone should be 6 mm or larger.

With surface ablation, the laser treatment is applied to the Bowman layer and the anterior stroma; in contrast, LASIK combines an initial lamellar incision with ablation of the underlying cornea, typically in the stromal bed (see Chapter 4 for further details of surgical technique). Flap thickness ranges from ultrathin (80–100 μm) to standard (120–180 μm). The thickness and diameter of the LASIK flap depend on instrumentation, corneal diameter, corneal curvature, and corneal thickness.

Treatments for myopia flatten the cornea by removing central corneal tissue, whereas those for hyperopia steepen the cornea by removing a doughnut-shaped portion of midperipheral tissue. Some lasers use a *multizone treatment algorithm* to conserve tissue by creating several concentric optical zones to achieve the total correction required. This method can provide the full correction centrally, while tapering peripheral zones can reduce symptoms created by abrupt transitions between ablated and nonablated cornea. It also allows higher degrees of myopia to be treated (Fig 1-22).

Care must be taken to ensure that enough stromal tissue remains after creation of the LASIK flap and ablation to maintain adequate corneal structure. The historical standard has been to leave a minimum of 250 μm of tissue in the stromal bed, although the exact amount of remaining tissue required to ensure biomechanical stability is not known and likely varies among individuals. See Chapters 2 and 5 for further discussion of these issues.

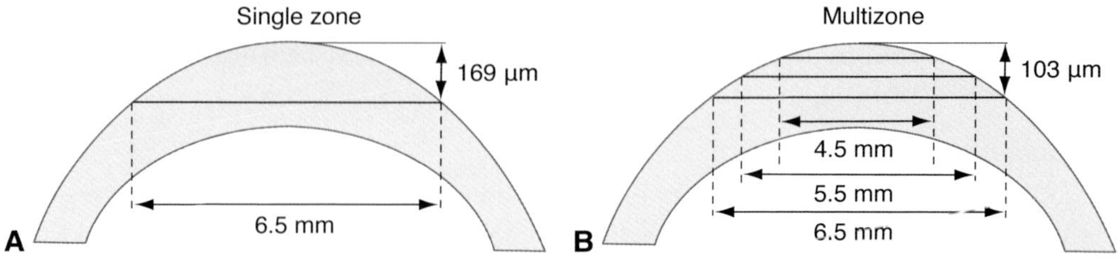

Figure 1-22 Schematic comparison of single and multizone keratectomies. **A,** Depth of ablation required to correct 12.00 D of myopia in a single pass. **B,** The diagram shows how the use of multiple ablation zones reduces the ablation depth required to treat 12.00 D of myopia: 6.00 D are corrected in a 4.5-mm optical zone, 3.00 D in a 5.5-mm optical zone, and 3.00 D in a 6.5-mm optical zone. Thus, the total 12.00 D correction is achieved centrally using a shallower ablation depth (103 µm versus 169 µm for a single pass). *(Illustrations by Cyndie C. H. Wooley.)*

Types of Photoablative Lasers

Photoablative lasers can be subdivided into broad-beam lasers, scanning-slit lasers, and flying spot lasers. *Broad-beam lasers* have larger-diameter beams and slower repetition rates and rely on optics or mirrors to create a smooth and homogeneous multimode laser beam of up to approximately 7 mm in diameter. These lasers have very high energy per pulse and require a small number of pulses to ablate the cornea. *Scanning-slit lasers* generate a narrow-slit laser beam that is scanned over the surface of the tissue to alter the photoablation profile, thus improving the smoothness of the ablated cornea and allowing for larger-diameter ablation zones. *Flying spot lasers* use smaller-diameter beams (approximately 0.5–2.0 mm) that are scanned at a higher repetition rate; they require use of a tracking mechanism for precise placement of the desired pattern of ablation. Broad-beam lasers and some scanning-slit lasers require a mechanical iris diaphragm or ablatable mask to create the desired shape in the cornea, whereas the rest of the scanning-slit lasers and the flying spot lasers use a pattern projected onto the surface to guide the ablation profile without masking. The majority of excimer lasers in current clinical practice use some form of variable or flying spot ablation profile.

Wavefront-optimized and wavefront-guided laser ablations

Because conventional laser treatment profiles have small blend zones and create a more oblate corneal shape following myopic corrections, they are likely to induce some degree of higher-order aberration, especially spherical aberration and coma. These aberrations occur because the corneal curvature is angled more peripherally in relation to laser pulses emanating from the central location; thus, the pulses hitting the peripheral cornea are relatively less effective than are the central pulses.

Wavefront-optimized laser ablation improves the postoperative corneal shape by taking the curvature of the cornea into account and increasing the number of peripheral pulses; this approach minimizes the induction of higher-order aberrations and often results in better-quality vision and fewer night-vision concerns because it maintains a more prolate corneal shape. As in conventional procedures, the patient's refraction alone is used to program the wavefront-optimized laser ablation. This technology does not directly address preexisting higher-order aberrations; however, recent studies have found that the vast majority of patients do not have substantial preoperative higher-order aberrations. It also has the advantages of being faster than wavefront-guided technology and avoiding the additional expense of an aberrometer.

In *wavefront-guided laser ablation,* information obtained from a wavefront-sensing aberrometer (which quantifies the aberrations) is transferred electronically to the treatment laser to program the ablation. This process differs from conventional excimer laser and wavefront-optimized laser treatments in which subjective refraction alone is used to program the laser ablation. The wavefront-guided laser is intended to treat both lower-order (ie, myopia or hyperopia and/or astigmatism) and higher-order aberrations by applying complex ablation patterns to the cornea to correct the wavefront deviations. The correction of higher-order aberrations requires non–radially symmetric patterns of ablation, which are often much smaller in magnitude than ablations needed to correct defocus and astigmatism.

The difference between the desired and the actual wavefront is used to generate a 3-dimensional map of the planned ablation. Accurate registration is required to ensure that the ablation treatment actually delivered to the cornea matches the intended pattern. Such registration is achieved by using marks at the limbus before obtaining the wavefront patterns or by employing iris registration, which matches reference points in the natural iris pattern to compensate for cyclotorsion and pupil centroid shift. The wavefront-guided laser then uses a pupil-tracking system, which helps maintain centration during treatment and allows accurate delivery of the customized ablation profile. Another potential advantage is that the planned laser treatment is transferred directly from the aberrometer and does not require manual entry, helping to avoid transcription errors.

The results for both wavefront-optimized and wavefront-guided ablations for myopia, hyperopia, and astigmatism are excellent, with well over 90% of eyes achieving 20/40 or better uncorrected distance visual acuity (UDVA). Although most visual acuity parameters are similar between conventional and customized treatments (including both wavefront-optimized and wavefront-guided treatments), most recent reports demonstrate improved vision quality when customized treatment profiles are used. Outcomes of wavefront-optimized treatments are similar to those of wavefront-guided treatments for most patients, except for those with substantial preoperative higher-order aberrations.

Miraftab M, Seyedian MA, Hashemi H. Wavefront-guided vs. wavefront-optimized LASIK: a randomized clinical trial comparing contralateral eyes. *J Refract Surg.* 2011;27(4):245–250.

Netto MV, Dupps W Jr, Wilson SE. Wavefront-guided ablation: evidence for efficacy compared to traditional ablation. *Am J Ophthalmol.* 2006;141(2):360–368.

Padmanabhan P, Mrochen M, Basuthkar S, Viswanathan D, Joseph R. Wavefront-guided versus wavefront-optimized laser in situ keratomileusis: contralateral comparative study. *J Cataract Refract Surg.* 2008;34(3):389–397.

Perez-Straziota CE, Randleman JB, Stulting RD. Visual acuity and higher-order aberrations with wavefront-guided and wavefront-optimized laser in situ keratomileusis. *J Cataract Refract Surg.* 2010;36(3):437–441.

Schallhorn SC, Farjo AA, Huang D, et al; American Academy of Ophthalmology. Wavefront-guided LASIK for the correction of primary myopia and astigmatism: a report by the American Academy of Ophthalmology. *Ophthalmology.* 2008;115(7):1249–1261.

Schallhorn SC, Tanzer DJ, Kaupp SE, Brown M, Malady SE. Comparison of night driving performance after wavefront-guided and conventional LASIK for moderate myopia. *Ophthalmology.* 2009;116(4):702–709.

Smith RG, Manche EE. One-year outcomes from a prospective, randomized, eye-to-eye comparison of wavefront-guided and wavefront-optimized PRK in myopia. *J Refract Surg.* 2020;36(3):160–168.

Stonecipher KG, Kezirian GM. Wavefront-optimized versus wavefront-guided LASIK for myopic astigmatism with the ALLEGRETTO WAVE: three-month results of a prospective FDA trial. *J Refract Surg.* 2008;24(4):S424–S430.

Topography-guided laser ablations

Topography-guided (TG) lasers are similar in concept to wavefront-guided lasers, but TG laser ablations use data from refraction and corneal topography rather than wavefront data from the whole eye. TG ablations have been successful in regularizing the cornea and improving vision in patients with decentered ablation, small optical zone, and irregular corneal surface. A TG laser is now approved for performing ablations in eyes with normal corneas, as well. Analysis of the visual outcomes reported to the FDA for 249 myopic eyes with or without astigmatism that underwent TG laser ablation with one system showed excellent outcomes in terms of safety, efficacy, accuracy, and stability. Postoperatively, 93% of eyes had UDVA of 20/20 or better, and 95% had a manifest refraction spherical equivalent within ±0.5 D of emmetropia. A significant increase in mesopic (41.3%) and photopic (31.9%) contrast sensitivity was found 6 months postoperatively.

Knorz MC, Jendritza B. Topographically-guided laser in situ keratomileusis to treat corneal irregularities. *Ophthalmology.* 2000;107(6):1138–1143.

Pasquali T, Krueger R. Topography-guided laser refractive surgery. *Curr Opin Ophthalmol.* 2012;23(4):264–268.

Zhang Y, Chen Y. A randomized comparative study of topography-guided versus wavefront-optimized FS-LASIK for correcting myopia and myopic astigmatism. *J Refract Surg.* 2019;35(9):575–582.

Corneal Wound Healing

All forms of keratorefractive surgery are exquisitely dependent on corneal wound healing to achieve the desired results. Satisfactory outcomes require either modifying the process of wound healing or exploiting normal wound healing for the benefit of the patient. For example, AK requires initial weakening of the cornea followed by permanent corneal healing, with replacement of the epithelial plugs by collagen and remodeling of the collagen to ensure stability and to avoid long-term hyperopic drift. In PRK, the epithelium is intended to heal quickly, with minimal stimulation of the underlying keratocytes, to avoid corneal scarring and haze. LASIK depends on intact epithelium and healthy endothelium early in the postoperative period to seal the flap. Later, the cornea must heal in the periphery to secure the flap in place and avoid late-term displacement while minimizing irregular astigmatism; moreover, the central cornea must remain devoid of significant healing to maintain a clear visual axis.

In addition to stromal healing, regeneration of the corneal nerves is crucial to maintaining a normal ocular surface and good visual function. Delay or difficulty in reinnervation can lead to decreased or abnormal corneal sensitivity, tear film instability, and dry eye symptoms.

The understanding of corneal wound healing has advanced tremendously with recognition of the multiple factors involved in the cascade of events initiated by corneal wounding. The cascade is somewhat dependent on the nature of the injury. Injury to the epithelium, for example, can lead to loss of underlying keratocytes from apoptosis. The remaining keratocytes respond by generating new glycosaminoglycans and collagen, depending in part on the duration of the epithelial defect and the depth of the stromal injury.

Dupps WJ Jr, Wilson SE. Biomechanics and wound healing in the cornea. *Exp Eye Res.* 2006;83(4):709–720.

Selected Complications

Corneal haze

In some cases, the cascade following injury can result in corneal haze that is localized in the subepithelial anterior stroma and which can persist for several years after surface ablation. Clinically significant haze, however, is present in only a small percentage of eyes. The tendency toward haze formation increases with deeper ablations, greater surface irregularity, and longer absence of the epithelium. Despite loss of the Bowman layer, normal or even enhanced numbers of hemidesmosomes and anchoring fibrils form to secure the epithelium to the stroma. Haze formation very rarely occurs in the central flap interface after LASIK, which may be related either to lack of significant epithelial injury and consequent subcellular signaling or to maintenance of some intact surface neurons.

Netto MV, Mohan RR, Sinha S, Sharma A, Dupps W, Wilson SE. Stromal haze, myofibroblasts, and surface irregularity after PRK. *Exp Eye Res.* 2006;82(5):788–797.

LASIK flap response

LASIK shows very little long-term evidence of healing between the disrupted lamellae and only typical stromal healing at the peripheral wound. The lamellae are initially held in position by negative stromal pressure generated by the endothelial cells aided by an intact epithelial surface. Even years after treatment, the lamellar interface can be broken and the flap lifted, indicating that only a minimal amount of healing occurs. LASIK flaps can also be dislodged secondary to trauma many years postoperatively.

Schmack I, Dawson DG, McCarey BE, Waring GO 3rd, Grossniklaus HE, Edelhauser HF. Cohesive tensile strength of human LASIK wounds with histologic, ultrastructural, and clinical correlations. *J Refract Surg.* 2005;21(5):433–445.

Drugs to Modulate Wound Healing

Controversy persists over the value of different drugs in modulating wound healing after surface ablation. In the United States, clinicians typically use a tapering regimen of corticosteroids to reduce inflammation after surgery. Mitomycin C has been applied to the stromal bed after excimer surface ablation to attempt to decrease haze formation (see Chapters 4 and 5). Vitamin C has been postulated to play a role in protecting the cornea from ultraviolet light damage by the excimer laser, but no randomized prospective clinical trial has yet been performed. Various growth factors that have been found to promote wound healing after PRK, including transforming growth factor β, may be useful in the future.

Majmudar PA, Schallhorn SC, Cason JB, et al. Mitomycin-C in corneal surface excimer laser ablation techniques: a report by the American Academy of Ophthalmology. *Ophthalmology.* 2015;122(6):1085–1095.

Emerging Technologies

Ocular Light Scatter Evaluation

Intraocular light scatter, or *straylight,* is a phenomenon caused by reflection, refraction, and diffraction of light from the cornea, lens, or retina, as well as from light penetrating through the sclera and iris. It decreases light transmission, reduces image contrast, and degrades retinal image quality. The scatter may be forward or backward. In *forward scatter* (ie, toward the retina), the scattered light is deviated less than 90° relative to the direction of incident light. It produces a veiling luminance on the retina, which reduces the contrast of the retinal image and causes glare. Scattered light that is deviated more than 90° is referred to as *backward scatter;* its main result is a reduction in the amount of light reaching the retina. Because forward light scatter directly affects visual performance, measuring this type of scatter is vital.

Several devices are commercially available to quantify forward light scatter. One of the most common methods is a double-pass technique that measures forward scatter caused by localized deviations of light on an objective scatter index (OSI). The OSI shows the objective amount of scattering caused by tear film irregularities and the loss of ocular transparency. OSI values range from 0 (no scatter) to a maximum of 25 (highly scattered system). Other approaches measure forward light scatter by quantifying optical straylight or by using psychophysical measurements.

Donnelly WJ 3rd, Applegate RA. Influence of exposure time and pupil size on a Shack-Hartmann metric of forward scatter. *J Refract Surg.* 2005;21(5):S547–S551.

Gouvea L, Waring GO 4th, Brundrett A, Crouse M, Rocha KM. Objective assessment of optical quality in dry eye disease using a double-pass imaging system. *Clin Ophthalmol.* 2019;13:1991–1996.

Koh S, Maeda N, Ikeda C, et al. Ocular forward light scattering and corneal backward light scattering in patients with dry eye. *Invest Ophthalmol Vis Sci.* 2014;55(10):6601–6606.

Spadea L, Maraone G, Verboschi F, Vingolo EM, Tognetto D. Effect of corneal light scatter on vision: a review of the literature. *Int J Ophthalmol.* 2016;9(3):459–464.

Corneal Epithelial Mapping

The corneal epithelium can alter its thickness profile to compensate for irregularities in the stromal surface. Thus, epithelial thickening is observed in areas of tissue loss. For

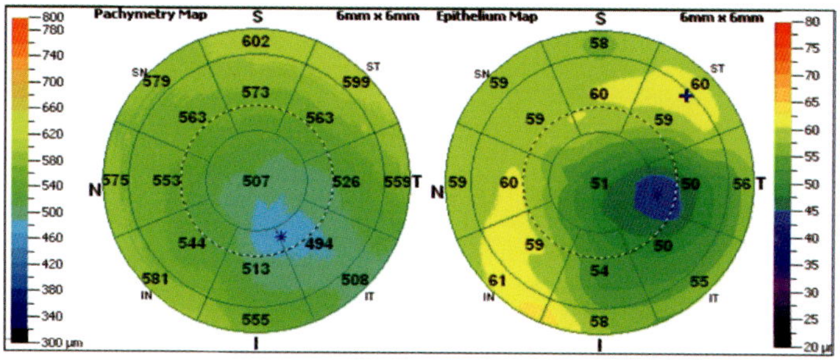

Figure 1-23 Spectral-domain optical coherence tomography epithelial mapping in keratoconus. Epithelial thickness profile shows localized zone of epithelial thinning over the region of the cone, surrounded by epithelial thickening. *(Courtesy of Karolinne Maia Rocha, MD, PhD.)*

example, in keratoconus, the epithelium tends to thin over the cone and to thicken over adjacent areas of stromal thinning (Fig 1-23). Similarly, after myopic LASIK, the magnitude of central epithelial thickening has been correlated to the degree of myopic refractive error ablated. Remodeling of the corneal epithelium may have a significant impact on corneal topography interpretation.

Corneal epithelial mapping can be performed with spectral-domain OCT or very high-frequency digital ultrasound. Epithelial thickness variations can be used to screen for early stages of corneal ectasia, to detect corneal warpage patterns, and to evaluate stability after laser vision correction.

Reinstein DZ, Gobbe M, Archer TJ, Silverman RH, Coleman DJ. Epithelial, stromal, and total corneal thickness in keratoconus: three-dimensional display with Artemis very-high frequency digital ultrasound. *J Refract Surg.* 2010;26(4):259–271.

Reinstein DZ, Silverman RH, Raevsky T, et al. Arc-scanning very high-frequency digital ultrasound for 3D pachymetric mapping of the corneal epithelium and stroma in laser in situ keratomileusis [published correction appears in *J Refract Surg.* 2001;17(1):4]. *J Refract Surg.* 2000;16(4):414–430.

Rocha KM, Krueger RR. Spectral-domain optical coherence tomography epithelial and flap thickness mapping in femtosecond laser-assisted in situ keratomileusis. *Am J Ophthalmol.* 2014;158(2):293–301.e1.

Rocha KM, Perez-Straziota CE, Stulting RD, Randleman JB. Epithelial and stromal remodeling after corneal collagen cross-linking evaluated by spectral-domain OCT. *J Refract Surg.* 2014;30(2):122–127.

Rocha KM, Perez-Straziota CE, Stulting RD, Randleman JB. SD-OCT analysis of regional epithelial thickness profiles in keratoconus, postoperative corneal ectasia, and normal eyes. *J Refract Surg.* 2013;29(3):173–179.

CHAPTER 2

Patient Evaluation

Highlights

- The preoperative history and examination determine whether a patient is an appropriate candidate for refractive surgery.
- A complete ocular and medical history, with special attention to stability of the refraction, contact lens wear, and previous ocular surgery, is important in determining candidacy.
- The eye examination should include uncorrected and corrected visual acuity for both distance and near, refraction, slit-lamp examination, and dilated fundus examination.
- Special testing, including scotopic pupil size, topography/tomography, pachymetry, wavefront analysis, and corneal biomechanics, contributes important information to the preoperative evaluation.

Aspects of Patient Evaluation

The preoperative patient evaluation is arguably the most critical component in achieving successful outcomes after refractive surgery. It is during this encounter that the surgeon develops an impression as to whether the patient is a good candidate for refractive surgery. Perhaps the most important goal of this evaluation, however, is to identify who should *not* have refractive surgery.

The evaluation actually begins before the physician sees the potential patient. Technicians or refractive surgical coordinators who interact with the individual may get a sense of his or her goals for refractive surgery. If the patient's interaction with staff is problematic or the technician has the impression that a patient may have unrealistic expectations, the surgeon should be informed. Such a patient may not be a good candidate for surgery.

Important parts of the preoperative refractive surgery evaluation include an assessment of the patient's expectations; the social, medical, and ocular history; manifest and cycloplegic refractions; a complete ophthalmic evaluation, including slit-lamp and dilated fundus examinations; and ancillary testing (Table 2-1). Because accurate test results are crucial to the success of refractive surgery, the surgeon must closely supervise office staff members who are performing the examination and ancillary testing during the preoperative evaluation and confirm that the instruments used are properly calibrated. If the patient is deemed to be a good candidate for surgery, the surgeon should discuss the benefits,

Table 2-1 Important Parts of the Preoperative Refractive Surgery Evaluation

Patient expectations and motivations
Assessment of specific patient expectations
Discussion of uncorrected distance versus reading vision
History
Social history, including vision requirements of profession and hobbies, tobacco and alcohol use
Medical history, including systemic medications and diseases such as diabetes mellitus and rheumatologic diseases
Ocular history, including history of contact lens wear
Ophthalmic examination
Uncorrected near and distance vision, ocular dominance
Manifest refraction (pushing plus)
Monovision demonstration, if indicated
External evaluation
Pupillary evaluation
Ocular motility
Slit-lamp examination, including intraocular pressure measurement
Corneal topography/tomography
Wavefront analysis, if indicated
Pachymetry
Cycloplegic refraction (refining sphere, not cylinder)
Dilated fundus examination
Informed consent
Discussion of findings
Discussion of medical and surgical alternatives and risks
Answering of patient questions
Having patient read informed consent document when undilated and unsedated, ideally before the day of procedure, and sign it prior to surgery

risks, and alternatives with the patient as part of the informed consent process (see the section Discussion of Findings and Informed Consent later in this chapter).

Patient Expectations

One of the most important aspects of the evaluation process is assessing the patient's expectations. Unrealistic expectations are probably the leading cause of patient dissatisfaction after refractive surgery. The results may be exactly what the surgeon expected, but if those expectations were not conveyed adequately to the patient before surgery, the patient may be disappointed.

The surgeon should explore expectations relating to both the refractive result and the emotional result (eg, improved self-esteem). Patients need to understand that the refractive surgery will not necessarily improve their corrected distance visual acuity (CDVA). In addition, they need to realize that the surgery will not alter the course of eventual presbyopia, nor will it prevent potential future ocular problems such as cataract, glaucoma, or retinal detachment. If the patient has clearly unrealistic goals, such as a guarantee of 20/20 uncorrected distance visual acuity (UDVA) or perfect uncorrected reading *and* distance vision despite presbyopia, the patient may need to be told that refractive surgery cannot currently fulfill his or her needs. The refractive surgeon should exclude such patients.

Social History

An accurate social and occupational history can uncover specific visual requirements of the patient's profession. Various occupations have differing visual needs. For example, it may be more important for an accountant to see numbers clearly on a computer screen than to have perfect UDVA. Others, such as military personnel, firefighters, or police officers, may have restrictions on minimum UDVA and CDVA and on the type of refractive surgery allowed. Knowledge of a patient's recreational activities may also help the surgeon to select the most appropriate refractive procedure or to determine whether that patient is even a good candidate for refractive surgery. For example, a surface laser procedure may be preferable to a lamellar procedure for a patient who is active and at high risk of ocular trauma. Someone with highly myopic and presbyopic vision who is used to examining objects a few inches from the eyes without the use of glasses (eg, a jeweler or stamp collector) may be dissatisfied with postoperative emmetropia.

Occupational or social factors unrelated to refractive status may also be relevant. Health care workers, for instance, may unknowingly be colonized with methicillin-resistant *Staphylococcus aureus;* appropriate prophylaxis may include the use of topical antibiotic drops such as polymyxin/trimethoprim. In addition, tobacco and alcohol use should be documented for all patients.

Solomon R, Donnenfeld ED, Holland EJ, et al. Microbial keratitis trends following refractive surgery: results of the ASCRS infectious keratitis survey and comparisons with prior ASCRS surveys of infectious keratitis following keratorefractive procedures. *J Cataract Refract Surg.* 2011;37(7):1343–1350.

Medical History

The medical history should include systemic conditions, previous surgical procedures, and current and prior medications. Certain systemic disorders, such as connective tissue disease or diabetes mellitus, can lead to poor healing after refractive surgery. An immunocompromised state—for example, from cancer or HIV infection and AIDS—can increase the risk of infection after refractive surgery (see Chapter 7). Medications that affect healing or the ability to fight infection, such as systemic corticosteroids or chemotherapy drugs, should be specifically noted. The use of corticosteroids increases the risk of cataract development, which could compromise the long-term postoperative visual outcome. Certain medications—including isotretinoin, amiodarone, and sumatriptan—have traditionally been thought to increase the risk of poor corneal healing or epithelial defects following photorefractive keratectomy (PRK) and laser in situ keratomileusis (LASIK), but there is no evidence for this association in the peer-reviewed literature. However, previous or current use of isotretinoin can damage the meibomian glands and predispose a patient to dry eye symptoms postoperatively.

Although laser manufacturers do not recommend excimer laser surgery for patients with cardiac pacemakers and implanted defibrillators, many such patients have undergone the surgery without problems. It may be advisable to check with the pacemaker and defibrillator manufacturer before laser surgery. Refractive surgery is also generally contraindicated in pregnant and breastfeeding women because of possible changes in refraction and corneal hydration status. Although newer studies have shown that minimal refractive changes occur during pregnancy, caution is warranted. Many surgeons recommend waiting at least 3 months after delivery and cessation of breastfeeding before performing the refractive surgery evaluation and procedure.

Hardten DR, Hira NK, Lombardo AJ. Triptans and the incidence of epithelial defects during laser in situ keratomileusis. *J Refract Surg.* 2005;21(1):72–76.

Kanellopoulos AJ, Vingopoulos F. Does pregnancy affect refractive and corneal stability or corneal epithelial remodeling after myopic LASIK? *J Refract Surg.* 2020;36(2):118–122.

Schallhorn JM, Schallhorn SC, Hettinger KA, et al. Outcomes and complications of excimer laser surgery in patients with collagen vascular and other immune-mediated inflammatory diseases. *J Cataract Refract Surg.* 2016;42(12):1742–1752.

Ocular History

The ocular history should focus on previous and current eye problems, such as dry eye symptoms, lagophthalmos, blepharitis, recurrent corneal erosions, glaucoma, and retinal tears or detachments, as well as use of ocular medications. A history of strabismus, amblyopia, or diplopia should be documented. In addition, potentially recurrent conditions, such as ocular herpes simplex virus infection, should be recognized so that preventive measures can be instituted. Prior ocular surgical procedures, such as radial keratotomy or penetrating keratoplasty, may affect clinical decision making in refractive surgery. A personal or family history of keratoconus may exclude a patient from consideration for traditional LASIK or PRK, although other refractive procedures (eg, crosslinking or intrastromal corneal ring segments) may be appropriate.

The patient's history of optical correction with glasses or contact lenses should be noted. The stability of the current refraction is a very important consideration. A change in prescription for glasses or contact lenses of more than 0.50 D in either sphere or cylinder, or a change in cylinder axis of more than 10 degrees, within the past year is thought to be significant. Information on contact lens wear should be recorded, including the type of lenses (soft or rigid gas-permeable [RGP]), the wearing schedule (daily wear or overnight), the cleaning and disinfecting agents used, and the age of the lenses.

Because contact lens wear can change the shape of the cornea (corneal warpage), it is recommended that patients stop using contact lenses before the refractive surgery evaluation as well as before the surgery. The exact length of time has not been established, but current clinical practice typically involves discontinuation of soft contact lenses for at least 3 days to 2 weeks (toric lenses may require longer) and of RGP lenses for at least 2–3 weeks. However, it may take months for the corneal curvature to return to normal in some long-term RGP lens wearers, and some surgeons keep patients out of rigid contact lenses for 1 month for every decade of contact lens wear. Before being considered for refractive surgery, patients with irregular or unstable corneas should discontinue their use of contact lenses for a longer period and then be reevaluated every few weeks until the refraction and corneal topography stabilize. For patients who wear RGP contact lenses and find glasses a hardship, some surgeons suggest changing to soft contact lenses for a period to aid stabilization and regularization of the corneal curvature.

Bower KS, Woreta F. Update on contraindications for laser-assisted in situ keratomileusis and photorefractive keratectomy. *Curr Opin Ophthalmol.* 2014;25(4):251–257.
de Rojas Silva V, Rodríguez-Conde R, Cobo-Soriano R, Beltrán J, Llovet F, Baviera J. Laser in situ keratomileusis in patients with a history of ocular herpes. *J Cataract Refract Surg.* 2007;33(11):1855–1859.

Patient Age, Presbyopia, and Monovision

The patient's age is a consideration in predicting postoperative patient satisfaction. The loss of near vision with aging should be discussed with all patients. Before 40 years of age, individuals with emmetropia generally do not require reading adds to see a near target. After this age, patients need to understand that if their eyes are made emmetropic through refractive surgery, they will require reading glasses for near vision. They must also understand that "near vision" tasks include all tasks performed up close, such as applying makeup, shaving, or seeing the computer or cell phone screen—not just reading. These points cannot be overemphasized for patients with myopia who are approaching 40 years of age. Before refractive surgery, these patients can read well with and without their glasses; some may even read well with their contact lenses. If their eyes are made emmetropic after surgery, many will not read well without reading glasses. The patient needs to understand this phenomenon and must be willing to accept this result before undergoing any refractive surgery that aims for emmetropia. In patients who wear glasses, a trial with contact lenses will simulate vision following refractive surgery and approximate the patient's reading ability after surgery.

A discussion of monovision (1 eye corrected for distance and the other eye for near/intermediate vision) often fits well into the evaluation at this point (see sidebar: Advantages and Disadvantages of Monovision). The monovision option should be discussed with all patients in the age groups approaching or affected by presbyopia. Many patients have successfully used monovision in contact lenses and want it after refractive surgery. Others have never tried it but would like to, and still others have no interest. If a patient has not used monovision before but is interested, the intended surgical result can first be demonstrated with glasses or temporary contact lenses at near and distance. Generally, the dominant eye is corrected for distance, and the nondominant eye is corrected to approximately −1.25 to −1.75 D. For most patients, such refraction allows good uncorrected distance and near vision without intolerable anisometropia. Some surgeons prefer a "mini-monovision" procedure, whereby the near-vision eye is corrected to approximately −0.75 D, which allows some near vision with better distance vision and less anisometropia. The exact amount of monovision depends on the desires of the patient. Blended vision would entail correction to achieve myopia in the range of −1.00 D to −1.50 D. Higher amounts of monovision (up to −2.50 D) can be used successfully in selected patients who want excellent postoperative near vision. However, in some patients with a higher degree of postoperative myopia, improving near vision may lead to unwanted adverse effects of loss of depth perception and anisometropia. It is advisable to have a patient simulate monovision with contact lenses before surgery (generally about 5 days to 1 week, but practices are variable) to ensure that distance and near vision and stereovision are acceptable and that no muscle imbalance is present, especially with higher degrees of monovision.

Advantages and Disadvantages of Monovision

Advantages:

- Monovision allows near vision without reading glasses for many near tasks such as reading newspaper headlines and looking at a cell phone or watch, while also providing acceptable distance correction.
- The difference between eyes is generally well tolerated, allowing patients to function spectacle free for most visual tasks.

Disadvantages:

- Depth perception for driving and for sports such as tennis may be compromised.
- Glasses may be needed for driving (distance) or for extended reading (near).
- The eye corrected for near may experience nighttime glare from unfocused light.

Caution must be exercised in patients with a history of strabismus; binocular summation is compromised.

Peng MY, Hannan S , Teenan D, Schallhorn SJ , Schallhorn JM . Monovision LASIK in emmetropic presbyopic patients. *Clin Ophthalmol.* 2018;12:1665–1671.

Although typically the nondominant eye is corrected for near, some patients prefer to have the dominant eye corrected for near. Of several methods for testing ocular dominance, one of the simplest is to have the patient point to a distant object, such as a small letter on an eye chart, with both eyes open and then close each eye to see which remains aligned better; this is the dominant eye. (Alternatively, the patient can make an "OK sign" with 1 hand and look at the examiner through the opening while closing each eye in turn.)

Durrie DS. The effect of different monovision contact lens powers on the visual function of emmetropic presbyopic patients (an American Ophthalmological Society thesis). *Trans Am Ophthalmol Soc.* 2006;104:366–401.

Examination

Uncorrected Visual Acuity, Manifest Refraction, and Cycloplegic Refraction

The refractive elements of the preoperative examination are extremely critical because they directly determine the amount of surgery to be performed. Visual acuity at distance and near should be measured. The current glasses prescription and visual acuity with those glasses should also be determined, and a manifest refraction should be performed. The sharpest visual acuity with the least amount of minus should be the endpoint. The duochrome test should not be used as the endpoint because it tends to overminus patients.

The best visual acuity obtainable should be documented, even if it is better than 20/20. An automated refraction with an autorefractor or wavefront aberrometer may be useful in providing a starting point for the manifest refraction.

A cycloplegic refraction is helpful to account for and measure latent hyperopia. Sufficient waiting time must be allowed between administration of the cycloplegic eyedrops and measurement of the refraction. Tropicamide 1% or cyclopentolate 1% are the most commonly used cycloplegic drops. For full cycloplegia, waiting at least 30 minutes (with tropicamide 1%) or 60 minutes (with cyclopentolate 1%) is recommended. The cycloplegic refraction should refine the sphere, but not the cylinder, from the manifest refraction, as it is done to neutralize accommodation. For eyes with a refractive error of more than 5.00 D, a vertex distance measurement is necessary to obtain the most accurate refraction.

When the difference between the manifest and cycloplegic refractions is greater than 0.50 D, a postcycloplegic manifest refraction may be helpful to recheck the original. In patients with myopia, such a large difference is often caused by an overminused manifest refraction. In patients with hyperopia, substantial latent hyperopia may be present, in which case the surgeon and patient need to decide exactly how much hyperopia to treat. If there is significant latent hyperopia, a pushed-plus spectacle or contact lens correction can be worn preoperatively to reduce the postoperative adjustment that may result from treating the true refraction.

Pupillary Examination

After the manifest refraction (but before dilating eyedrops are administered), the external and anterior segment examinations are performed. Specific attention should be given to the pupillary examination. The pupil size should be evaluated in bright room light and in dim illumination, and the surgeon should look for an afferent pupillary defect. Various techniques are available for measuring pupil size in low-light conditions, including use of a near card with pupil sizes on the edge (with the patient fixating at distance) or a pupillometer. The dim-light measurement should be taken using an amount of light that closely approximates the amount that enters the eye during normal nighttime activities, such as night driving, and not necessarily in completely dark conditions.

Pupil measurements should be standardized as much as possible. Measuring the scotopic pupil diameter preoperatively and using that measurement to direct surgery remains a controversial approach. Conventional wisdom suggests that the optical zone should be larger than the pupil diameter to minimize visual disturbances such as glare and halos. However, current evidence does not support an association between preoperative pupil size and an increased incidence of either glare or halo concerns 1 year postoperatively. It is not clear, therefore, that pupil size can be used to predict which patients are more likely to have such symptoms. However, a thorough and documented discussion with the patient is required. The size of the effective optical zone—which is related to the ablation profile and the level of refractive error—may be more important in minimizing visual adverse effects than is the scotopic pupil diameter.

When asked, patients often note that they had glare in dim-light conditions even before undergoing refractive surgery. Thus, it is helpful for patients to become aware of their glare and halo symptoms preoperatively, as this knowledge may minimize postoperative concerns or misunderstanding.

Chan A, Manche EE. Effect of preoperative pupil size on quality of vision after wavefront-guided LASIK. *Ophthalmology.* 2011;118(4):736–741.

Edwards JD, Burka JM, Bower KS, Stutzman RD, Sediq DA, Rabin JC. Effect of brimonidine tartrate 0.15% on night-vision difficulty and contrast testing after refractive surgery. *J Cataract Refract Surg.* 2008;34(9):1538–1541.

Myung D, Schallhorn S, Manche EE. Pupil size and LASIK: a review. *J Refract Surg.* 2013;29(11):734–741.

Pop M, Payette Y. Risk factors for night vision complaints after LASIK for myopia. *Ophthalmology.* 2004;111(1):3–10.

Schallhorn SC, Kaupp SE, Tanzer DJ, Tidwell J, Laurent J, Bourque LB. Pupil size and quality of vision after LASIK. *Ophthalmology.* 2003;110(8):1606–1614.

Schmidt GW, Yoon M, McGwin G, Lee PP, McLeod SD. Evaluation of the relationship between ablation diameter, pupil size, and visual function with vision-specific quality-of-life measures after laser in situ keratomileusis. *Arch Ophthalmol.* 2007;125(8):1037–1042.

Ocular Motility and Confrontation Visual Fields

Ocular motility should be carefully evaluated before surgery. In patients with asymptomatic tropia or phoria, symptoms may develop after refractive surgery if the change in refraction leads to a breakdown in ocular alignment. If there is a history of strabismus (see Chapter 7) or a concern about postoperative ocular alignment, a trial with contact lenses can be considered before surgery. Monovision may not be appropriate for such patients, as binocular summation and fusion may be compromised. A sensory motor evaluation can be obtained preoperatively if strabismus is an issue. Confrontation visual field tests are generally performed as part of the basic ophthalmic examination.

Intraocular Pressure

The intraocular pressure (IOP) should be checked after the manifest refraction is completed and corneal topography measurements are taken. A history of glaucoma is noteworthy because IOP can be dramatically elevated in some refractive surgical procedures, potentially exacerbating preexisting optic nerve damage (see Chapter 7). Also, topical corticosteroids are used after most refractive surgery procedures and, after a surface ablation procedure, may be continued for months. Long-term use of topical corticosteroids may cause marked elevation of IOP in corticosteroid responders.

Ahmad M, Chocron I, Shrivastava A. Considerations for refractive surgery in the glaucoma patient. *Curr Opin Ophthalmol.* 2017;28(4):310–315.

Slit-Lamp Examination

A complete slit-lamp examination of the eyelids and anterior segment is necessary. The cornea and conjunctiva are examined specifically for scarring, conjunctivochalasis, pterygium, and chemosis. These abnormalities may cause problems in achieving good suction, whether using a microkeratome or docking with a femtosecond laser. Corneal scars have been associated with vertical gas breakthrough when a femtosecond laser is used to create LASIK flaps. The cornea is evaluated for surface abnormalities such as decreased tear breakup time (Fig 2-1) and punctate epithelial erosions (Fig 2-2). Significant blepharitis (Fig 2-3), meibomitis, and dry eye syndrome can be addressed before refractive surgery, as they are associated with increased postoperative discomfort and decreased vision; and dry eye symptoms frequently worsen postoperatively.

A careful examination for epithelial basement membrane dystrophy (EBMD; Fig 2-4) is required because its presence increases the risk of flap complications during LASIK. Thus, patients with EBMD may be better candidates for surface ablation not only because of possible

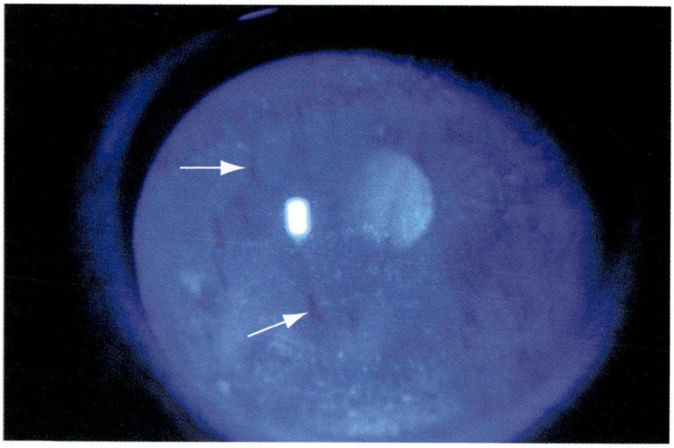

Figure 2-1 Slit-lamp photograph showing decreased tear breakup time. After fluorescein dye is instilled, the patient keeps the eye open for 10 seconds, and the tear film is examined with cobalt blue light. Breaks, or dry spots, in the tear film *(arrows)* are visible in this image. Punctate epithelial erosions are also present. *(Courtesy of Christopher J. Rapuano, MD.)*

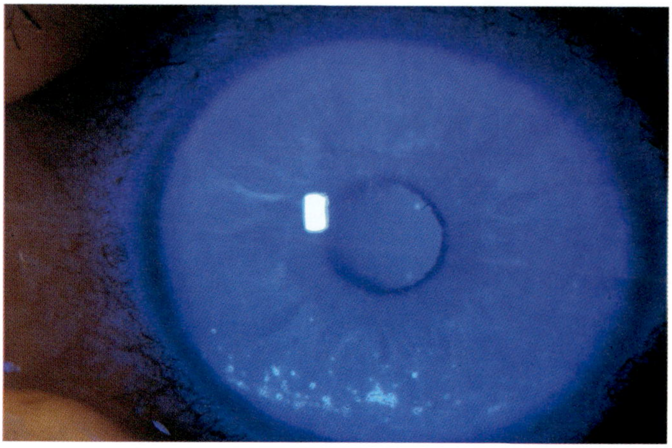

Figure 2-2 Slit-lamp photograph showing punctate epithelial erosions. Inferior punctate fluorescein staining can be seen in this patient with moderately dry eyes. *(Courtesy of Christopher J. Rapuano, MD.)*

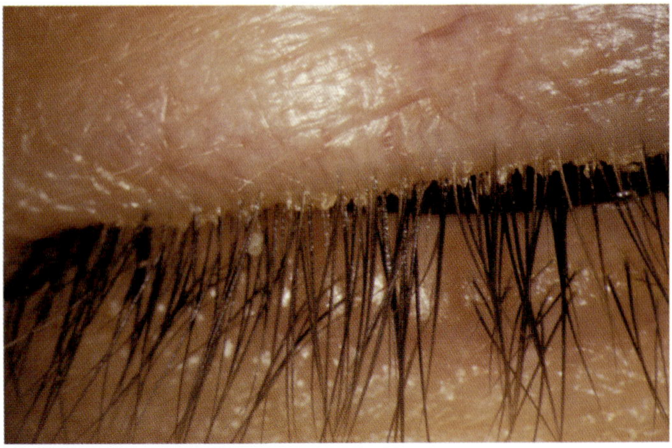

Figure 2-3 Example of blepharitis. Moderate crusting is apparent at the base of the lashes in this patient with seborrheic blepharitis. *(Courtesy of Christopher J. Rapuano, MD.)*

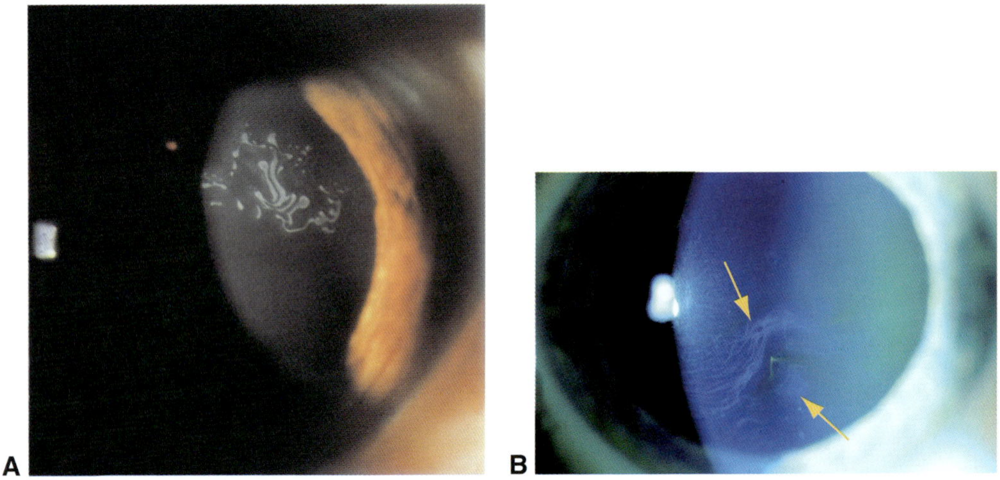

Figure 2-4 Epithelial basement membrane dystrophy. Epithelial map changes can be obvious **(A)** or more subtle **(B)**. *Arrows* show geographic map lines. *(Part A courtesy of Vincent P. deLuise, MD; part B courtesy of Christopher J. Rapuano, MD.)*

LASIK flap complications but also because removal of the abnormal epithelium may be palliative. Signs of keratoconus, such as iron rings and corneal thinning or steepening, may also be found. Keratoconus is typically a contraindication to incisional or ablative refractive surgery (see Chapter 7). The endothelium should be examined carefully for signs of cornea guttata and other dystrophies. Poor visual results have been reported in patients with cornea guttata and a family history of Fuchs dystrophy. Corneal edema is generally considered a contraindication to refractive surgery. The deposits of granular and Avellino corneal dystrophies may increase substantially in size and number in the flap interface after LASIK, resulting in poor vision.

Evaluation of the anterior chamber, iris, and crystalline lens completes the slit-lamp examination. A shallow anterior chamber may be a contraindication for use of certain phakic intraocular lenses (see Chapter 9). Careful evaluation of the crystalline lens for clarity is essential in both the undilated and dilated state, especially in patients older than 50 years. Progressive myopia due to nuclear sclerosis is not uncommon. Mild lens changes may become visually significant in the future, independent of refractive surgery. In patients with moderate lens opacities, cataract extraction with IOL implantation is probably the best form of refractive surgery.

Alió JL, Grzybowski A, Romaniuk D. Refractive lens exchange in modern practice: when and when not to do it? *Eye Vis (Lond).* 2014;1:10.

dos Santos AM, Torricelli AA, Marino GK, et al. Femtosecond laser–assisted LASIK flap complications. *J Refract Surg.* 2016;32(1):52–59.

Kim TI, Kim T, Kim SW, Kim EK. Comparison of corneal deposits after LASIK and PRK in eyes with granular corneal dystrophy type II. *J Refract Surg.* 2008;24(4):392–395.

Moshirfar M, Feiz V, Feilmeier MR, Kang PC. Laser in situ keratomileusis in patients with corneal guttata and family history of Fuchs' endothelial dystrophy. *J Cataract Refract Surg.* 2005;31(12):2281–2286.

Dilated Fundus Examination

A dilated fundus examination is performed before refractive surgery to ensure that the posterior segment is normal. Special attention should be given to the macula, optic nerve (for glaucoma, optic nerve drusen), and peripheral retina (for retinal breaks, detachment). Patients and surgeons should realize that highly myopic eyes are naturally at increased risk of retinal detachment (see Chapter 7), unrelated to refractive surgery.

Kanclerz P, Grzybowski A. Does corneal refractive surgery increase the risk of retinal detachment? A literature review and statistical analysis. *J Refract Surg.* 2019;35(8):517–524.

Ancillary Tests

Corneal Topography

The corneal curvature must be evaluated. Although manual keratometry readings can be quite informative, they have largely been replaced by computerized corneal topographic analyses. Several different methods are available to analyze the corneal curvature, including Placido disk–based topography, scanning slit-beam imaging, rotating Scheimpflug photography, high-frequency ultrasound, and optical coherence tomography (OCT) techniques. (See also the discussion of corneal topography in Chapter 1.) These techniques image the cornea and provide color maps showing corneal power and/or elevation. Patients with visually significant irregular astigmatism are generally not good candidates for corneal refractive surgery. Early keratoconus (Fig 2-5) and contact lens warpage are potential causes of visually significant irregular astigmatism. Irregular astigmatism secondary to contact lens warpage usually resolves over time after the lenses are discontinued, although the process may take months. Serial corneal topographic studies are helpful to document the resolution of visually significant irregular astigmatism before any refractive surgery is undertaken.

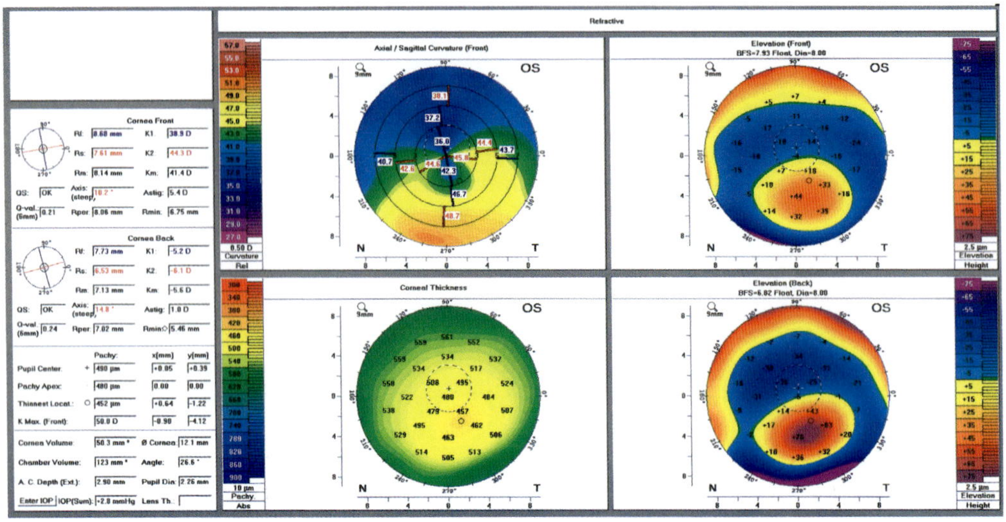

Figure 2-5 Pentacam images of eye with keratoconus displaying inferior corneal steepening, corneal thinning, and irregular astigmatism. *(Courtesy of Michael J. Taravella, MD.)*

Unusually steep or unusually flat corneas can increase the risk of poor flap creation with the microkeratome (see the section Special Considerations for LASIK). Femtosecond laser flap creation theoretically may avoid these risks. When keratometric or corneal topographic measurements reveal an amount or an axis of astigmatism that differs significantly from that determined through refraction, the refraction should be rechecked for accuracy. Lenticular astigmatism or posterior corneal curvature may account for the difference between refractive and keratometric or topographic astigmatism. Most surgeons will treat the amount and axis of the refractive astigmatism, as long as the patient understands that after any future cataract surgery, some astigmatism may reappear (after the astigmatism contributed by the natural lens has been eliminated).

Pachymetry

The thickness of the cornea is an important factor in determining whether the patient is a candidate for refractive surgery and in identifying the optimal refractive procedure. Corneal thickness can be measured with ultrasound, Scheimpflug tomography, and OCT systems. Modern topography/tomography systems provide a pachymetry profile map showing the relative thickness of the cornea at various locations. This can be helpful in ascertaining the location of the thinnest part of the cornea, which is not always central.

Measurement of corneal thickness is also necessary for calculating the residual stromal bed to help assess ectasia risk (see the section Special Considerations for LASIK). In a study of 896 eyes undergoing LASIK, the mean central corneal thickness was 550 μm ± 33 μm (range, 472–651 μm). Patients with thin corneas (beyond 2 standard deviations) may not be ideal candidates for laser ablative procedures. If there is suspicion that endothelial dysfunction is causing an abnormally thick cornea, specular microscopy can be helpful in assessing the health of the endothelium.

Price FW Jr, Koller DL, Price MO. Central corneal pachymetry in patients undergoing laser in situ keratomileusis. *Ophthalmology.* 1999;106(11):2216–2220.

Wavefront Analysis

Wavefront analysis is a technique that can provide an objective refraction measurement (see also Chapter 1). Certain excimer lasers can use this wavefront analysis information directly to design the ablation profile, a procedure called *wavefront-guided,* or *custom, ablation.* Some surgeons use wavefront analysis to document preoperative higher-order aberrations. Refraction data from the wavefront analysis unit can also be used to refine the manifest refraction. If the manifest refraction and the wavefront analysis refraction are very dissimilar, the patient may not be a good candidate for wavefront treatment. Note that a custom wavefront ablation generally removes more tissue than does a standard ablation in the same eye. The range of treatment approved by the US Food and Drug Administration (FDA) for wavefront-guided ablations is more restrictive than that for traditional laser treatments.

Kligman BE, Baartman BJ, Dupps WJ. Errors in treatment of lower-order aberrations and induction of higher-order aberrations in laser refractive surgery. *Int Ophthalmol Clin.* 2016;56(2):19–45.

Patient Selection for Photoablation

Special Considerations for Surface Ablation

In general, any condition that significantly delays epithelial healing is a relative contraindication to surface ablation. Although keloid scar formation was listed as a contraindication to PRK in FDA trials, 1 study found that African Americans with a history of keloids did well after PRK, and keloid formation is no longer considered a contraindication to surface ablation or LASIK.

As noted earlier, patients with EBMD are better candidates for surface ablation than for LASIK because surface ablation may be therapeutic, reducing epithelial irregularity and improving postoperative quality of vision while enhancing epithelial adhesion. It is important to note that even after surface ablation, loose epithelium may recur. In contrast, LASIK may cause a frank epithelial defect in eyes with EBMD, especially when performed with a mechanical microkeratome, and in rare cases may lead to vertical gas breakthrough in femtosecond laser flaps.

Any patient undergoing excimer laser photoablation should have a pachymetric and topographic evaluation. Younger patients and patients with thin corneas, low predicted residual stromal bed (RSB) thickness, or irregular topography may be at increased risk for the development of ectasia with LASIK. As such, these patients may be better candidates for surface ablation. Patients with subtle topographic pattern abnormalities need to be evaluated on a case-by-case basis. In some circumstances, patients who are stable may be offered surface ablation but with a clear acknowledgment, as well as a signed informed consent form, that they understand there may still be a risk of progression to corneal ectasia. (See sidebar on p. 56: Risk Factors for Ectasia.)

Specific algorithms have been developed from elevation-based topography and tomography metrics that aid in identifying patients who have keratoconus and are at risk for developing post-LASIK ectasia (eg, the Belin/Ambrósio Enhanced Ectasia Display). Such algorithms, although helpful, may be device specific and do not guarantee that eyes with "normal" topographic patterns will not develop ectasia following LASIK or PRK (Figs 2-6, 2-7).

Duncan JK, Belin MW, Borgstrom M. Assessing progression of keratoconus: novel tomographic determinants. *Eye Vis (Lond).* 2016;3:6.

Kosekahya P, Koc M, Caglayan M, Kiziltoprak H, Atilgan CU, Yilmazbas P. Repeatability and reliability of ectasia display and topometric indices with the Scheimpflug system in normal and keratoconic eyes. *J Cataract Refract Surg.* 2018;44(1):63–70.

A

B

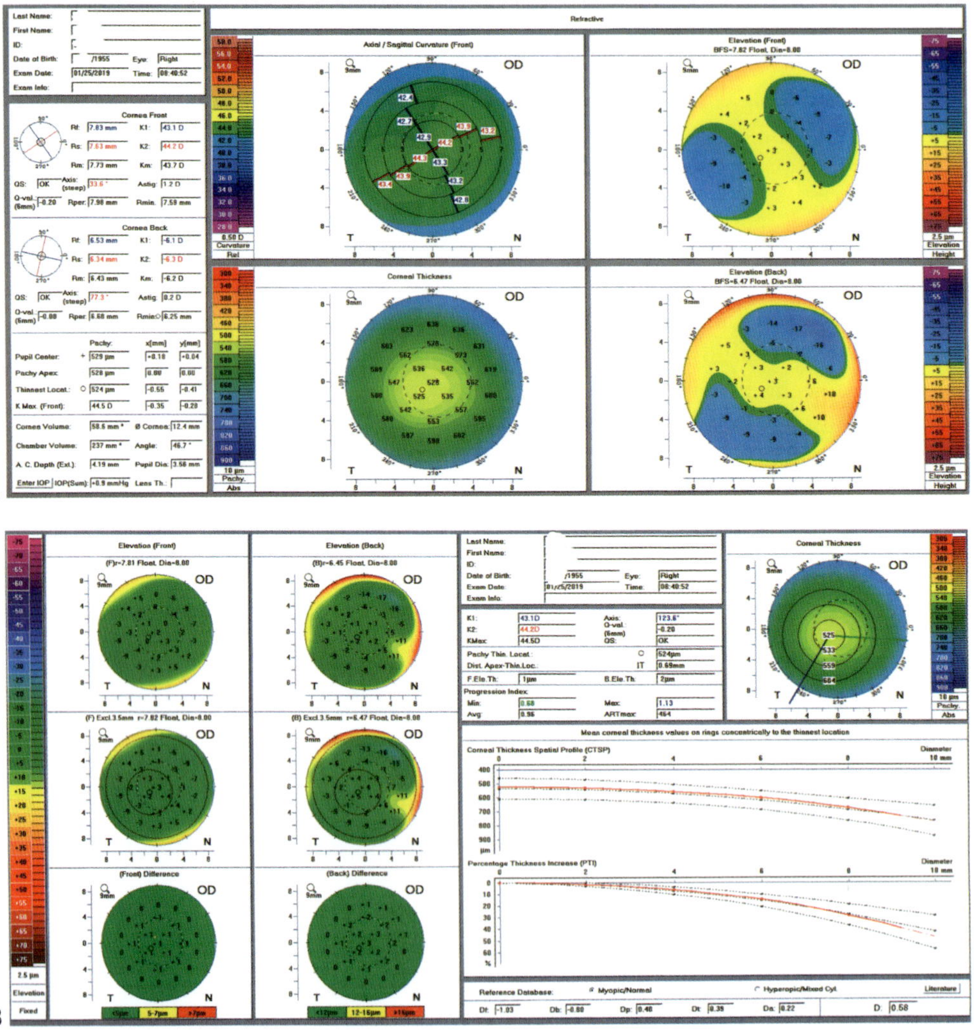

Figure 2-6 Normal cornea. **A,** Pentacam images showing normal corneal curvature and thickness. **B,** Belin/Ambrósio Enhanced Ectasia Display of the same eye. *(Courtesy of Michael J. Taravella, MD.)*

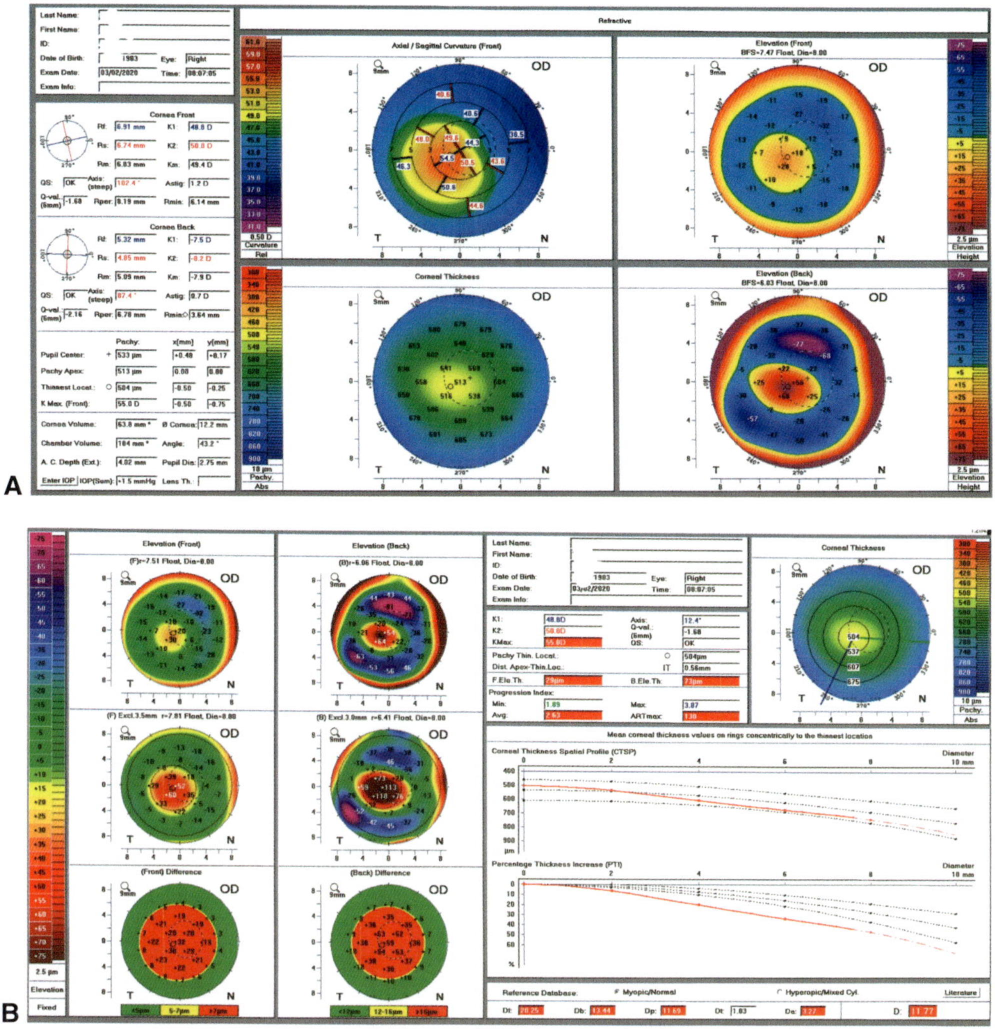

Figure 2-7 Keratoconus. **A,** Pentacam images of an eye with keratoconus demonstrating inferior corneal steepening and thinning. **B,** Belin/Ambrósio Enhanced Ectasia Display of the same eye. The numbers in red indicate an abnormal cornea consistent with keratoconus. *(Courtesy of Michael J. Taravella, MD.)*

Ribeiro GC, Krueger RR. Management of bilateral gas-bubble breakthrough during femtosecond LASIK in the presence of anterior basement membrane dystrophy. *J Cataract Refract Surg.* 2014;40(10):1736–1739.

Special Considerations for LASIK

Calculation of residual stromal bed thickness after LASIK

A lamellar laser refractive procedure such as LASIK involves creating and lifting a corneal flap, ablating the stromal bed, and replacing the flap. The postoperative strength and integrity

Risk Factors for Ectasia

Ectasia is a biomechanical weakening of the cornea that shares many structural and morphologic similarities with keratoconus. In 2008, Randleman and coauthors reported on a series of patients in whom post-LASIK ectasia developed. They analyzed multiple risk factors including age, degree of myopia at the time of surgery, corneal thickness, RSB, and preoperative topography patterns. Ectasia cases were, on average, younger, more myopic, and more likely to have abnormal topography; in addition, they had thinner corneas before surgery and less RSB thickness after. The most significant factor that distinguished cases from controls was abnormal topography. From these data, Randleman and colleagues developed a point system that is useful in screening patients for risk of ectasia.

Another helpful and simple metric is percent tissue altered (PTA); greater than 40% PTA is associated with a higher risk of ectasia. PTA is calculated by the following equation:

$$\text{PTA} = [(\text{LASIK flap thickness} + \text{ablation depth in } \mu\text{m}) / \text{total corneal thickness } (\mu\text{m})] \times 100$$

Randleman JB, Woodward M, Lynn MJ, Stulting RD. Risk assessment for ectasia after corneal refractive surgery. *Ophthalmology.* 2008;115(1):37–50.

of the cornea depend greatly on maintaining a sufficiently thick RSB; thus, it is an important factor in assessing the risk of complications such as ectasia. Thickness of the RSB is calculated by subtracting the sum of the flap thickness and the calculated laser ablation depth from the preoperative corneal thickness.

$$\text{RSB} = \text{Central Corneal Thickness} - \text{Thickness of Flap} - \text{Depth of Ablation}$$

For example, if the central corneal thickness is 550 μm, the flap thickness is estimated to be 140 μm, and the ablation depth for the patient's refraction is 50 μm, the RSB would be 550 μm − (140 μm + 50 μm) = 360 μm. When the surgeon determines the RSB, the amount of tissue estimated to be removed should be based on the actual intended refractive correction, not on the nomogram-adjusted number entered into the laser (see sidebar: What Is a Nomogram?).

Most surgeons believe that the RSB should be at least 250 μm. Others prefer the RSB to be greater than 50% of the original corneal thickness. If the calculation reveals a thinner RSB than desired, LASIK may not be the best surgical option. In these cases, a surface ablation procedure may be preferable, as it will result in a thicker RSB postoperatively. Further, patients with thinner corneas or higher corrections may not be candidates for future LASIK enhancements because of an inadequate RSB. These patients may be better candidates for surface ablation enhancements if needed.

Determining flap thickness and RSB via intraoperative pachymetry provides the most accurate data. This is accomplished by measuring the central corneal thickness at the beginning of the procedure, creating the LASIK flap with the surgeon's instrument

What Is a Nomogram?

A nomogram is a method of adjusting for differences in individual surgeon outcomes for refractive surgery, especially laser vision correction. Differences in outcomes can be attributed to variations in techniques, minor differences between lasers, patient age, the amount of correction attempted, and environmental factors such as temperature and humidity. For instance, low humidity can cause drying of the exposed cornea after epithelial removal or LASIK flap creation. This, in turn, can lead to overcorrections in PRK and LASIK because more tissue will be removed per pulse of laser than in high-humidity environments. After analysis of the surgeon's results, an adjustment factor can be applied to the refractive correction entered into the laser. If, on average, entering the patient's full correction as suggested by the manifest refraction leads to overcorrections of 10%, then a 10% reduction can be applied. In this example, for a 10.00 D patient with myopia, a 10% reduction (1.00 D) would be applied, and −9.00 D would be entered. However, the same amount of tissue (approximately 128 μm at an optical zone of 6.5 mm) will be removed by ablation to achieve full correction, regardless of how the laser is programmed.

of choice, lifting the flap, measuring the untreated stromal bed, and subtracting the intended thickness of corneal ablation from the stromal bed to ascertain the actual RSB. Flap thickness is then calculated by subtracting the untreated stromal bed measurement from the initial central corneal thickness. It is important to measure the corneal bed thickness quickly after making the flap in order to avoid corneal thinning from exposure to the air.

Other considerations in the evaluation for LASIK

The preoperative evaluation of patients for LASIK is similar to that for surface ablation. However, orbital anatomy has a greater impact in LASIK and should be assessed. A narrow palpebral fissure and a prominent brow with deep-set globes increase the difficulty of creating a successful corneal flap because of inadequate exposure. Placement of a microkeratome or docking with a femtosecond laser can be problematic in such eyes, and these anatomical features may lead a surgeon to consider surface ablation over LASIK.

Many patients seek laser vision correction because of contact lens intolerance and related dry eye. A transient sensation of dry eye can be expected early in the healing period after laser vision correction. Although uncommon, a number of reports in the literature indicate that ongoing postoperative dry eye may be more prevalent with LASIK than with PRK. Superior hinge placement during LASIK may exacerbate symptoms because the corneal nerves entering at the 3-o'clock and 9-o'clock positions are interrupted during flap creation. This difference between LASIK and surface ablation is important to remember when considering refractive surgery in a patient with advanced dry eye syndrome.

As with PRK, corneal topography/tomography is performed to assess corneal astigmatism and rule out the presence of ectatic disorders, such as keratoconus, or contact lens–induced corneal warpage. Steep corneas (>48.00 D) are more prone to buttonholes (central perforation of the flap), whereas flat corneas (<40.00 D) are more likely to have smaller-diameter or free flaps due to transection of the hinge when a mechanical microkeratome is used.

Many ophthalmologists believe that excessive corneal flattening or steepening after LASIK may reduce vision quality and increase aberrations; however, no established guidelines are available on the specific values to avoid. The surgeon can estimate the postoperative keratometry by calculating a flattening of 0.80 D for every diopter of myopia treated and a steepening of 1.00 D for every diopter of hyperopia treated. In clinical practice, it is generally recommended to maintain an intended corneal power of less than 49 D after a hyperopic ablation. Flat corneas (hyperoblate) tend to be tolerated much better than steep corneas (hyperprolate).

If wavefront-guided laser ablation is planned, wavefront error is measured preoperatively (see Chapter 1). Although wavefront data are used to program the laser, the surgeon must still compare these data to the manifest refraction before surgery to prevent data-input errors. Substantial differences between the manifest refraction and the wavefront refraction (which may be due to accommodation or dry eye) must be reconciled. A wavefront-adjusted manifest refraction may be helpful in such instances. This is performed by placing the wavefront refraction in the phoropter and adjusting the sphere only with a pushed-plus technique.

Durairaj VD, Balentine J, Kouyoumdjian G, et al. The predictability of corneal flap thickness and tissue laser ablation in laser in situ keratomileusis. *Ophthalmology.* 2000;107(12):2140–2143.

Flanagan G, Binder PS. Estimating residual stromal thickness before and after laser in situ keratomileusis. *J Cataract Refract Surg.* 2003;29(9):1674–1683.

Giri P, Azar DT. Risk profiles of ectasia after keratorefractive surgery. *Curr Opin Ophthalmol.* 2017;28(4):337–342.

Kim WS, Jo JM. Corneal hydration affects ablation during laser in situ keratomileusis surgery. *Cornea.* 2001;20(4):394–397.

Randleman JB, Hebson CB, Larson PM. Flap thickness in eyes with ectasia after laser in situ keratomileusis. *J Cataract Refract Surg.* 2012;38(5):752–757.

Randleman JB, Woodward M, Lynn MJ, Stulting RD. Risk assessment for ectasia after corneal refractive surgery. *Ophthalmology.* 2008;115(1):37–50.

Salib GM, McDonald MB, Smolek M. Safety and efficacy of cyclosporine 0.05% drops versus unpreserved artificial tears in dry-eye patients having laser in situ keratomileusis. *J Cataract Refract Surg.* 2006;32(5):772–778.

Santhiago MR, Wilson SE, Smadja D, Chamon W, Krueger RE, Randleman JB. Validation of the percent tissue altered as a risk factor for ectasia after LASIK. *Ophthalmology.* 2019;126(6):908–909.

Williams LB, Dave SB, Moshirfar M. Correlation of visual outcome and patient satisfaction with preoperative keratometry after hyperopic laser in situ keratomileusis. *J Cataract Refract Surg.* 2008;34(7):1083–1088.

Discussion of Findings and Informed Consent

After completing the evaluation, the surgeon analyzes the information and discusses the findings with the patient. If the patient is a candidate for refractive surgery, the discussion must include the risks and benefits of the medical and surgical alternatives, as well as other refractive options such as glasses and contact lenses. Table 2-2 summarizes contraindications to LASIK and PRK, while Table 2-3 provides an overview of the most common refractive surgery procedures, their typical refractive ranges, and their key limitations. Important discussion points include the following:

- expected visual outcome
- possible need for glasses
- chance of needing an enhancement
- risk of severe vision loss
- night-vision problems such as glare and halos
- possible dry eye postoperatively
- potential for flap complications such as displacement, striae, or epithelial ingrowth

In addition, the patient should understand that the laser ablation procedure may be aborted in case of intraoperative flap complications. The risks of bilateral versus unilateral surgery should be discussed. For example, the rare possibility of infection or laser malfunction may be more consequential in bilateral procedures, while serial unilateral surgery may result in temporary anisometropia and may be more inconvenient. Patients should be given the opportunity to decide which is best for them.

Ideally, patients considering refractive surgery are given the informed consent document to take home and review and will have an opportunity to discuss questions related to surgery or the consent form with the surgeon preoperatively. It is optimal to have the

Table 2-2 Excimer Laser Photoablation: Contraindications, Warnings, and Precautions

Age younger than 18 years
Connective tissue disease
Rheumatoid arthritis
Sjögren syndrome
Systemic lupus erythematosus
Granulomatosis with polyangiitis (formerly, Wegener granulomatosis)
Corneal ectatic disorders (keratoconus)
Corneal stromal dystrophies
Diabetic retinopathy
Dry eye syndrome
Fuchs corneal dystrophy
Monocular status
Neurotrophic corneas
Pregnancy or lactation
Previous herpes simplex infection
Previous herpes zoster ophthalmicus
Thyroid eye disease
Uncontrolled diabetes mellitus
Unreasonable patient expectations

Table 2-3 Limitations of the Most Common Refractive Surgery Procedures

Procedure	Spherical Range	Cylinder Range	Limitations
LASIK[a]	−14.00 to +5.00 D	Up to 5.00 D	Thin corneas (thin residual stromal bed); epithelial basement membrane dystrophy; small palpebral fissures; preoperative severe dry eye; certain medications. Unusually flat or steep corneas may predispose to flap complications. Wavefront-guided ablations have more restricted FDA-approved treatment parameters.
Surface ablation[a]	−12.00 to +6.00 D	Up to 4.00 D	Preoperative severe dry eye; certain medications. Postoperative haze may occur at high end of treatment range but range may be extended with the use of mitomycin C. Longer vision-recovery time and more postoperative discomfort compared with LASIK.
Phakic intraocular lenses[a]	−3.00 to −20.00 D	Up to 4.00 D (toric lens)	FDA approved for myopia; intraocular surgery; potential for long-term complications such as glaucoma, iritis, cataract, pupil distortion, and corneal edema.
Refractive lens exchange	All ranges; multifocal and extended depth of field lenses possible	Up to 4.00 D	Not FDA approved; same complications as with cataract extraction with a lens implant.
SMILE	Up to −6.00 D	Less than 1.00 D	Only 1 femtosecond platform currently approved for this procedure. Enhancements may require PRK. Limited range of cylinder.

FDA = US Food and Drug Administration; LASIK = laser in situ keratomileusis; NA = not applicable; SMILE = small-incision lenticule extraction.

[a] FDA-approved range; age restrictions apply as well. In general, patients must be 21 years or older for most procedures. Different laser platforms may have a different FDA-approved range and age restrictions. Other restrictions may apply and are part of the labeling of individual devices and lasers.

consent form signed preoperatively, prior to sedation, and not when the patient is dilated. For sample informed consent forms, see the website of the Ophthalmic Mutual Insurance Company (www.omic.com/risk-management/consent-forms/).

Emerging Technologies

While the essentials of the preoperative examination are unchanged, screening for refractive procedures has been streamlined with the advent of new technologies that allow many preoperative tests to be performed with a touch of a button. It is now possible to obtain wavefront refraction, topography/tomography, corneal thickness profile, and pupil measurements with 1 or 2 devices, helping to minimize the ophthalmic technician's and physician's time and improve the patient experience. Some of these devices (wavefront units and topographers) couple directly with the lasers used for treatment, potentially improving the efficacy of laser vision correction. It is anticipated that the continued integration of multiple devices into a single platform will improve the speed and accuracy of the preoperative workup.

Schallhorn JM, Seifert S, Schallhorn SC. SMILE, topography-guided LASIK, and wavefront-guided LASIK: review of clinical outcomes in premarket approval FDA studies. *J Refract Surg*. 2019;35(11):690–698.

CHAPTER 3

Incisional Corneal Surgery

This chapter includes related videos. Go to www.aao.org/bcscvideo_section13 or scan the QR codes in the text to access this content.

Highlights

- Radial keratotomy is now an obsolete procedure, but it is important to understand the refractive principles because of its effect on corneal biomechanics and its consequences in subsequent cataract surgery.
- Incisional correction of astigmatism can be performed in various ways, as a standalone procedure or in combination with cataract surgery.
- Coupling is an important concept in treating astigmatism, as the optical power, or spherical equivalent, of the cornea is unchanged in most peripheral incisional procedures.
- The correction of astigmatism requires an accurate reference axis from which to guide the placement of the incisions.

Current Role of Incisional Procedures

Incisional refractive surgery for the treatment of myopia has largely been replaced by other modalities. However, incisional procedures are still used to treat primary astigmatism in combination with cataract surgery and to manage residual astigmatism after cataract or keratorefractive surgery and following penetrating keratoplasty. In fact, astigmatism management by means of incisional techniques, both traditional and intrastromal, has increased substantially with the advent of refractive cataract surgery.

Radial Keratotomy for Myopia

Although radial keratotomy (RK) is now considered an obsolete procedure, it played an important role in the history of refractive surgery. RK differs from surface ablation, or photorefractive keratectomy (PRK), and laser in situ keratomileusis (LASIK) in that it does not involve removal of tissue from the central cornea; rather, radial incisions are used to redistribute power from the center to the periphery of the cornea.

To evaluate the safety and efficacy of RK, the Prospective Evaluation of Radial Keratotomy (PERK) study was initiated in 1982 for patients with myopia from −2.00 D to −8.75 D (mean, −3.875 D). Ten years after the procedure, 53% of the 435 study patients had 20/20 or better uncorrected distance visual acuity (UDVA; also called *uncorrected visual acuity, UCVA*), and 85% had 20/40 or better. In addition, the older the patient, the greater the effect achieved with the same surgical technique. The most important finding in the 10-year PERK study was the continuing long-term instability of the procedure. A hyperopic shift of 1.00 D or greater was found in 43% of eyes between 6 months and 10 years postoperatively. This hyperopic shift can have implications in refractive targeting for cataract surgery in patients who have undergone RK.

Waring GO 3rd, Lynn MJ, McDonnell PJ. Results of the Prospective Evaluation of Radial Keratotomy (PERK) study 10 years after surgery. *Arch Ophthalmol.* 1994;112(10):1298–1308.

Postoperative Effects of Radial Keratotomy

Radial corneal incisions sever collagen fibrils in the corneal stroma. This produces a wound gape with midperipheral bulging of the cornea, compensatory central corneal flattening, and decreased refractive power, thereby decreasing myopia (Fig 3-1).

RK changes not only the curvature of the central cornea but also its overall topography, creating an oblate cornea—flatter in the center and steeper in the periphery—which reduces myopia but increases spherical aberration. After RK, there is less correlation among the parameters of refraction, central keratometry, and UDVA, presumably because the altered corneal curvature creates a more complex, multifocal optical system. As a consequence, keratometric readings might show degrees of astigmatism that differ from those detected by refraction. In addition, central corneal flattening affects intraocular lens (IOL) power calculations for cataract surgery (discussed later in this chapter and in Chapter 8).

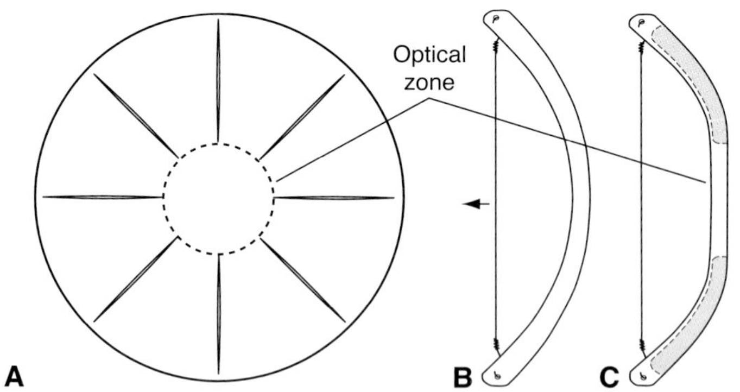

Figure 3-1 Schematic diagrams of the effect of radial incisions. **A,** 8-incision radial keratotomy (RK) with circular central optical zone *(dashed circle),* which shows the limit of the inner incision length. **B,** Cross-sectional view of the cornea before RK. **C,** After RK, the corneal periphery is steepened, and flattening is induced in the central cornea. *(Modified from Troutman RC, Buzard KA. Corneal Astigmatism: Etiology, Prevention, and Management. Mosby-Year Book; 1992.)*

Stability of refraction

Diurnal fluctuation of vision and a progressive flattening effect after surgery can be persistent, resulting in refractive instability. *Diurnal fluctuation* is caused by hypoxic edema of the incisions when the eyelids are closed during sleep. This edema leads to flattening of the central cornea (and hyperopic shift) upon awakening, followed by steepening later in the day. In a subset of the PERK study at 10 years, the mean change in the spherical equivalent of refraction between the morning (waking) and evening examinations was an increase of 0.31 ± 0.58 D in minus power. The *progressive flattening effect* of surgery was one of the major untoward results described in the PERK study. Greater hyperopic shift was noted with smaller optical zones. The potential stabilizing effect of corneal collagen crosslinking in post-RK eyes is currently being studied, but no consensus has been reached on its efficacy.

Elbaz U, Yeung SN, Ziai S, et al. Collagen crosslinking after radial keratotomy. *Cornea.* 2014;33(2):131–136.

Mazzotta C, Baiocchi S, Denaro R, Tosi GM, Caporossi T. Corneal collagen cross-linking to stop corneal ectasia exacerbated by radial keratotomy. *Cornea.* 2011;30(2):225–228.

Complications

Many patients reported the appearance of starburst, glare, or halo effects around lights at night after RK. Treatment with drugs that promote pupillary constriction, such as pilocarpine, or decrease pupillary dilation, such as brimonidine, may reduce symptoms by keeping the pupillary diameter within the central optical clear zone. Other complications included fluctuation in vision, loss of corrected distance visual acuity, induced astigmatism due to epithelial plugs and wound gape (Fig 3-2), vascularization of stromal scars, and nonprogressive endothelial disruption beneath the incisions.

Potentially blinding complications occurred only rarely after RK, usually secondary to corneal perforation and the possible sequelae of endophthalmitis, epithelial downgrowth, and traumatic cataract. The postoperative use of contact lenses often resulted in vascularization of the incisions, with subsequent scarring and irregular astigmatism. Scleral contact lenses have proved to be successful in managing irregular astigmatism and ametropia after RK. The incisions remain a point of weakness, and rupture of RK wounds secondary to blunt trauma has been reported as much as 13 years after the procedure.

A 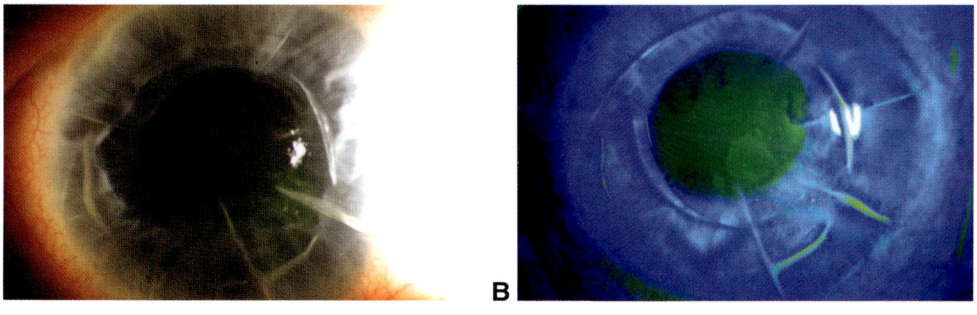 B

Figure 3-2 Incision complications. **A,** Crossed RK and arcuate keratotomy incisions with epithelial plugs in a patient who had intraoperative corneal perforation. **B,** Fluorescein study demonstrates gaping of the incisions, causing persistent ocular irritation. *(Courtesy of Jayne S. Weiss, MD.)*

Ocular Surgery After Radial Keratotomy

Laser refractive procedures

It is not uncommon for RK patients to present years later with hyperopia. LASIK and PRK have been shown to be effective in correcting low amounts of hyperopia and myopia after RK. However, PRK may be preferable, as creation of a LASIK flap may result in irregular astigmatism, splaying of the incisions, and epithelial ingrowth, as well as loss of sections of the flap, which can be challenging to treat. Surface ablation avoids the LASIK-related risks after RK but increases the risk of postoperative corneal haze. The off-label (in the United States) use of mitomycin C, 0.02% (0.2 mg/mL), applied to the stroma after laser ablation for 12–30 seconds has dramatically reduced corneal haze after RK and other corneal surgical procedures (eg, corneal transplant and LASIK). The drug should be copiously irrigated from the eye to reduce its toxic effects.

Patients undergoing laser vision correction for refractive errors after RK need to understand that the laser procedure will not remove scars resulting from RK incisions, so symptoms of glare or fluctuation may remain. In addition, some patients may continue to experience hyperopic progression.

Anbar R, Malta JB, Barbosa JB, Leoratti MC, Beer S, Campos M. Photorefractive keratectomy with mitomycin-C for consecutive hyperopia after radial keratotomy. *Cornea.* 2009;28(4): 371–374.

Joyal H, Grégoire J, Faucher A. Photorefractive keratectomy to correct hyperopic shift after radial keratotomy. *J Cataract Refract Surg.* 2003;29(8):1502–1506.

Linebarger EJ, Hardten DR, Lindstrom RL. Laser-assisted in situ keratomileusis for correction of secondary hyperopia after radial keratotomy. *Int Ophthalmol Clin.* 2000;40(3):125–132.

Majmudar PA, Schallhorn SC, Cason JB, et al. Mitomycin-C in corneal surface excimer laser ablation techniques: a report by the American Academy of Ophthalmology. *Ophthalmology.* 2015;122(6):1085–1095.

Nassaralla BA, McLeod SD, Nassaralla JJ Jr. Prophylactic mitomycin C to inhibit corneal haze after photorefractive keratectomy for residual myopia following radial keratotomy. *J Refract Surg.* 2007;23(3):226–232.

Keratoplasty

In patients with endothelial dystrophy, corneal infection, irregular astigmatism, severe visual fluctuations, or starburst effects, keratoplasty may be necessary to restore visual functioning. Keratoplasty should be avoided if the patient's visual problems can be corrected with glasses or contact lenses (see the section Corneal Transplantation After Refractive Surgery in Chapter 8). If keratoplasty is deemed necessary, the RK incisions may need to be stabilized with sutures before trephination, outside the trephine cut. This minimizes the chance of their opening and allows adequate suturing of the donor corneal graft to the recipient bed.

Cataract surgery

Results may be variable for cataract extraction with IOL implantation after RK. In addition, IOL power calculation can be problematic and may result in ametropia. Most experts favor using third- or fourth-generation IOL formulas and aiming for a slightly myopic result (−0.5 to −1 D) to help counteract the ongoing hyperopic shift after RK (see Chapter 8).

A useful online resource for calculating IOL power in a post-RK patient is the post–refractive surgery IOL power calculator available through the website of the American Society of Cataract and Refractive Surgery, www.ascrs.org, and directly at http://iolcalc.ascrs.org (see Chapter 8). In addition, modalities such as intraoperative wavefront aberrometry can be used to obtain real-time IOL calculations that may help improve refractive outcomes.

Incision placement and construction are vital when performing cataract surgery in a post-RK patient. Scleral tunnel incisions are often preferred because clear corneal incisions increase the risk of the blade transecting the RK incision, which can cause the incisions to splay and induce irregular astigmatism. To help reduce preoperative corneal astigmatism, the surgeon may consider placing the cataract incision in the steep astigmatic meridian of the cornea. Toric IOLs can be used in patients with regular astigmatism, but multifocal IOLs should be avoided. Recently, some surgeons have obtained good refractive results and patient satisfaction with the use of extended depth of focus IOLs in post-RK patients. The surgeon should have an extensive preoperative discussion with the patient about the unpredictable refractive outcomes with our current understanding of biometry in post-RK eyes and the introduction of another potential source of dysphotopsia.

At the conclusion of surgery, care should be taken to prevent overhydration of the cataract incisions, which could lead to rupture of the RK incisions. There should be a low threshold for placing a suture to close and stabilize the surgical incisions.

In the early postoperative period, corneal edema may result in temporary hyperopia. It may take several months for the refraction to stabilize in these patients; thus, stability of refraction and vision should be confirmed before additional refractive procedures such as PRK or an IOL exchange are considered.

Baartman BJ, Karpuk K, Eichhorn B. Extended depth of focus lens implantation after radial keratotomy. *Clin Ophthalmol.* 2019;13:1401–1408.

Hemmati HD, Gologorsky D, Pineda R 2nd. Intraoperative wavefront aberrometry in cataract surgery. *Semin Ophthalmol.* 2012;27(5–6):100–106.

IOL power calculations: post radial keratotomy (RK). doctor-hill.com. Accessed October 6, 2021. https://www.doctor-hill.com/iol-main/postRK.htm

Shammas HJ. Intraocular lens power calculation in patients with prior refractive surgery. *Focal Points: Clinical Modules for Ophthalmologists.* American Academy of Ophthalmology; 2013, module 6.

Wang L, Hill WE, Koch DD. Evaluation of intraocular lens power prediction methods using the American Society of Cataract and Refractive Surgeons post–keratorefractive intraocular lens power calculator. *J Cataract Refract Surg.* 2010;36(9):1466–1473.

Arcuate Keratotomy and Limbal Relaxing Incisions for Astigmatism

Several techniques of incisional surgery have been used to correct astigmatism. The most commonly used are *arcuate* (curved) *keratotomy (AK),* in which incisions are typically placed in the cornea at the 7-mm optical zone, and *limbal relaxing incisions (LRIs),* which are placed at the limbus. *Tangential* (transverse/straight) *keratotomy* was formerly used in combination with RK to correct myopic astigmatism but now is seldom performed. Along with LRIs, AK is used to correct astigmatism during or after cataract surgery and IOL implantation, as well as after refractive surgery procedures such as LASIK and PRK (Video 3-1). AK is also used to correct postkeratoplasty astigmatism. Several femtosecond laser platforms have been approved for incisional keratotomies.

VIDEO 3-1 Femtosecond laser–assisted astigmatic keratotomy in the setting of LASIK.
Courtesy of George O. Waring IV, MD.

The Coupling Principle

When a single meridian is flattened as a result of an astigmatic incision, a compensatory steepening occurs in the meridian 90° away. This phenomenon is known as *coupling* (Fig 3-3). When the *coupling ratio* (the amount of flattening in the meridian of the incision divided by the induced steepening in the opposite meridian) is 1.0, the spherical equivalent remains unchanged. When the coupling ratio is greater than 1.0, a hyperopic shift occurs. The type of incision (arcuate versus tangential) and the length and number of parallel incisions can influence the coupling ratio. Long, straight, and tangential incisions tend to induce a coupling ratio greater than 1.0, unlike short, arcuate incisions. With a correction less than 2.00 D of astigmatism, the coupling ratio is typically 1.0; however, with a correction greater than 2.00 D of astigmatism, the ratio tends to be greater than 1.0. In general, LRIs do not change the spherical equivalent.

Rowsey JJ, Fouraker BD. Corneal coupling principles. *Int Ophthalmol Clin.* 1996;36(4):29–38.

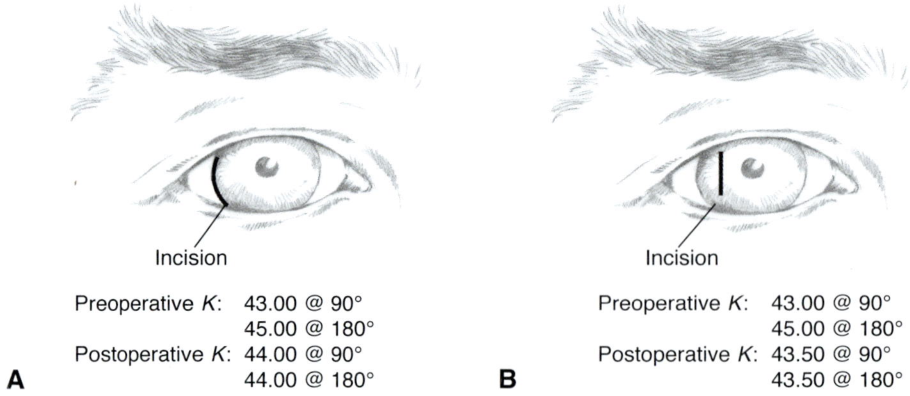

Figure 3-3 Coupling effect of astigmatic incisions. **A,** A limbal relaxing incision has a coupling ratio of 1.0, and the spherical equivalent and average corneal power are not changed. **B,** A transverse incision has a coupling ratio greater than 1.0, which causes a hyperopic change in refraction by decreasing the average corneal power. *(Illustration by Cyndie C. H. Wooley.)*

Surgical Considerations and Techniques

Arcuate keratotomy is an incisional surgical procedure in which arcuate incisions of approximately 95% depth are made in the steep meridians of the midperipheral cornea at the 7–9-mm optical zone and no closer than 3.5 mm from the center of the pupil to avoid induced glare and aberrations. LRIs are incisions placed just anterior to the limbus, with the depth set at approximately 600 µm, or 50 µm less than the thinnest pachymetry measurement at the limbus (Video 3-2).

VIDEO 3-2 Manual LRI at the time of cataract surgery.
Courtesy of Sumit (Sam) Garg, MD.

AKs differ from LRIs in their midperipheral location and greater relative corneal depth. However, these procedures are similar in that both have coupling ratios of 1.0 and, therefore, correct astigmatism without inducing a substantial hyperopic shift. Increasing the length of an LRI increases the magnitude of the astigmatic correction. For AK, the amount of cylindrical correction is increased by increasing the length or depth of the incision, using multiple incisions, or reducing the optical zone (see Tables 3-1, 3-2 later in the chapter). Older patient age is associated with greater effect of astigmatic incisions. When astigmatism is being corrected in the context of cataract surgery, most surgeons recommend using incisional techniques for low amounts of astigmatism, while relying on toric IOLs for higher corrections.

Instrumentation

The instruments used in AK and LRIs are similar. Both are performed with diamond blades: adjustable blades are used more often in AK, whereas preset blades are more common in LRIs, although adjustable blades are sometimes used in the latter procedure as well (Fig 3-4). Toric axis markers are used to specify the length of the planned incision (Fig 3-5).

A femtosecond laser is commonly used to create peripheral arcuate incisions. These incisions can be programmed to a specific depth and can be titrated, with only part of the incision opened initially, followed by a larger opening later if needed for greater astigmatic correction. In addition, femtosecond lasers allow for nonpenetrating intrastromal astigmatic keratotomies, which have shown efficacy and safety in early results.

Day AC, Lau NM, Stevens JD. Nonpenetrating femtosecond laser intrastromal astigmatic keratotomy in eyes having cataract surgery. *J Cataract Refract Surg.* 2016;42(1):102–109.

Surgical planning and nomograms

It is essential for the surgeon to accurately determine the steep meridian when planning for astigmatism correction. The plus cylinder axis of the manifest refraction is generally used, as this measurement takes into account both corneal and lenticular astigmatism, which are "manifest" in the refraction. However, when astigmatism is being treated with AKs or LRIs at the time of cataract surgery, the correction should be based on the steep meridian and magnitude as measured by corneal topography or keratometry, as the lenticular portion of the astigmatism will be nullified when the lens is removed. In addition, a

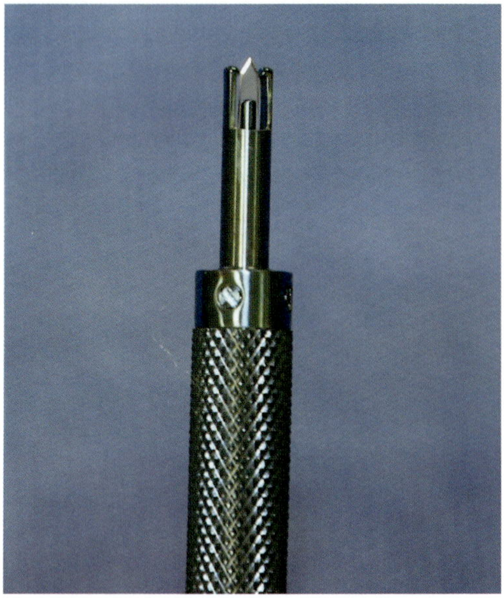

Figure 3-4 A 600-µm adjustable diamond knife for creating limbal relaxing incisions. *(Courtesy of Sumit [Sam] Garg, MD.)*

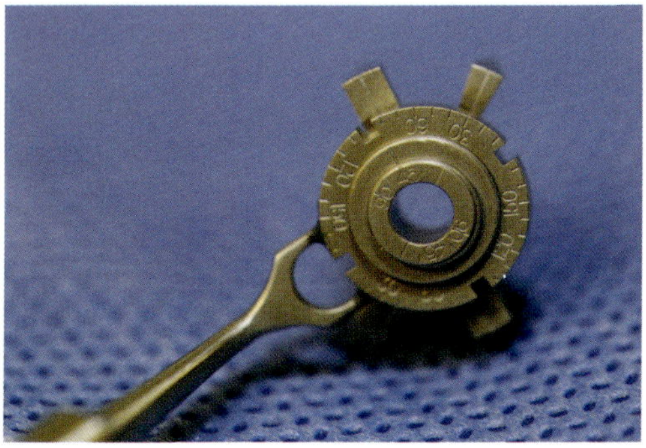

Figure 3-5 Adjustable toric axis marker. *(Courtesy of Sumit [Sam] Garg, MD.)*

prerequisite for combining LRIs with cataract surgery is the use of astigmatically predictable phacoemulsification incisions.

It is prudent to establish the correct reference (ie, 0°–180°) for the astigmatic treatment. There are many methods to achieve this, including pen marking, automated marking, and use of thermal or digital markers. Marking should be done with the patient in a seated position, looking straight ahead, to avoid reference-mark error due to cyclotorsion (Fig 3-6). Studies have demonstrated that up to 15° of cyclotorsion can occur when patients move from an upright to a supine position.

Intraoperative keratoscopy, aberrometry (Video 3-3), and automated guidance can be helpful in determining incision location and effect. The amount of treatment for a given degree of astigmatism employing LRIs can be determined from one of several nomograms, such as those shown in Tables 3-1 and 3-2. In addition, many nomograms are now available online to help guide astigmatic treatments (eg, www.lricalculator.com, www.laserarcs.com). It is important to note whether the nomogram has been developed for manual or femtosecond

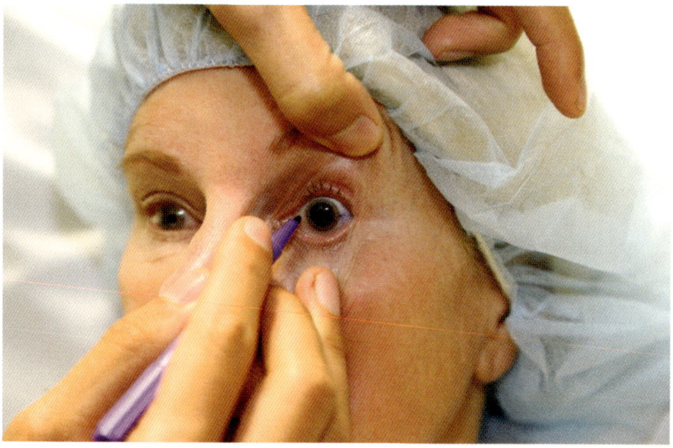

Figure 3-6 Marking the 3- to 9-o'clock axis at the limbus, with the patient sitting upright and looking straight ahead. *(Courtesy of Sumit [Sam] Garg, MD.)*

Table 3-1 Donnenfeld LRI Nomogram

Astigmatism (Diopters)	LRI and Arc Length[a]
0.50	1 incision, 45°
0.75	2 incisions, 30° each
1.50	2 incisions, 60° each
3.00	2 incisions, 90° each

LRI = limbal relaxing incision.

[a] For against-the-rule astigmatism, increase arc length by 5°. For younger patients, increase arc length by 5°. For older patients, decrease arc length by 5°.

Note: Most surgeons generally do not perform arcuate incision >45°. LRIs are generally reserved for lower amounts of corneal astigmatism, and toric IOLs are used to treat higher amounts of astigmatism. *Also note:* This nomogram is for manual LRIs; femtosecond astigmatic incisions require modifications.

Information from LRI Calculator website. Accessed October 7, 2020. www.lricalculator.com

laser incisions. Manual LRIs are typically made more peripherally (larger optical zone) and their depth is estimated, whereas femtosecond laser incisions typically have a smaller optical zone and are set for a specified depth (typically 90% of the OCT-measured corneal thickness). As such, it is recommended to "back off" the planned treatment when using a traditional nomogram for a femtosecond laser case, as the optical zone will be smaller, and the depth will be deeper, both producing a greater effect from the incision (Video 3-4).

VIDEO 3-3 Manual LRI using intraoperative aberrometry at the time of cataract surgery.
Courtesy of Sumit (Sam) Garg, MD.

VIDEO 3-4 Femtosecond laser–assisted astigmatic keratotomy at the time of cataract surgery.
Courtesy of Sumit (Sam) Garg, MD.

Table 3-2 Nichamin Age- and Pachymetry-Adjusted LRI Nomogram

With-the-Rule[a]

Preoperative Cylinder (Diopters)	Age 20–30 y	Age 31–40 y	Age 41–50 y	Age 51–60 y	Age 61–70 y	Age 71–80 y
0.75	40°	35°	35°	30°	30°	25°
1.00	45°	40°	40°	35°	35°	30°
1.25	55°	50°	45°	40°	35°	35°
1.50	60°	55°	50°	45°	40°	40°
1.75	65°	60°	55°	50°	45°	45°
2.00	70°	65°	60°	55°	50°	45°
2.25	75°	70°	65°	60°	55°	50°
2.50	80°	75°	70°	65°	60°	55°
2.75	85°	80°	75°	70°	65°	60°
3.00	90°	90°	85°	80°	70°	65°

Against-the-Rule[b]

Preoperative Cylinder (Diopters)	Age 20–30 y	Age 31–40 y	Age 41–50 y	Age 51–60 y	Age 61–70 y	Age 71–80 y
0.75	45°	40°	40°	35°	35°	30°
1.00	50°	45°	45°	40°	40°	35°
1.25	55°	55°	50°	45°	40°	35°
1.50	60°	60°	55°	50°	45°	40°
1.75	65°	65°	60°	55°	50°	45°
2.00	70°	70°	65°	60°	55°	50°
2.25	75°	75°	70°	65°	60°	55°
2.50	80°	80°	75°	70°	65°	60°
2.75	85°	85°	80°	75°	70°	65°
3.00	90°	90°	85°	80°	75°	70°

Blade depth is set to 90% of the thinnest pachymetry.
[a] Steep corneal meridian at 45°–135°.
[b] Steep corneal meridian at 0°–44° or 136°–180°.

Note: Most surgeons generally do not perform arcuate incision >45°. LRIs are generally reserved for lower amounts of corneal astigmatism, and toric IOLs are used to treat higher amounts of astigmatism. *Also note:* This nomogram is for manual LRIs; femtosecond astigmatic incisions require modifications.

Data from LRI Calculator website. Accessed October 7, 2020. www.lricalculator.com

Chang JSM. Femtosecond laser-assisted astigmatic keratotomy: a review. *Eye Vis (Lond).* 2018;5:6.

Nichamin LD. Nomogram for limbal relaxing incisions. *J Cataract Refract Surg.* 2006;32(9):1048.

Visco DM, Bedi R, Packer M. Femtosecond laser–assisted arcuate keratotomy at the time of cataract surgery for the management of preexisting astigmatism [published correction appears in *J Cataract Refract Surg.* 2020;46(4):658]. *J Cataract Refract Surg.* 2019;45(12):1762–1769.

Outcomes

The outcome of AK and LRI surgery depends on several variables, including patient age; the distance separating the incision pairs (optical zone); and the length, depth, and number of incisions. Few large prospective trials have been performed. The Astigmatism Reduction Clinical Trial (ARC-T) of AK, which used a 7-mm optical zone and varying arc lengths, showed a reduction in astigmatism of 1.6 ± 1.1 D in patients with preoperative, naturally occurring astigmatism of 2.8 ± 1.2 D. Other studies of AK have shown a final UDVA of 20/40 in 65%–80% of eyes. Overcorrections have been reported in 4%–20% of patients.

Studies of LRIs are limited, but these incisions are frequently used with apparently good results in astigmatic patients undergoing cataract surgery. One study showed an absolute change in refractive astigmatism of 1.72 ± 0.81 D after LRIs in patients with mixed astigmatism. Astigmatism was decreased by 0.91 D, or 44%, in another series of LRIs in 22 eyes of 13 patients. Femtosecond laser astigmatic incisions have shown safety and efficacy in several studies. Incisions in the horizontal meridian have been reported to cause approximately twice as much astigmatic correction as those in the vertical meridian (see Table 3-2). There can be a loss of effect of incisional astigmatic treatment with time. In cases where the treatment was successful and a regression has occurred, it is possible to reopen the AK or LRI incisions at the slit lamp with sharp or blunt dissection.

Faktorovich EG, Maloney RK, Price FW Jr. Effect of astigmatic keratotomy on spherical equivalent: results of the Astigmatism Reduction Clinical Trial. *Am J Ophthalmol.* 1999;127(3):260–269.

Price FW, Grene RB, Marks RG, Gonzales JS. Astigmatism Reduction Clinical Trial: a multicenter prospective evaluation of the predictability of arcuate keratotomy. Evaluation of surgical nomogram predictability. ARC-T Study Group [published correction appears in *Arch Ophthalmol.* 1995;113(5):577]. *Arch Ophthalmol.* 1995;113(3):277–282.

Complications

Irregular astigmatism may occur after either AKs or LRIs; however, it is more common with the former, presumably because LRIs are farther from the corneal center, thus mitigating any effects of irregular incisions. Off-axis AKs can lead to undercorrection or even worsening of preexisting astigmatism. To avoid creating an edge of cornea that swells and cannot be epithelialized, arcuate incisions and LRIs should not intersect other incisions (see Figure 3-2). Corneal infection and perforation have been reported.

Ocular Surgery and Arcuate Keratotomy or Limbal Relaxing Incisions

Arcuate keratotomy and LRIs can be combined with or performed after cataract surgery (see the section "Surgical planning and nomograms" earlier in the chapter), PRK, and LASIK. Better predictability can be obtained if astigmatic correction is performed after the refraction is stable.

AK can be used to correct astigmatism after penetrating keratoplasty. In such cases, the AK incisions are often made in the graft or in the graft–host junction, but care must be taken to avoid perforation. AK incisions in a corneal graft may require compression sutures at the meridian 90° away, and an initial overcorrection is desired in order to compensate for wound healing. When AK incisions are made in the host cornea, the effect is significantly reduced.

Penetrating keratoplasty can be done after extensive AK, but the wounds may have to be sutured before trephination, as discussed earlier for RK.

Bayramlar HH, Dağlioğlu MC, Borazan M. Limbal relaxing incisions for primary mixed astigmatism and mixed astigmatism after cataract surgery. *J Cataract Refract Surg.* 2003;29(4):723–728.

Dick HB, Gerste RD, Schultz T. Femtosecond laser-assisted cataract surgery. *Focal Points: Clinical Modules for Ophthalmologists.* American Academy of Ophthalmology; 2015, module 4.

Gills JP. Treating astigmatism at the time of cataract surgery. *Curr Opin Ophthalmol.* 2002;13(1):2–6.

Rubenstein JB, Raciti M. Management of astigmatism: LRIs. *Int Ophthalmol Clin.* 2012;52(2):31–40.

Yeu E, Rubenstein JB. Management of Astigmatism in Lens-Based Surgery. *Focal Points: Clinical Modules for Ophthalmologists.* American Academy of Ophthalmology; 2008, module 2.

CHAPTER 4

Photoablation: Techniques and Outcomes

This chapter includes related videos. Go to www.aao.org/bcscvideo_section13 or scan the QR codes in the text to access this content.

Highlights

- Photoablation is possible with the 193-nm argon-fluoride (ArF) excimer laser because the cornea has an extremely high absorption coefficient at that wavelength.
- The excimer laser is used for both surface ablation (eg, photorefractive keratectomy [PRK]) and stromal ablation under a flap (laser in situ keratomileusis [LASIK]).
- The popularity of PRK declined after the advent of LASIK, but newer surface ablation procedures—laser subepithelial keratomileusis (LASEK) and epipolis laser in situ keratomileusis (epi-LASIK)—have been introduced.
- Different excimer laser ablation profiles such as wavefront-guided, wavefront-optimized, and topography-guided profiles are available, and each offers distinct advantages.
- The femtosecond laser has become an important technology for creating the corneal flap in LASIK.
- Residual ametropia after excimer keratorefractive surgery can be improved through re-treatment (enhancement) by means of surface ablation or flap lifting with stromal ablation, depending on the primary procedure.

Excimer Laser

Fundamentals

The excimer laser uses a high-voltage electrical charge to transiently combine atoms of excited argon and fluorine; when the molecule, or *dimer,* reverts to its separate atoms, a charged photon is emitted. The word *excimer* comes from "*exc*ited d*imer*." Srinivasan, an IBM engineer, was studying the far-ultraviolet (193-nm) ArF excimer laser for photoetching of computer chips. He and Trokel, an ophthalmologist, not only showed that the excimer laser could remove corneal tissue precisely with minimal adjacent corneal damage but also recognized its potential for use in refractive and therapeutic corneal surgery.

Photoablation, the removal of corneal tissue with minimal adjacent corneal damage, is possible because the cornea has an extremely high absorption coefficient at 193 nm. A single 193-nm photon has sufficient energy to directly break carbon–carbon and carbon–nitrogen bonds that form the peptide backbone of the corneal collagen molecules. Excimer laser radiation ruptures the collagen polymer into small fragments, expelling a discrete volume and depth of corneal tissue from the surface with each pulse of the laser (Fig 4-1) without significantly damaging adjacent tissue.

Srinivasan R. Ablation of polymers and biological tissue by ultraviolet lasers. *Science.* 1986;234(4776):559–565.

Trokel SL, Srinivasan R, Braren B. Excimer laser surgery of the cornea. *Am J Ophthalmol.* 1983;96(6):710–715.

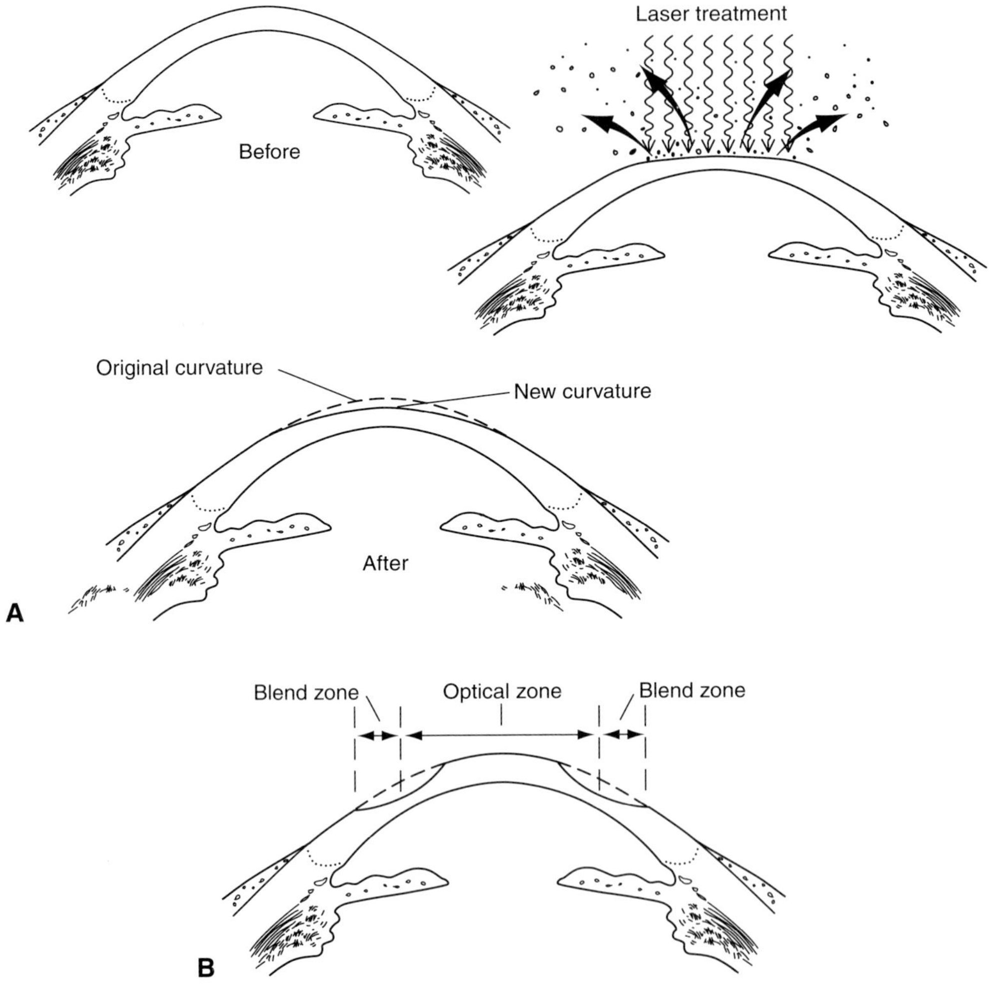

Figure 4-1 Schematic illustrations of corneal recontouring by the excimer laser. **A,** Correction of myopia by flattening the central cornea. **B,** Correction of hyperopia by steepening the central corneal optical zone and blending the periphery.

(Continued)

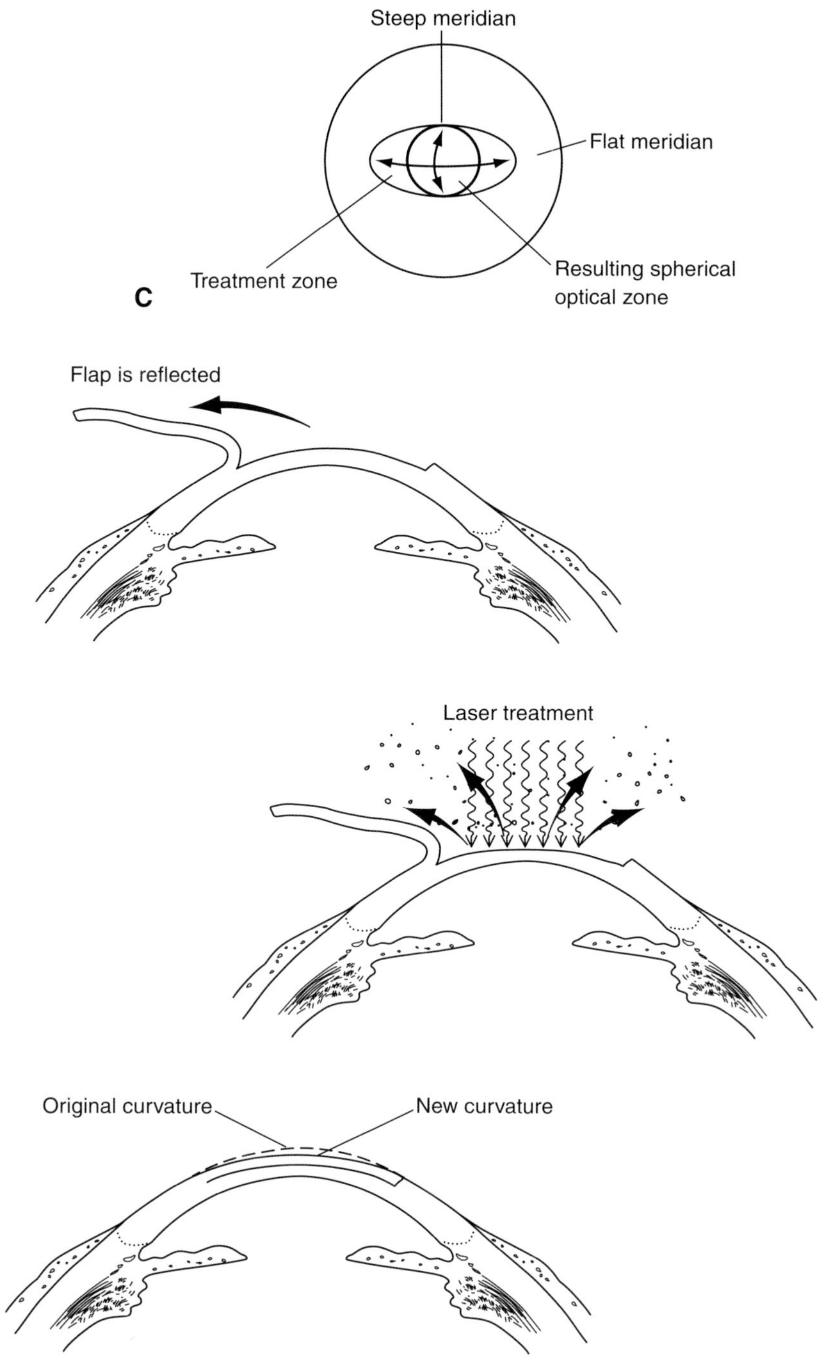

Figure 4-1 *(continued)* **C,** Correction of astigmatism by differential tissue removal 90° apart. Note that in correction of myopic astigmatism, the steeper meridian with more tissue removal corresponds to the smaller dimension of the ellipse. **D,** In LASIK, a corneal flap is reflected back, the excimer laser ablation is performed on the exposed stromal bed, and the flap is then reposited. The altered corneal contour of the bed produces the same alteration in the anterior surface of the flap. *(Illustrations by Jeanne Koelling.)*

Role of the Excimer Laser in Keratorefractive Surgery

The ArF excimer laser treats refractive error by ablating the anterior corneal stroma to create a new radius of curvature. Two major refractive surgical techniques use excimer laser ablation: surface ablation and LASIK. *Surface ablation* techniques include photorefractive keratectomy (PRK), laser subepithelial keratomileusis (LASEK), and epipolis laser in situ keratomileusis (epi-LASIK). In these techniques, the Bowman layer is exposed either by debriding the epithelium through various methods or by loosening and moving—but attempting to preserve—the epithelium. In LASIK, the excimer laser ablation is performed under a lamellar flap that is created with either a femtosecond laser or mechanical microkeratome. Excimer laser ablation algorithms can be classified generally as conventional, wavefront optimized, wavefront guided, and topography guided.

Surface Ablation

Surface ablation procedures were initially performed as PRK, the sculpting of the de-epithelialized corneal stroma to alter refractive power, and they underwent extensive preclinical investigation before being applied to sighted human eyes. Results of early animal studies provided evidence of relatively normal wound healing in laser-ablated corneas.

The popularity of PRK decreased in the late 1990s when LASIK became available because of the faster recovery of vision and reduced postoperative discomfort with LASIK. Although more LASIK than surface ablation procedures are still being performed, the number of surface ablations has increased in recent years. PRK remains an especially attractive alternative for specific indications, including irregular or thin corneas; epithelial basement membrane disease (often called *map-dot-fingerprint dystrophy*); previous corneal surgery, such as penetrating keratoplasty (PKP) and radial keratotomy (RK); and treatment of some LASIK flap complications, such as incomplete or buttonholed flaps. Surface ablation eliminates the potential for stromal flap–related complications and may have a decreased incidence of postoperative dry eye compared with LASIK. Corneal haze, the major risk of PRK, has decreased markedly with the off-label use of adjunctive mitomycin C (MMC); consequently, the use of PRK for higher levels of myopia has increased.

Majmudar PA, Forstot SL, Dennis RF, et al. Topical mitomycin-C for subepithelial fibrosis after refractive corneal surgery. *Ophthalmology.* 2000;107(1):89–94.

LASIK

The term *keratomileusis* comes from the Greek words for "cornea" *(kerato)* and "to carve" *(mileusis). Laser in situ keratomileusis,* which combines keratomileusis with excimer laser stromal ablation, is currently the most frequently performed keratorefractive procedure because of its safety, efficacy, quick recovery of vision, and minimal patient discomfort. LASIK combines 2 techniques: creation of a stromal flap and excimer laser stromal ablation.

Wavefront-Guided, Wavefront-Optimized, and Topography-Guided Ablations

Conventional excimer laser ablation treats *lower-order,* or *spherocylindrical, aberrations* such as myopia, hyperopia, and astigmatism. These lower-order aberrations constitute approximately 90% of all aberrations. *Higher-order aberrations* make up the remainder; such aberrations cannot be treated with glasses. It is important to note that the visual impact of higher-order aberrations decreases as the refractive error (myopia, hyperopia, astigmatism) increases. Some ophthalmologists believe that small amounts of higher-order aberrations, which are commonly found in patients with excellent uncorrected vision, may not adversely affect vision. Higher-order aberrations are also a by-product of excimer laser ablation. Some higher-order aberrations can cause symptoms—such as loss of contrast sensitivity and induced nighttime halos and glare—that decrease the quality of vision. The aberrations most commonly associated with these visual concerns are spherical aberration and coma. See Chapter 1 for more detailed discussion of higher-order aberrations.

In an effort to reduce preexisting aberrations and minimize the induction of new aberrations, *wavefront-guided* ablation creates ablation profiles that are customized for the individual patient. In addition to correcting the lower-order aberrations of spherical error and astigmatism, wavefront-guided treatments can address higher-order aberrations.

Wavefront-optimized lasers do not use patient-specific wavefront data. Instead, they adjust the ablation profile of conventional treatments to create a more prolate corneal shape, with additional peripheral ablation in the myopic patient, to reduce spherical aberration; however, they have no effect on other higher-order aberrations.

Compared with conventional excimer laser ablation, wavefront-guided and wavefront-optimized ablations appear to offer better contrast sensitivity and induce fewer postoperative higher-order aberrations. Although advances in aberrometry and registration systems have led to improved outcomes, patients who undergo photoablation may still have more higher-order aberrations postoperatively than they did preoperatively. In general, wavefront-guided ablations remove more tissue than conventional ablations for the same preoperative refraction.

Wavefront-guided ablation appears to have clear-cut benefit compared with wavefront-optimized ablation only for patients with significant preoperative higher-order aberrations. The procedure is not suitable for all patients and may be inappropriate for use after cataract surgery. Intraocular lenses, especially multifocal intraocular lenses, interfere with capturing the wavefront scan and could result in the delivery of an inaccurate treatment. In addition, wavefront data may be impossible to obtain in highly irregular corneas or in eyes with small pupils.

Topography-guided ablations have been approved by the US Food and Drug Administration (FDA) since late 2013. Topography-guided systems use corneal topography data to create ablation profiles that treat existing corneal shape irregularities and optimize corneal curvature. Topography-guided ablations have gained traction outside the United States in the treatment of corneas with irregular surfaces, such as those with small or decentered optical zones from prior excimer ablations, LASIK flap complications, or post-RK corneal irregularities. Data from a recent FDA clinical trial demonstrated that topography-guided ablations may result in excellent outcomes even for routine laser vision correction cases in previously unoperated eyes.

Nuijts RM, Nabar VA, Hament WJ, Eggink FA. Wavefront-guided versus standard laser in situ keratomileusis to correct low to moderate myopia. *J Cataract Refract Surg.* 2002; 28(11):1907–1913.

Stonecipher KG, Kezirian GM. Wavefront-optimized versus wavefront-guided LASIK for myopic astigmatism with the ALLEGRETTO WAVE: three-month results of a prospective FDA trial. *J Refract Surg.* 2008;24(4):S424–S430.

Stulting RD, Fant BS; T-CAT Study Group, et al. Results of topography-guided laser in situ keratomileusis custom ablation treatment with a refractive excimer laser. *J Cataract Refract Surg.* 2016;42(1):11–18.

Surgical Techniques for Photoablation

Many of the steps in keratorefractive surgery are identical for surface ablation and LASIK. These include calibration and programming of the laser and patient preparation. The major difference between the 2 techniques is preparation for ablation: exposure of the Bowman layer for surface ablation and of the midstroma for LASIK. A list of FDA-approved lasers for refractive surgery can be found on the FDA website.

US Food & Drug Administration. List of FDA-approved lasers for LASIK. Medical Devices website. Updated September 6, 2018. Accessed October 6, 2021. https://www.fda.gov /medical-devices/lasik/list-fda-approved-lasers-lasik

Laser Calibration, Preoperative Planning, and Laser Programming

At the start of each surgery day and between patients, the technician should check the excimer laser for proper homogeneous beam profile, alignment, and power output, according to the manufacturer's instructions. As part of preoperative planning, the laser is programmed with the appropriate refraction. Often, the patient's manifest and cycloplegic refractions differ, or the amount and axis of astigmatism differ between the topographic evaluation and refractive examination. Thus, it may be unclear which refractive data to enter into the laser. The surgeon's decision about whether to use the manifest or the cycloplegic refraction is based on his or her individual nomogram and technique, although most surgeons use the manifest refraction, with a possible adjustment based on the cycloplegic refraction. The manifest refraction is more accurate in determining cylinder axis and amount. If the refractive cylinder is confirmed to be different from the topographic cylinder, lenticular astigmatism or posterior corneal curvature is assumed to be the cause. In this case, the laser is still programmed with the axis and amount of cylinder noted on refraction, which may differ from cylinder correction in cataract surgery. The surgeon should take particular care to check the axis obtained on the refraction with the value programmed into the laser. Entering an incorrect value is a potential source of error, particularly when converting between plus and minus cylinder formats.

Before each surgery, the surgeon and the technician should review a checklist of information, confirming the patient's name, the eye on which surgery is to be performed, the refraction, and any adjustments. In wavefront procedures, the treatment should correspond to the patient's refraction, and adjustments may be required to compensate for accommodation.

For many laser models, the surgeon also must enter the size of the optical zone and indicate whether a blend of the ablation zone should be performed. The *blend zone* is an area of peripheral asphericity designed to reduce the possible undesirable effects of an abrupt transition from the optical zone to the untreated cornea, resulting in spherical aberration (see Figure 4-1B). A prolate blend zone reduces the risk of glare and halo after excimer laser photoablation.

Special considerations for wavefront-guided techniques

Several wavefront mapping systems and wavefront-guided lasers are commercially available. Wavefront mapping systems are specific to the particular wavefront-guided laser used. Calibration should be performed according to the manufacturer's specifications.

For wavefront-guided ablations, the wavefront maps are taken with the patient sitting up at an aberrometer under scotopic conditions; the mapping results are then applied to the cornea in the laser suite with the patient lying down under the operating microscope. Some systems require pupillary dilation to capture wavefront data. The wavefront refraction indicated on wavefront analysis is then compared with the manifest refraction. If the difference between them exceeds 0.75 D, the manifest refraction and the wavefront analysis may need to be repeated. The data are either electronically transferred to the laser or downloaded to a portable drive and then transferred to the laser. Unlike conventional or wavefront-optimized excimer laser treatment, in which the manifest or cycloplegic refraction is used to program the laser, wavefront-guided laser treatment uses programmed wavefront data to create a custom ablation pattern.

Preoperative Patient Preparation

Many surgeons administer topical antibiotic prophylaxis preoperatively. The patient's skin is prepared with povidone-iodine 5%–10% or alcohol wipes before or after the patient enters the laser suite, and povidone-iodine solution 5% is sometimes applied as drops to the ocular surface and then irrigated out for further antisepsis. There is no consensus about the utility of these measures. When preparing the patient, the surgeon should take care to avoid irritation of the conjunctiva, which could lead to swelling of the conjunctiva and difficulties with suction.

In addition, patients should be informed before laser treatment about the sounds and smells they will experience during the treatment. They may receive an oral antianxiety medication such as diazepam.

If substantial astigmatism is being treated, some surgeons mark the cornea at the horizontal or vertical axis while the patient is sitting up to ensure accurate alignment under the laser. This step is done to compensate for the cyclotorsion that commonly occurs when the patient changes from a sitting to a lying position. A 15° offset in the axis of treatment can decrease the effective cylinder change and result in a significant axis shift. There are multiple methods for marking the cornea or limbus. Several platforms have iris registration to account for cyclotorsion.

Before any procedure, the surgical team should take a "time-out," during which the identity of the patient, the eye(s) to be treated, and the treatment to be performed are confirmed. After the patient is positioned under the laser, a sterile drape may be placed over the skin and eyelashes according to the surgeon's preference. Topical anesthetic drops are placed in the eye; for LASIK patients, care should be taken to ensure that the drops are not instilled too early, as doing so may loosen the epithelium substantially. An eyelid speculum is placed in the eye to be treated, and an opaque patch is placed over the fellow eye to avoid cross-fixation. A gauze pad may be taped over the temple between the eye to be treated and the ear to absorb any excess fluid.

The patient is asked to fixate on the laser centration light while the surgeon reduces ambient illumination from the microscope, focuses on the cornea, and centers the laser. It is important for the plane of the eye to remain parallel to the plane of the laser, for the patient to maintain fixation, and for the surgeon to control centration even when using lasers with tracking systems. For most patients, voluntary fixation during photoablation produces more accurate centration than globe immobilization by the surgeon.

Preparation of the Bowman Layer or Stromal Bed for Ablation

The next surgical step for all excimer photoablation procedures is preparation of the cornea for ablation. With surface ablation procedures, such preparation consists of epithelial removal to expose the Bowman layer. With LASIK, preparation involves the creation of a lamellar flap with a mechanical microkeratome or a femtosecond laser to expose the central stroma.

Epithelial debridement techniques for surface ablation

The epithelium can be removed with

- a sharp blade
- a blunt spatula
- a rotary corneal brush
- application of 20% absolute alcohol to the corneal surface for 10–45 seconds to loosen the epithelium with Weck-Cel sponge debridement (Video 4-1)
- a mechanical microkeratome with an epi-LASIK blade
- transepithelial ablation from the excimer laser itself

Figure 4-2 shows de-epithelialization techniques. In both transepithelial ablation and epi-LASIK, the peripheral margin of the de-epithelialization is defined by the laser or epikeratome itself. For other epithelial debridement techniques, the surgeon often defines the outer limit of de-epithelialization with an optical zone marker and then debrides from the periphery toward the center. An ophthalmic surgical cellulose sponge can be brushed uniformly over the surface of the cornea to remove any residual epithelium and provide a smooth surface. The epithelium should be removed efficiently and consistently to prevent hydration changes in the stroma, because excessive corneal stromal dehydration may increase the amount of tissue removed and lead to overcorrection. Care should be taken to not disturb peripheral epithelium to avoid recurrent erosion in the future. The laser treatment zone must be free of epithelial cells, debris, and excess fluid before ablation.

VIDEO 4-1 Photorefractive keratectomy procedure.
Courtesy of George O. Waring IV, MD.

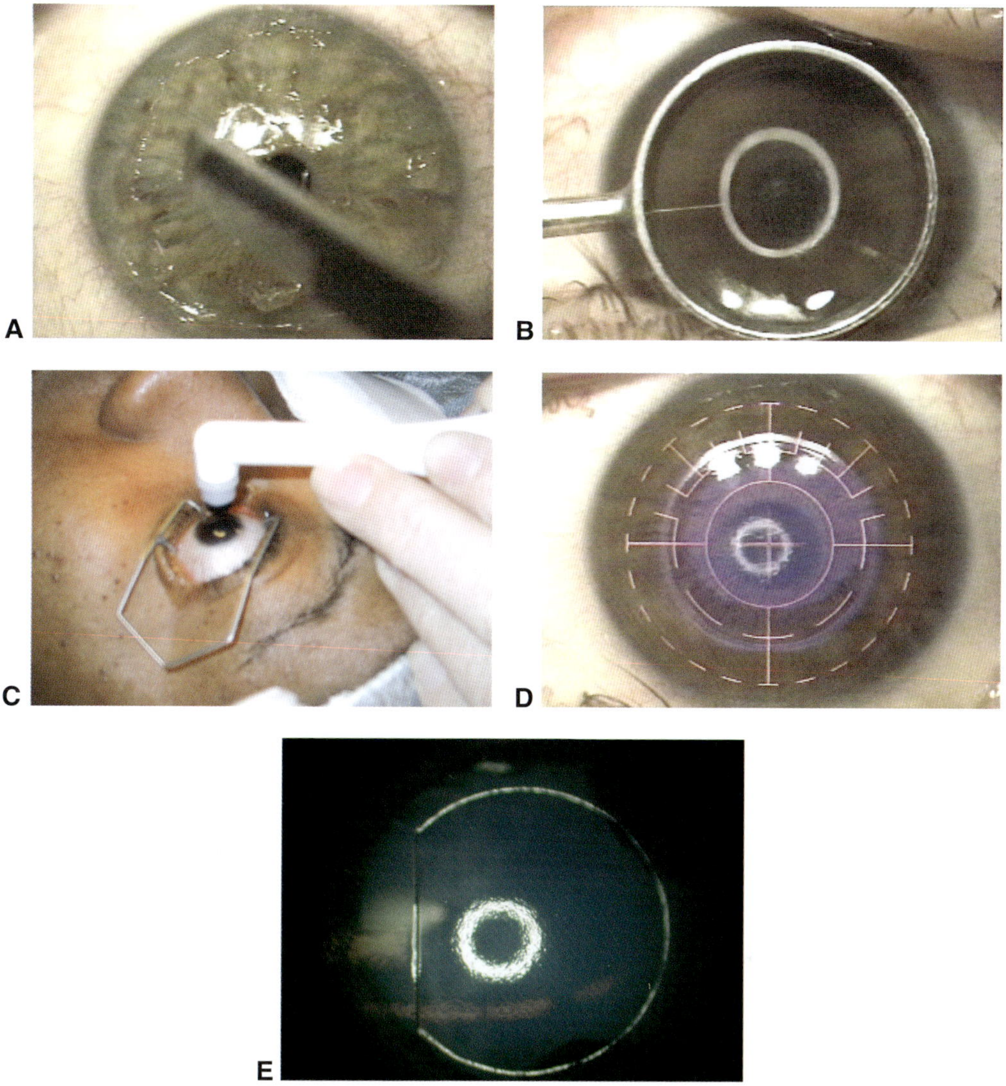

Figure 4-2 Techniques of de-epithelialization for surface ablation. **A,** Scraping with a blade. **B,** 20% dilution of absolute ethanol in an optical zone marker well. **C,** Rotary brush debridement. **D,** "Laser scrape," in which a broad-beam laser exposes the entire treatment zone to ablation pulses; these pulses remove most of the epithelium that is fluorescing brightly, after which the basal epithelial layer is removed by scraping with a blade. **E,** Epi-LASIK with a mechanical microkeratome (the epithelial flap may be removed or retained). *(Parts A, B, and D courtesy of Roger F. Steinert, MD; part C courtesy of Steven C. Schallhorn, MD; part E courtesy of Eric D. Donnenfeld, MD.)*

Epithelial preservation techniques

LASEK In the LASEK variant of surface ablation, the goal is to preserve the patient's epithelium. Instead of debriding and discarding the epithelium or ablating the epithelium with the excimer laser, the surgeon loosens the epithelium with 20% alcohol for 20 seconds and folds back an intact sheet of epithelium.

Epi-LASIK In epi-LASIK, an epithelial flap is fashioned with a microkeratome fitted with a blunt epi-keratome and a thin applanation plate that mechanically separates the epithelium.

Although the goal of LASEK and epi-LASIK is to reduce postoperative pain, speed the recovery of vision, and decrease postoperative haze formation compared with PRK, controlled studies have reported mixed results. In addition, the epithelial flap may not remain viable and may slough off, actually delaying healing and visual recovery. To date, epi-LASIK and LASEK have not proved to be superior to PRK in reducing corneal haze and are used less commonly.

Ambrósio R Jr, Wilson S. LASIK vs LASEK vs PRK: advantages and indications. *Semin Ophthalmol.* 2003;18(1):2–10.

Matsumoto JC, Chu YS. Epi-LASIK update: overview of techniques and patient management. *Int Ophthalmol Clin.* 2006;46(3):105–115.

Stevens SX, Bowyer BL. Corneal modulators and their use in excimer laser phototherapeutic keratectomy. *Int Ophthalmol Clin.* 1996;36(4):119–125.

Flap creation for LASIK

Lamellar flap creation can be performed using a femtosecond laser or a mechanical microkeratome. Many surgeons make asymmetric sterile ink marks in the corneal periphery, away from the intended flap hinge, just before placement of the suction ring. These marks can aid in alignment of the flap at the end of surgery and in proper orientation in the rare event of a free cap.

Femtosecond laser The femtosecond laser is the most commonly used technology for making a lamellar corneal flap within the stroma. Each laser pulse creates a discrete area of photodisruption of the collagen, with adjacent plasma pulses inducing a lamellar dissection within the corneal stroma. The greater the number of laser spots and the more the spots overlap, the more easily the tissue will separate when lifted and the more uniform the stromal bed will be. The femtosecond laser allows adjustments for several variables involved in making the flap, including flap thickness, flap diameter, hinge location, hinge angle, bed energy, and spot separation. Although the goal is to try to minimize the total energy used in flap creation, a certain level of power is necessary to ensure complete photodisruption. With the computer programmed for flap diameter, depth, and hinge location and size, thousands of adjacent pulses are scanned across the cornea in a controlled pattern that results in creation of a flap. Potential advantages of the femtosecond laser include

- excellent depth control
- reduction of complications such as buttonhole perforations
- precise control of flap dimensions, location, and centration
- creation of a non-meniscus planar flap
- ability to make pockets and channels within the cornea

Moreover, use of the femtosecond laser allows the geometry of the side cut to be modified in a manner that may reduce the incidence of epithelial ingrowth and flap slippage.

Femtosecond laser complications can occur, however. One study of 208 eyes showed that 1.9% had a loss of suction during femtosecond laser–assisted flap creation but that all

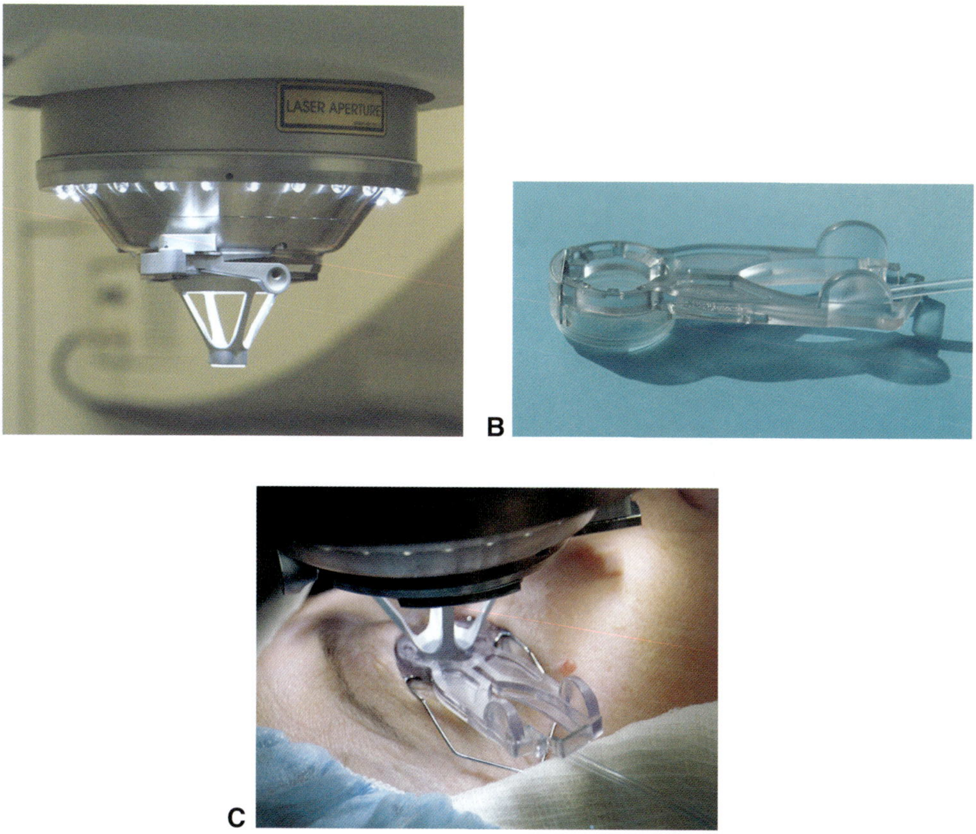

A B C

Figure 4-3 Example of 1 model of femtosecond laser (IntraLase; other types are also available). **A,** Femtosecond laser with cone attached. **B,** Suction ring. **C,** Docking of cone with suction ring positioned on the eye. *(Reproduced with permission from Feder RS, Rapuano CJ.* The LASIK Handbook: A Case-Based Approach. *Lippincott Williams & Wilkins; 2007:45–46. Images courtesy of Robert Feder, MD.)*

had successful flap creation after re-applanation of the eye. Occasionally, an opaque bubble layer may develop from gas expansion into the stroma adjacent to the flap interface and lead to improper flap creation. To prevent formation of an opaque bubble layer, most lasers now make a pocket deep within the cornea to disperse the gas away from the flap interface.

Although some variation exists between femtosecond lasers, all systems require centration and vacuum adherence to the patient's cornea. Complete applanation of the cornea must be achieved, or an incomplete flap or incomplete side cut may result. Figure 4-3 depicts some components of the femtosecond laser. Figure 4-4 illustrates the different stages of femtosecond laser–assisted flap creation. Video 4-2 demonstrates the use of a femtosecond laser for flap creation and subsequent treatment with the excimer laser.

VIDEO 4-2 Femtosecond LASIK procedure.
Courtesy of George O. Waring IV, MD.

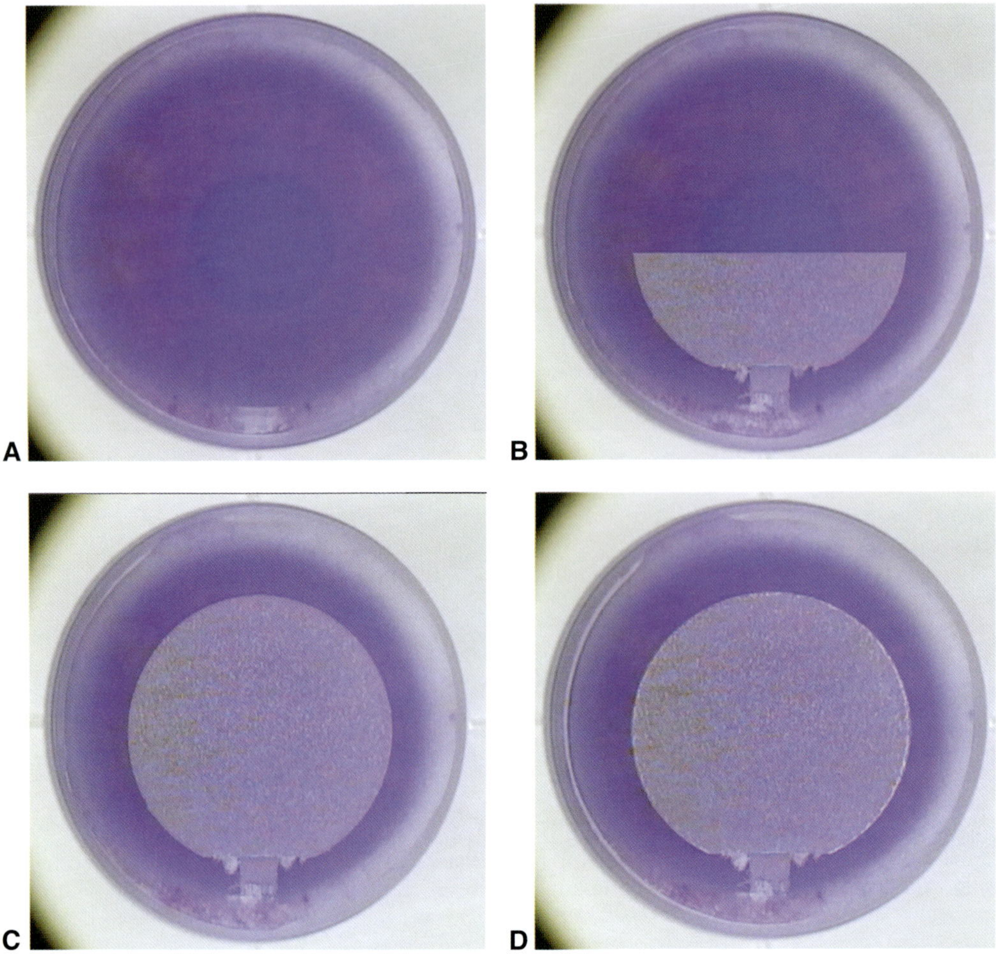

Figure 4-4 Femtosecond laser–assisted flap creation. **A,** Initiation of patient interface suction. **B,** Half of the lamellar interface created. **C,** Entire lamellar interface created. **D,** Creation of side cut. *(Courtesy of George O. Waring IV, MD.)*

Once centration is confirmed on the laser, the surgeon administers the femtosecond laser treatment. The vacuum is then released, the suction ring is removed, and the patient is positioned under the excimer laser. Figure 4-5 shows the basic technique of lifting a LASIK flap. A LASIK spatula is used to identify and enter the lamellar interface at the flap edge near the hinge. The instrument is then passed across the flap along the base of the hinge, and the flap is lifted by sweeping inferiorly and separating the flap interface, dissecting one-third of the flap at a time and thus reducing the risk of tearing. Figure 4-6 depicts the step-by-step process.

Several studies have compared the results of the mechanical microkeratome with those of femtosecond lasers for creating flaps. It has generally been shown that femtosecond lasers yield greater precision and accuracy of flap architecture, which may reduce rare complications (Table 4-1).

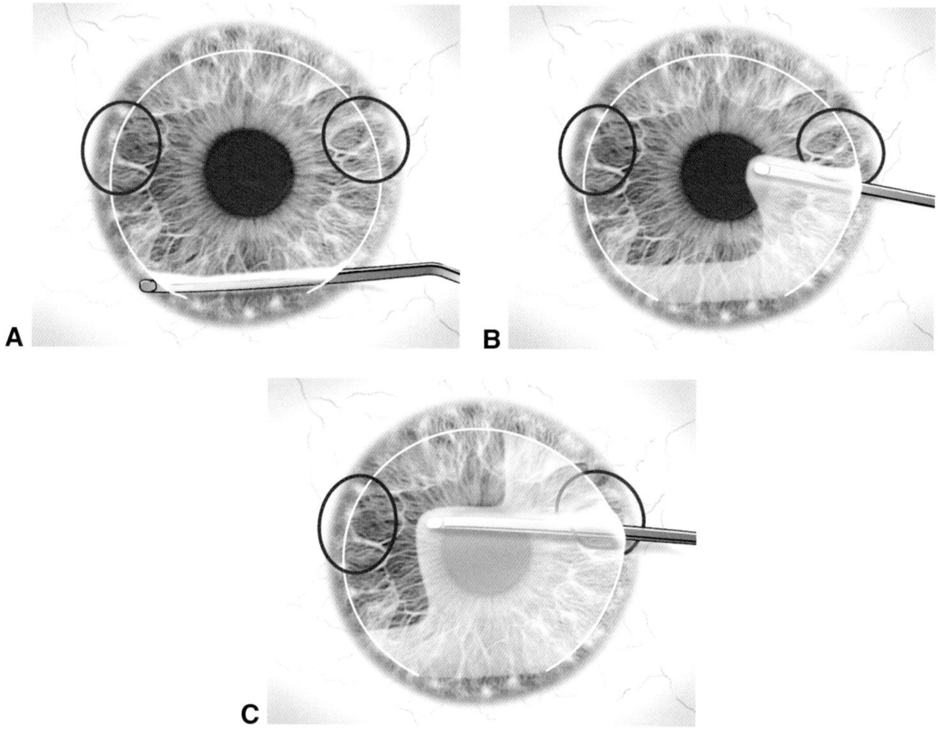

Figure 4-5 Flap-lift technique following application of the femtosecond laser. **A,** After the flap edge is scored near the hinge on either side *(black ovals)*, a spatula is passed across the flap. **B,** The interface is separated by starting at the superior hinge and sweeping inferiorly. **C,** Dissecting one-third of the flap at a time reduces the risk of tearing the hinge. *(Reproduced with permission from Feder RS, Rapuano CJ.* The LASIK Handbook: A Case-Based Approach. *Lippincott Williams & Wilkins; 2007:48. Image courtesy of Robert Feder, MD.)*

Bryar PJ, Hardten DR, Vrabec M. Femtosecond laser flap creation. In: Feder RS, ed. *The LASIK Handbook: A Case-Based Approach.* 2nd ed. Lippincott Williams & Wilkins; 2013:chap 5.

Chen S, Feng Y, Stojanovic A, Jankov MR 2nd, Wang Q. IntraLase femtosecond laser vs mechanical microkeratomes in LASIK for myopia: a systematic review and meta-analysis. *J Refract Surg.* 2012;28(1):15–24.

Davison JA, Johnson SC. Intraoperative complications of LASIK flaps using the IntraLase femtosecond laser in 3009 cases. *J Refract Surg.* 2010;26(11):851–857.

Holzer MP, Rabsilber TM, Auffarth GU. Femtosecond laser–assisted corneal flap cuts: morphology, accuracy, and histopathology. *Invest Ophthalmol Vis Sci.* 2006;47(7):2828–2831.

Slade SG, Durrie DS, Binder PS. A prospective, contralateral eye study comparing thin-flap LASIK (sub-Bowman keratomileusis) with photorefractive keratectomy. *Ophthalmology.* 2009;116(6):1075–1082.

Zhang ZH, Jin HY, Suo Y, et al. Femtosecond laser versus mechanical microkeratome laser in situ keratomileusis for myopia: metaanalysis of randomized controlled trials. *J Cataract Refract Surg.* 2011;37(12):2151–2159.

Microkeratome The basic principles of the microkeratome and the role of the suction ring and cutting head are illustrated in Figure 4-7. The surgeon should be aware that

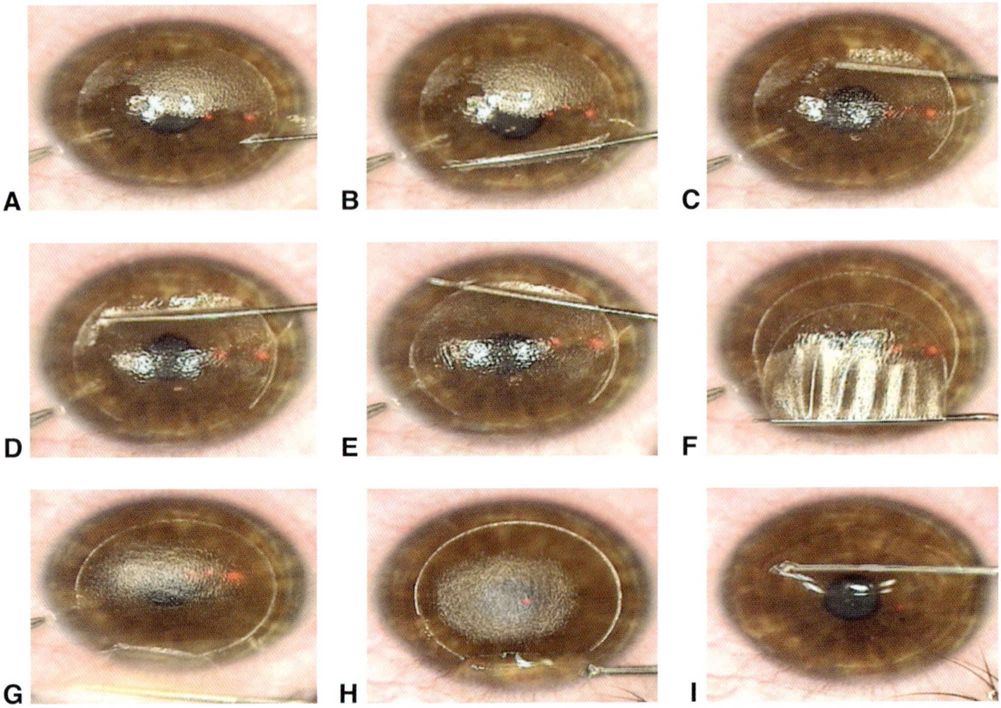

Figure 4-6 Steps in lifting a femtosecond laser flap. **A,** Initiation of the lamellar interface with a LASIK spatula. **B,** Advancing the spatula superiorly near the hinge and exiting the side cut. **C,** Dissecting the first third of the lamellar interface. **D,** Dissecting the second portion of the lamellar interface. **E,** Exiting the side cut while dissecting the side cut and the final third of the lamellar interface. **F,** Reflecting the flap from the stromal bed. **G,** Folding the flap in a "taco" technique in preparation for the excimer ablation. **H,** Unfolding the flap with a LASIK balanced salt solution cannula. **I,** Irrigating the interface before replacement of the flap. *(Courtesy of George O. Waring IV, MD.)*

Table 4-1 Advantages and Disadvantages of the Femtosecond Laser for Flap Creation

Advantages	Disadvantages
More customizable flap parameters	More flap manipulation
Size and thickness of flap less dependent on keratometry	Opaque bubble layer may interfere with excimer ablation
Centration easier to control	Bubbles in the anterior chamber may interfere with tracking and registration
Epithelial defects on flap are rare	Difficulty lifting flap after 6 months
Less risk of free cap and buttonhole	Increased risk of transient light sensitivity
More reliable flap thickness	Higher cost
Planar flaps	Delayed photosensitivity or good acuity plus photosensitivity
Hemorrhage from limbal vessels less likely	
Ability to re-treat immediately if incomplete femtosecond laser ablation	

Modified with permission from Feder RS, Rapuano CJ. *The LASIK Handbook: A Case-Based Approach.* Lippincott Williams & Wilkins; 2007.

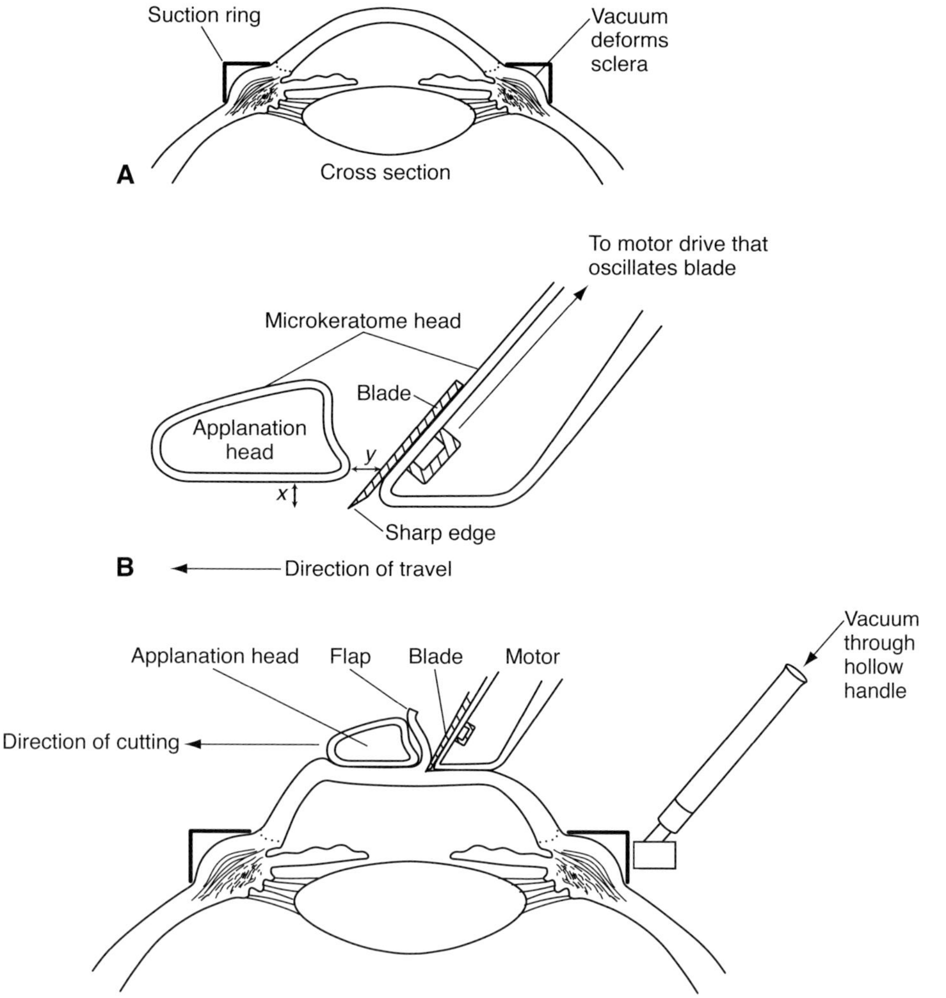

Figure 4-7 Schematic illustrations of microkeratome use. **A,** The suction ring serves as a platform for the microkeratome head, gripping the conjunctiva and sclera adjacent to the limbus. **B,** Simplified cross-sectional schematic of a typical microkeratome head. **C,** Creation of the flap. When the microkeratome head passes across the cornea, the applanating surface of the head flattens the cornea in advance of the blade. *(Illustration by Jeanne Koelling.)*

regardless of the label describing the flap thickness with a specific device, the actual flap thickness varies with the type of microkeratome, patient age, preoperative corneal thickness, preoperative keratometry reading, preoperative astigmatism, corneal diameter, and translation speed of the microkeratome pass. It is important to maintain a steady translation speed to avoid creating irregularities in the stromal bed.

Corneas steeper than 48.00 D are more likely to have thin flaps or frank buttonholes (central perforation of the flap) with procedures using mechanical microkeratomes. Corneas flatter than 40.00 D are more likely to have smaller-diameter flaps and are at increased risk for creation of a free cap due to transection of the hinge with mechanical microkeratomes. These concerns are avoided with the use of a femtosecond laser for flap creation.

Barequet IS, Hirsh A, Levinger S. Effect of thin femtosecond LASIK flaps on corneal sensitivity and tear function. *J Refract Surg.* 2008;24(9):897–902.

Calvillo MP, McLaren JW, Hodge DO, Bourne WM. Corneal reinnervation after LASIK: prospective 3-year longitudinal study. *Invest Ophthalmol Vis Sci.* 2004;45(11):3991–3996.

Hardten DR, Feder RS, Rosenfeld SI. Mechanical microkeratomes. In: Feder RS, ed. *The LASIK Handbook: A Case-Based Approach.* 2nd ed. Lippincott Williams & Wilkins; 2013:chap 4.

Kumano Y, Matsui H, Zushi I, et al. Recovery of corneal sensation after myopic correction by laser in situ keratomileusis with a nasal or superior hinge. *J Cataract Refract Surg.* 2003;29(4):757–761.

Application of Laser Treatment

Tracking, centration, and ablation

For surface ablation, the exposed Bowman layer should be inspected and found to be smooth, uniformly dry, and free of debris and residual epithelial islands. For LASIK, the flap must be lifted and reflected, and the stromal bed must be uniformly dry before treatment. Fluid or blood accumulation on the stromal bed should be avoided, as it can lead to an irregular ablation.

Current excimer lasers use open-loop tracking systems, which have improved clinical outcomes compared with earlier devices. The tracker uses video technology to monitor the location of an infrared image of the pupil and to shift the laser beam accordingly.

The laser is centered and focused according to the manufacturer's recommendations. Tracking systems, although effective, do not lessen the importance of keeping the reticule centered on the patient's entrance pupil. If the patient is unable to maintain fixation, the illumination of the operating microscope should be reduced. If decentration occurs and the ablation does not stop automatically, the surgeon should immediately stop the treatment until adequate refixation is achieved. It is still important for the surgeon to monitor for excessive eye movement, which can result in decentration despite the tracking device. In addition, the fellow eye should be covered to avoid cross-fixation.

The change in illumination and patient position (ie, from sitting to lying down) can cause pupil centroid shift and cyclotorsion. In most patients, the pupil moves nasally and superiorly when it is constricted. *Registration* is a technique in which a fixed landmark is used at the time of wavefront aberrometry and treatment to apply the ablation to the correct area of the cornea and account for cyclotorsion; it relies on iris landmarks and not on the pupil for laser centration (Fig 4-8). Once the patient confirms that the fixation light of the excimer laser is still visible and that he or she is looking directly at it, ablation begins. Neither tracking nor iris registration is a substitute for accurate patient fixation. It is important to initiate stromal ablation promptly, before excessive stromal dehydration takes place. During larger-diameter ablations, a flap protector may be needed to shield the underside of the LASIK flap near the hinge from the laser pulses. In addition, it is important to remove the excessive fluid that can accumulate during treatment, especially in patients undergoing high corrections.

Donnenfeld E. The pupil is a moving target: centration, repeatability, and registration. *J Refract Surg.* 2004;20(5):S593–S596.

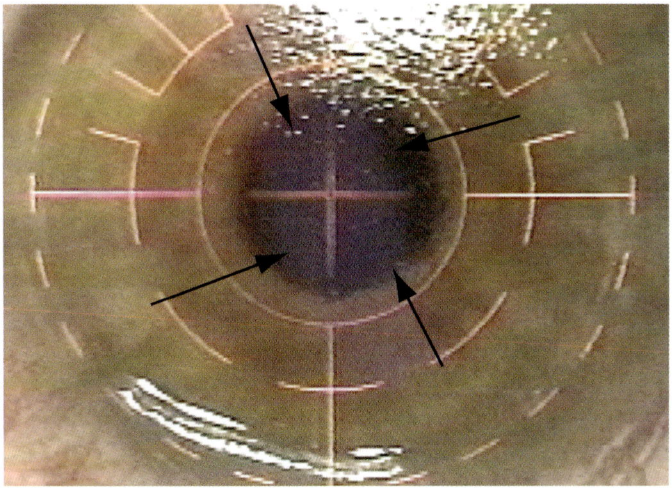

Figure 4-8 Excimer laser ablation of the stromal bed. Note the faint blue fluorescence of the stromal bed from the laser pulse *(arrows)*. The rectangular shape of the exposure by this broad-beam laser indicates that the laser is correcting the cylindrical portion of the treatment. (Photograph is enhanced to increase fluorescence; the surgeon usually sees minimal or no fluorescence through the operating microscope.) *(Courtesy of Roger F. Steinert, MD.)*

Moshirfar M, Chen MC, Espandar L, et al. Effect of iris registration on outcomes of LASIK for myopia with the VISX CustomVue platform. *J Refract Surg.* 2009;25(6):493–502.

Immediate Postablation Measures

Surface ablation

One of the major potential complications of surface ablation is corneal haze, especially in eyes with previous corneal surgery such as PRK, LASIK, PKP, RK, or primary surface ablations for moderate to high ametropia or deeper ablation depths. To decrease the chance of corneal haze formation, a pledget soaked in MMC (usually 0.02% or 0.2 mg/mL) can be placed on the ablated surface for approximately 12 seconds to 2 minutes at the end of the laser exposure (off-label use). The concentration and duration of MMC application varies by diagnosis and surgeon preference; however, most surgeons tend toward shorter durations of MMC exposure. Application of MMC for 12 seconds appears to be as effective for prophylaxis as more prolonged times. Some surgeons reduce the amount of treatment when applying MMC in surface ablation because of reports of potential endothelial cell toxicity. The cornea is then copiously irrigated with balanced salt solution to remove excess MMC. To avoid damage to limbal stem cells, the surgeon should take care to protect the limbus and conjunctiva from MMC. Confocal microscopy studies of human eyes have shown a reduced keratocyte population and less haze in eyes that received MMC.

Some surgeons apply sterile, chilled, balanced salt solution or a frozen cellulose sponge before and/or after the surface ablation procedure in the belief that cooling reduces pain and haze formation. However, the advantage of this practice has not been substantiated in a controlled study. Care should be taken to not expose the eye to tap water, which may result in infectious contamination.

Antibiotic, corticosteroid, and, occasionally, nonsteroidal anti-inflammatory drugs (NSAIDs) are then placed on the eye, followed by a bandage contact lens. Some NSAIDs and antibiotics can be placed directly on the corneal bed, whereas others should be placed only on the surface of the contact lens, as they have been associated with poor corneal healing. If the patient cannot tolerate a bandage contact lens, a pressure patch may be used.

Of note, the American Society of Cataract and Refractive Surgery released a clinical alert on February 14, 2013, discussing the postoperative risks posed by certain medications used topically prior to or during LASIK or PRK (see sidebar: Medication Alert for LASIK and PRK). The medications listed in this statement have the potential to cause flap slippage and/or diffuse lamellar keratitis (DLK) following LASIK surgery and poor epithelial healing following PRK.

Carones F, Vigo L, Scandola E, Vacchini L. Evaluation of the prophylactic use of mitomycin-C to inhibit haze formation after photorefractive keratectomy. *J Cataract Refract Surg.* 2002;28(12):2088–2095.

Lee DH, Chung HS, Jeon YC, Boo SD, Yoon YD, Kim JG. Photorefractive keratectomy with intraoperative mitomycin-C application. *J Cataract Refract Surg.* 2005;31(12):2293–2298.

Virasch VV, Majmudar PA, Epstein RJ, Vaidya NS, Dennis RF. Reduced application time for prophylactic mitomycin C in photorefractive keratectomy. *Ophthalmology.* 2010;117(5):885–889.

LASIK

After the ablation is completed, the flap is replaced onto the stromal bed. The interface is irrigated until all interface debris is eliminated (which is apparent more readily with oblique than with coaxial illumination). The surface of the flap is gently stroked with a smooth instrument, such as an irrigation cannula or a moistened microsurgical spear sponge, from the hinge, or center, to the periphery. This approach helps to ensure that wrinkles are eliminated and that the flap settles back into its original position, as indicated by realignment of the corneal marks made earlier. The peripheral gutters should be symmetric and even. The physiologic dehydration of the stroma by the endothelial pump will begin to secure the flap in position within several minutes. If a significant epithelial defect or a large, loose sheet of epithelium is present, a bandage contact lens should be put in place. Once the flap is adherent, the eyelid speculum is removed carefully so as not to disturb the flap. Most surgeons apply varying combinations of antibiotic, NSAID, and corticosteroid drops on the eye at the conclusion of the procedure. The flap is usually rechecked at the slit lamp before the patient leaves to confirm its proper alignment. A clear shield or protective goggles are often placed to guard against accidental trauma that could displace the flap. Patients are instructed not to rub or squeeze their eyes.

Lui MM, Silas MA, Fugishima H. Complications of photorefractive keratectomy and laser in situ keratomileusis. *J Refract Surg.* 2003;19(Suppl 2):S247–S249.

Price FW Jr. LASIK. *Focal Points: Clinical Modules for Ophthalmologists.* American Academy of Ophthalmology; 2000, module 3.

Schallhorn SC, Amesbury EC, Tanzer DJ. Avoidance, recognition, and management of LASIK complications. *Am J Ophthalmol.* 2006;141(4):733–739.

Medication Alert for LASIK and PRK

The Cornea and Refractive Surgery Clinical Committees of the American Society of Cataract and Refractive Surgery issued a joint alert regarding the use of the following topical medications immediately prior to or intraoperatively during LASIK and PRK. These medications contain advanced vehicles designed to deliver consistent dosage of medication, increase contact time on the eye, stabilize the ocular surface, and reduce dosing frequency.

- Azithromycin 1% ophthalmic solution with a vehicle of polycarbophil, edetate disodium, sodium chloride (Azasite; Merck)
- Besifloxacin 0.6% ophthalmic suspension with a vehicle of polycarbophil, edetate disodium, sodium chloride (Besivance; Bausch + Lomb)
- Cyclosporine ophthalmic emulsion 0.05% with a vehicle that includes castor oil (Restasis; Allergan)
- Difluprednate ophthalmic emulsion 0.05% with a vehicle that includes castor oil (Durezol; Alcon)
- Ketorolac 0.45% ophthalmic solution with a vehicle of carboxymethylcellulose sodium (Acuvail; Allergan)
- Loteprednol 0.5% ophthalmic gel with a vehicle that includes glycerin, polycarbophil, propylene glycol, tyloxapol (Lotemax Gel drop; Bausch + Lomb)
- Moxifloxacin 0.5% ophthalmic solution with a vehicle that includes xanthan gum and tyloxapol (Moxeza; Alcon)
- Nepafenac 0.3% ophthalmic suspension with a vehicle that includes mannitol, carbomer 974P, sodium chloride, tyloxapol, edetate disodium (Nevanac; Alcon)
- Nepafenac 0.3% ophthalmic suspension with a vehicle that includes propylene glycol, carbomer 974P, guar gum, and carboxymethylcellulose sodium (Ilevro; Alcon)

These medications contain vehicles that have the potential to be sequestered beneath a LASIK flap or a bandage contact lens following PRK and not absorbed.

There have been no problems documented with the use of these medications after the flap has been properly positioned. There have also been documented cases of poor epithelial healing when topical ophthalmic medications with these advanced vehicles have been instilled on the stromal bed following PRK prior to placement of a bandage contact lens.

The use of these medications with advanced vehicles following routine LASIK and PRK has not been associated with increased adverse events and may provide benefits in the postoperative period. We would note that ketorolac, loteprednol, moxifloxacin, and nepafanac are also FDA approved in solution or suspension formulations without these advanced vehicles.

Modified with permission from ASCRS Cornea and Refractive Surgery Clinical Committees. Medication alert for LASIK and PRK. *EyeWorld Online.* March 2013. Accessed January 9, 2021. https://www.eyeworld.org/article-medication-alert-for-lasik-and-prk

Postoperative Care

Surface ablation

After surface ablation, patients may experience variable degrees of pain, from minimal to severe, and some may need oral NSAID, narcotic, or neuropathic pain medications. Studies have shown that topical NSAID drops reduce postoperative pain, although they may also slow the rate of re-epithelialization and promote sterile infiltrates (see Chapter 5). Corneal melting and stromal scarring have been described after the use of some topical NSAIDs. If the cornea is not healing normally after surface ablation, the use of any topical NSAID should be discontinued. Preservative-free artificial tears should be used liberally for several months postoperatively.

Patients should be monitored closely until the epithelium is completely healed, which usually occurs within 4–5 days. As long as the bandage contact lens is in place, patients are treated with topical broad-spectrum antibiotics and corticosteroids, usually 4 times daily. Once the epithelium is healed, the bandage contact lens, antibiotic drops, and NSAID drops (if used) may be discontinued. In addition, most clinicians recommend that patients refrain from swimming or using hot tubs for at least 2 weeks postoperatively to reduce the risk of infection.

The use of topical corticosteroids to modulate postoperative wound healing, reduce anterior stromal haze, and decrease regression of the refractive effect remains controversial. Although some studies have demonstrated that corticosteroids have no significant long-term effect on corneal haze or visual outcome after PRK, others have shown that corticosteroids are effective in limiting haze and myopic regression after PRK, particularly after higher myopic corrections. Some surgeons who advocate use of topical corticosteroids after the removal of the bandage contact lens restrict them to patients with higher levels of myopia (eg, greater than −4.00 or −5.00 D). When used after removal of the bandage contact lens, corticosteroid drops are typically tapered over a 1-month period, depending on the patient's corneal haze and refractive outcome. Patients who received MMC at the time of surgery have a reduced risk of haze formation and thus may have a shorter duration of corticosteroid use. Patients who had PRK for hyperopia may experience prolonged epithelial healing because of the larger epithelial defect resulting from the larger ablation zone, as well as a temporary reduction in corrected distance visual acuity in the first week to month, which usually improves with time. Many patients with hyperopia also experience a temporary myopic overcorrection, which regresses over several weeks to months. In the absence of complications, routine follow-up examinations are typically scheduled at approximately 1 day, 4–7 days for bandage contact lens removal, 2–4 weeks, 2–3 months, 6 months, and 12 months postoperatively and perhaps more frequently, depending on the steroid taper used.

LASIK

Many surgeons instruct their patients to use topical antibiotics and corticosteroids postoperatively for 7 days. It is very important for the surface of the flap to be kept well lubricated in the early postoperative period. Patients may be told to use the protective shield for 1–7 days when they shower or sleep and to avoid swimming or using hot tubs for 2 weeks. Patients are examined 1 day after surgery to ensure that the flap has remained in proper alignment and that there is no evidence of infection or excessive inflammation. Surgeons should have a low threshold for refloating flaps that have clinically significant microstriae, macrostriae, or interface debris on the first postoperative day. In the absence of complications, the next examinations are typically scheduled at approximately 1 week, 1 month, 3 months, 6 months, and 12 months postoperatively.

Santhiago MR, Kara-Junior N, Waring GO 4th. Microkeratome versus femtosecond flaps: accuracy and complications. *Curr Opin Ophthalmol.* 2014;25(4):270–274.

Santhiago MR, Wilson SE. Cellular effects after laser in situ keratomileusis flap formation with femtosecond lasers: a review. *Cornea.* 2012;31(2):198–205.

Refractive Outcomes

As the early broad-beam excimer laser systems improved and surgeons gained experience, the results achieved with surface ablation and LASIK improved markedly. The ablation zone diameter was enlarged because it was found that small ablation zones, originally intended to limit depth of tissue removal, produced more haze and regression in surface ablation treatments and concerns about subjective glare and halos for both surface ablation and LASIK. The larger treatment diameters currently used, including those for optical zones and for gradual aspheric peripheral blend zones, improve optical quality and refractive stability in both myopic and hyperopic treatments. Central island elevations have become less common with improvements in beam quality, vacuums to remove the ablation plume, and development of scanning and variable-spot-size excimer lasers.

Solomon KD, Fernández de Castro LE, Sandoval HP, et al; Joint LASIK Study Task Force. LASIK world literature review: quality of life and patient satisfaction. *Ophthalmology.* 2009;116(4):691–701.

Outcomes for Myopia

Initial FDA clinical trials of conventional excimer laser treatments limited to myopia of 6.00 D or less revealed that 56%–86% of eyes treated with either PRK or LASIK achieved uncorrected distance visual acuity (UDVA) of at least 20/20, 88%–100% achieved UDVA of at least 20/40, and 82%–100% were within 1.00 D of emmetropia. Up to 2.1% of eyes lost 2 or more lines of best-corrected visual acuity (BCVA). Reports since 2000 have demonstrated significantly improved outcomes and safety profiles, with fewer than 0.6% of eyes losing 2 or more lines of BCVA.

el Danasoury MA, el Maghraby A, Klyce SD, Mehrez K. Comparison of photorefractive keratectomy with excimer laser in situ keratomileusis in correcting low myopia (from –2.00 to –5.50 diopters): a randomized study. *Ophthalmology.* 1999;106(2):411–420.

Luger MH, Ewering T, Arba-Mosquera S. Influence of patient age on high myopic correction in corneal laser refractive surgery. *J Cataract Refract Surg.* 2013;39(2):204–210.

Sugar A, Rapuano CJ, Culbertson WW, et al. Laser in situ keratomileusis for myopia and astigmatism: safety and efficacy: a report by the American Academy of Ophthalmology. *Ophthalmology.* 2002;109(1):175–187.

Tole DM, McCarty DJ, Couper T, Taylor HR. Comparison of laser in situ keratomileusis and photorefractive keratectomy for the correction of myopia of −6.00 diopters or less. Melbourne Excimer Laser Group. *J Refract Surg.* 2001;17(1):46–54.

Outcomes for Hyperopia

In myopic ablations, the central cornea is flattened, whereas in hyperopic ablations, more tissue is removed from the midperiphery than from the central cornea, resulting in an effective steepening (see Figure 4-1B). To ensure that the size of the central hyperopic treatment zone is adequate, a large ablation area is required. Most studies have employed hyperopic treatment zones with transition zones out to 9.0–9.5 mm. FDA clinical trials of PRK and LASIK for hyperopia up to +6.00 D reported that 46%–59% of eyes had postoperative UDVA of 20/20 or better, 92%–96% had UDVA of 20/40 or better, and 84%–91% were within 1.00 D of emmetropia; loss of more than 2 lines of BCVA occurred in 1.00%–3.50%. The VISX FDA clinical trial of hyperopic astigmatic PRK up to +6.00 D sphere and +4.00 D cylinder reported an approximate postoperative UDVA of 20/20 or better in 50% of eyes, UDVA of 20/40 or better in 97%, and 87% within 1.00 D of emmetropia, with loss of more than 2 lines of BCVA in 1.5%. For the same amount of correction, the period from surgery to postoperative stabilization is longer for hyperopic than for myopic corrections. Overall, studies with larger ablation zones have demonstrated good results for refractive errors up to +4.00 D for conventional treatments, but predictability and stability are markedly reduced with LASIK treatments for hyperopia above this level. Consequently, most refractive surgeons do not treat up to the highest levels of hyperopia that have been approved by the FDA for conventional treatments.

Gil-Cazorla R, Teus MA, de Benito-Llopis L, Mikropoulos DG. Femtosecond laser vs mechanical microkeratome for hyperopic laser in situ keratomileusis. *Am J Ophthalmol.* 2011;152(1):16–21.

Llovet F, Galal A, Benitez-del-Castillo JM, Ortega J, Martin C, Baviera J. One-year results of excimer laser in situ keratomileusis for hyperopia. *J Cataract Refract Surg.* 2009;35(7): 1156–1165.

Salz JJ, Stevens CA; LADARVision LASIK Hyperopia Study Group. LASIK correction of spherical hyperopia, hyperopic astigmatism, and mixed astigmatism with the LADARVision excimer laser system. *Ophthalmology.* 2002;109(9):1647–1656.

Tabbara KF, El-Sheikh HF, Islam SM. Laser in situ keratomileusis for the correction of hyperopia from +0.50 to +11.50 diopters with the Keracor 117C laser. *J Refract Surg.* 2001;17(2):123–128.

Varley GA, Huang D, Rapuano CJ, Schallhorn S, Boxer Wachler BS, Sugar A; Ophthalmic Technology Assessment Committee Refractive Surgery Panel. LASIK for hyperopia, hyperopic astigmatism, and mixed astigmatism: a report by the American Academy of Ophthalmology. *Ophthalmology.* 2004;111(8):1604–1617.

Williams L, Moshirfar M, Dave S. Preoperative keratometry and visual outcomes after hyperopic LASIK. *J Refract Surg.* 2009;25(12):1052.

Wavefront-Guided, Wavefront-Optimized, and Topography-Guided Treatment Outcomes

Wavefront-guided or wavefront-optimized LASIK coupled with sophisticated eye-tracking systems has greatly improved the accuracy and reproducibility of results, allowing even higher percentages of patients to obtain UDVA of 20/20 and 20/40. In wavefront-guided LASIK for myopic astigmatism, for example, up to about −10.00 to −12.00 D, 79%–95% of patients obtained 20/20 UDVA, and 96%–100% obtained 20/40 UDVA. In wavefront-guided LASIK for hyperopic astigmatism up to +6.00 D, 55%–59% of patients obtained 20/20 UDVA, and 93%–97% obtained 20/40 UDVA. In wavefront-guided LASIK for mixed astigmatism with up to +5.00 D of cylinder, 56%–61% of patients obtained 20/20 UDVA, and 95% obtained 20/40 UDVA. A recent study found that the visual acuity results for the vast majority of patients were equivalent between wavefront-guided and wavefront-optimized LASIK.

Recent clinical trial data on topography-guided ablations demonstrated that for corrections up to −9.00 D of spherical equivalent myopia with up to −8.00 D spherical and −3.00 D astigmatic components, 93% of eyes had UDVA of 20/20 or better. The data also showed that 32% of eyes achieved 20/12.5 or better and 69% achieved 20/16 or better. In 30% of patients, postoperative UDVA improved 1 line or more compared to preoperative BCVA.

Fares U, Otri AM, Al-Aqaba MA, Faraj L, Dua HS. Wavefront-optimized excimer laser in situ keratomileusis for myopia and myopic astigmatism: refractive outcomes and corneal densitometry. *J Cataract Refract Surg.* 2012;38(12):2131–2138.

Keir NJ, Simpson T, Jones LW, Fonn D. Wavefront-guided LASIK for myopia: effect on visual acuity, contrast sensitivity, and higher order aberrations. *J Refract Surg.* 2009;25(6): 524–533.

Randleman JB, Perez-Straziota CE, Hu MH, White AJ, Loft ES, Stulting RD. Higher-order aberrations after wavefront-optimized photorefractive keratectomy and laser in situ keratomileusis. *J Cataract Refract Surg.* 2009;35(2):260–264.

Schallhorn SC, Farjo AA, Huang D, et al; American Academy of Ophthalmology. Wavefront-guided LASIK for the correction of primary myopia and astigmatism: a report by the American Academy of Ophthalmology. *Ophthalmology.* 2008;115(7):1249–1261.

Tan J, Simon D, Mrochen M, Por YM. Clinical results of topography-based customized ablations for myopia and myopic astigmatism. *J Refract Surg.* 2012;28(Suppl 11):S829–S836.

Re-treatment

Although excimer laser ablation reduces refractive error and improves UDVA in almost all cases, some patients have residual refractive errors and would benefit from re-treatment (enhancement). The degree of refractive error that warrants re-treatment varies depending on the patient's lifestyle and expectations. Re-treatment rates vary from 1% to 11% depending on the amount of correction attempted, postoperative UDVA, patient's tolerance of residual refractive error, surgeon's experience, and the laser and nomograms used. Typically, the rates are higher in patients treated for hyperopia and for high astigmatism than for other indications. Rates are also higher for patients with residual astigmatism and those older than 40 years. The surgeon should be cautious about performing an enhancement for a myopic shift in a patient older than 50 years, as this shift may be lens induced rather than due to post–corneal refractive surgery regression.

One advantage of LASIK over surface ablation is that refractive stability generally occurs earlier, allowing earlier enhancements, typically within the first 3 months after LASIK. With surface ablation, the ongoing activation of keratocytes and the risk of haze after enhancement usually require a wait of 3–6 months before an enhancement is performed.

Techniques for Re-treatment

Re-treatment after surface ablation is similar to primary surface ablation treatment, whereas LASIK re-treatment can be accomplished either by lifting the preexisting lamellar flap and applying additional ablation to the stromal bed or by performing surface ablation on the LASIK flap. In most cases, the flap can be lifted many years after the original procedure. However, because of the safety of surface ablation after LASIK and the increased risk of epithelial ingrowth with flap lifts, many surgeons now prefer to perform surface ablation re-treatment if the primary LASIK was performed more than 2–3 years earlier. Creating a new flap is possible but generally not recommended because free slivers of tissue, irregular stromal beds, and irregular astigmatism may be produced.

Flap-lift procedures

When a preexisting flap is lifted, it is important to minimize epithelial disruption. A jeweler's forceps, Sinskey hook, or 27-gauge needle can be used to locate the edge of the flap. Because the edge of the flap can be seen more easily with the slit lamp than with the diffuse illumination of the laser operating microscope, some surgeons find it easier to begin a flap lift at the slit lamp and complete it at the excimer laser. Alternatively, the surgeon can often visualize the edge of the flap under the diffuse illumination of the operating microscope by applying pressure with a small Sinskey hook or similar device; the edge of the flap will dimple and disrupt the light reflex (Fig 4-9). A careful circumferential

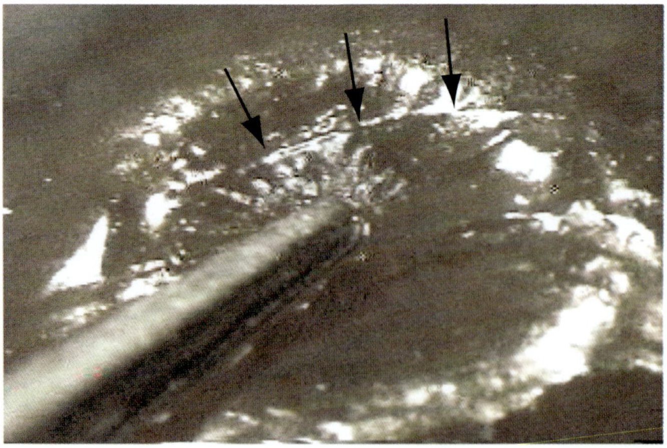

Figure 4-9 Indenting the cornea with forceps to visualize the edge of the flap *(arrows)* through an operating microscope prior to an enhancement procedure. *(Courtesy of Roger F. Steinert, MD.)*

epithelial dissection is performed so that the flap can then be lifted without tearing the epithelial edges. Smooth forceps, iris spatulas, and several instruments specifically designed for dissecting the flap edge can be used to lift the original flap.

Once the ablation has been performed, the flap is reposited and the interface is irrigated, as in the initial LASIK procedure. Special care must be taken to ensure that no loose epithelium is trapped beneath the edge of the flap that could lead to epithelial ingrowth; the risk of epithelial ingrowth is greater after re-treatment than after primary treatment. Many surgeons recommend placement of a bandage contact lens after LASIK enhancements to provide comfort and to possibly enhance regular reepithelialization.

Caster AI, Friess DW, Schwendeman FJ. Incidence of epithelial ingrowth in primary and retreatment laser in situ keratomileusis. *J Cataract Refract Surg.* 2010;36(1):97–101.

Davis EA, Hardten DR, Lindstrom M, Samuelson TW, Lindstrom RL. LASIK enhancements: a comparison of lifting to recutting the flap. *Ophthalmology.* 2002;109(12):2308–2313.

Rubinfeld RS, Hardten DR, Donnenfeld ED, et al. To lift or recut: changing trends in LASIK enhancement. *J Cataract Refract Surg.* 2003;29(12):2306–2317.

Santhiago MR, Smadja D, Zaleski K, Espana EM, Armstrong BK, Wilson SE. Flap relift for retreatment after femtosecond laser–assisted LASIK. *J Refract Surg.* 2012;28(7):482–487.

Surface ablation

Surface ablation may also be considered to enhance a previous primary LASIK treatment. Surface ablation performed on a LASIK flap carries an increased risk of haze formation and irregular astigmatism. However, it is an appealing alternative when the residual stromal bed (RSB) is insufficient for further ablation, when the LASIK was performed by another surgeon and the flap thickness or RSB is not known, or when conditions such as a buttonhole or incomplete flap are present; it also reduces the risk of epithelial ingrowth. When removing the epithelium over a flap, the surgeon must take care to avoid inadvertently lifting or dislocating the flap. Applying 20% ethanol for 20–30 seconds inside a corneal well will loosen the epithelium, after which epithelial removal techniques are performed, extending from the hinge toward the periphery. A rotating brush should not be used to remove the epithelium from a LASIK flap. The risk of postoperative haze due to surface ablation over a previous LASIK flap may be avoided or reduced by administering intraoperative topical MMC 0.02% and postoperative topical corticosteroids.

Conventional versus wavefront-guided treatment

It has not yet been established whether conventional or wavefront-guided treatment is preferable for enhancing vision in patients who have previously undergone conventional LASIK. Some studies report better results in both safety and efficacy with conventional LASIK re-treatment. The risk of overcorrection, particularly in patients with high spherical aberrations, may be greater with wavefront-guided re-treatments. Caution should be exercised in evaluating the degree of higher-order aberrations and the planned depth of the ablation when deciding between conventional and wavefront-guided treatments.

Carones F, Vigo L, Carones AV, Brancato R. Evaluation of photorefractive keratectomy retreatments after regressed myopic laser in situ keratomileusis. *Ophthalmology.* 2001;108(10): 1732–1737.

Hersh PS, Fry KL, Bishop DS. Incidence and associations of retreatment after LASIK. *Ophthalmology.* 2003;110(4):748–754.

Jin GJ, Merkley KH. Conventional and wavefront-guided myopic LASIK retreatment. *Am J Ophthalmol.* 2006;141(4):660–668.

Randleman JB, White AJ Jr, Lynn MJ, Hu MH, Stulting RD. Incidence, outcomes, and risk factors for retreatment after wavefront-optimized ablations with PRK and LASIK. *J Refract Surg.* 2009;25(3):273–276.

Vaddavalli PK, Diakonis VF, Canto AP, et al. Complications of femtosecond laser–assisted re-treatment for residual refractive errors after LASIK. *J Refract Surg.* 2013; 29(8):577–580.

Weisenthal RW, Salz J, Sugar A, et al. Photorefractive keratectomy for treatment of flap complications in laser in situ keratomileusis. *Cornea.* 2003;22(5):399–404.

Emerging Technologies

Most innovation in photoablation is in the area of higher-speed excimer laser technology with faster treatment times and, therefore, more rapid eye trackers. Smaller form factor excimer lasers with internal nomograms are in US FDA clinical trials. Ray-tracing technologies for both diagnostic and excimer ablation profiles are in development.

CHAPTER 5

Photoablation: Complications and Adverse Effects

This chapter includes a related video. Go to www.aao.org/bcscvideo_section13 or scan the QR code in the text to access this content.

Highlights

- With proper management, almost all complications and adverse effects of LASIK and surface ablation can resolve with a good patient outcome.
- Most LASIK complications arise from creation of the flap, while most surface ablation problems result from the presence of a large iatrogenic epithelial defect.
- Technological improvements have led to a decrease in many of the most serious complications.

General Complications Related to Laser Ablation

Photorefractive keratectomy (PRK) and laser in situ keratomileusis (LASIK), 2 of the most common types of refractive surgery, are safe and effective procedures. As with all surgery, however, there are potential risks and complications, so it is important to understand how to avoid, diagnose, and treat the complications of refractive surgery. Both comprehensive ophthalmologists and refractive surgeons should be knowledgeable about these postoperative problems given the fact that hundreds of thousands of patients undergo refractive surgery each year.

Overcorrection

Overcorrection can occur if significant stromal dehydration develops before initiation of the excimer treatment, as more stromal tissue will be ablated per pulse. Dehydration may result from delayed ablation after removal of the epithelium in surface ablation or lifting of the flap in LASIK. Controlling the humidity and temperature in the laser suite within the recommended excimer laser guidelines may decrease variability and improve refractive outcomes, although studies have failed to demonstrate this consistently. Overcorrection tends to occur more often in older individuals, as their wound-healing response is less vigorous and their corneas ablate more rapidly for reasons not fully understood.

Myopic or hyperopic surface ablation typically undergoes some degree of refractive regression for at least 3–6 months. In general, patients with higher degrees of myopia and any degree of hyperopia require more time to attain refractive stability, which must be achieved before any decision is made regarding possible re-treatment of the overcorrection. The terms *overcorrection* and *undercorrection* usually apply to residual refractive error during this initial healing period, as opposed to longer-term drift away from the target.

Various modalities are available for treating small amounts of overcorrection. Myopic regression can be induced after surface ablation by abrupt discontinuation of corticosteroids. If further laser vision correction (LVC) is needed, patients with consecutive hyperopia (ie, hyperopia due to overcorrection of myopia) or consecutive myopia (myopia due to overcorrection of hyperopia) require less treatment than previously untreated eyes. When re-treating such patients, the surgeon should take care not to overcorrect a second time because they are overresponders. With conventional ablation, surgeons often reduce the ablation by 20%–25% for consecutive treatments. For wavefront procedures, a review of the depth of the ablation and the amount of higher-order aberration helps titrate the re-treatment. In general, re-treatment for over- or undercorrection after surface ablation is performed with another surface procedure. LASIK enhancements usually are performed by relifting the flap if its initial construction was normal.

Undercorrection

Undercorrection occurs much more commonly with treatment of higher degrees of ametropia. Patients with regression after treatment of their first eye have an increased likelihood of regression in their second eye. Topical mitomycin C, administered at the time of initial surface ablation, can be used to modulate the response, especially in patients with higher levels of ametropia. Sometimes the regression may be reversed with aggressive administration of topical corticosteroids. The patient may undergo a re-treatment generally no sooner than 3 months postoperatively, assuming that the refraction has stabilized. If LASIK was initially performed, the flap is usually relifted for the enhancement.

A patient with significant corneal haze and regression after surface ablation is at higher risk after re-treatment for further regression, recurrence, or worsening of the corneal haze, as well as loss of corrected distance visual acuity (CDVA). It is prudent to wait at least 6–12 months for the haze to improve before repeating surface ablation. If the haze fails to clear spontaneously or if the patient has residual myopia, removal of the haze with adjunctive use of mitomycin C without a refractive treatment will commonly improve the refractive outcome.

Before re-treating patients with delayed and ongoing regression, it is important to evaluate for irregular astigmatism that may indicate ectasia. In an older patient, the refractive shift may signify cataract, which should instead be treated with phacoemulsification.

Dry Eye

Temporary exacerbation of dry eye is a common adverse effect of excimer LVC. Although patients generally return to at least their baseline level of dryness by postoperative month 6, some symptoms may uncommonly persist. Surgeons should consider ocular surface optimization before and after LVC (see Chapter 7). PROWL-1 and PROWL-2 were prospective observational studies of patients undergoing LASIK that enrolled military and civilian populations, respectively. Approximately 5% of patients with normal Ocular Surface Disease Index (OSDI, a dry eye questionnaire) scores preoperatively had moderate or severe OSDI scores after surgery, but overall, the percentage of patients with normal OSDI scores significantly increased. Surgery satisfaction scores were 91%–93%, with 2% dissatisfied. The amount of dissatisfaction was moderately associated with more complaints on the OSDI.

Eydelman M, Hilmantel G, Tarver ME, et al. Symptoms and satisfaction of patients in the Patient-Reported Outcomes With Laser In Situ Keratomileusis (PROWL) studies. *JAMA Ophthalmol.* 2017;135(1):13–22.

Optical Aberrations

After undergoing surface ablation or LASIK, some patients report symptoms related to optical aberrations, including glare, ghost images, and halos. These symptoms are most prevalent after treatment with smaller ablation zones (<6.0 mm in diameter), after attempted higher spherical and cylindrical correction, and in patients who had similar symptoms preoperatively. These problems seem to be worse in dim light, when the pupil enlarges. Wavefront mapping can reveal higher-order aberrations associated with these subjective concerns. In general, a larger, more uniform, and better-centered optical zone provides better quality of vision, especially at night.

Night-vision complaints are often the result of spherical aberration, although other higher-order aberrations also contribute. The cornea and lens have inherent spherical aberration. In addition, excimer laser ablation increases positive spherical aberration in the midperipheral cornea. Wavefront-guided and wavefront-optimized corneal treatment patterns are designed to reduce existing aberrations and to help prevent the creation of new aberrations, with the goal of achieving a better quality of vision after laser ablation.

In both the first and second PROWL studies, visual symptoms such as halos and starbursts did not correspond to optical aberrations or reduced UDVA, unlike in multiple earlier studies. In approximately 45% of patients, new visual symptoms developed, so surgeons should discuss this possibility preoperatively. Very few patients reported that these symptoms caused significant difficulty, and the percentage of patients with symptoms decreased after laser surgery.

Excimer laser photoablation is the cause of most post-LASIK changes in lower- and higher-order aberrations (Fig 5-1). Creation of a flap with a microkeratome also has been reported to cause aberrations, but other studies have demonstrated minimal to no induced aberration with use of the femtosecond laser.

Pallikaris IG, Kymionis GD, Panagopoulou SI, Siganos CS, Theodorakis MA, Pallikaris AI. Induced optical aberrations following formation of a laser in situ keratomileusis flap. *J Cataract Refract Surg.* 2002;28(10):1737–1741.

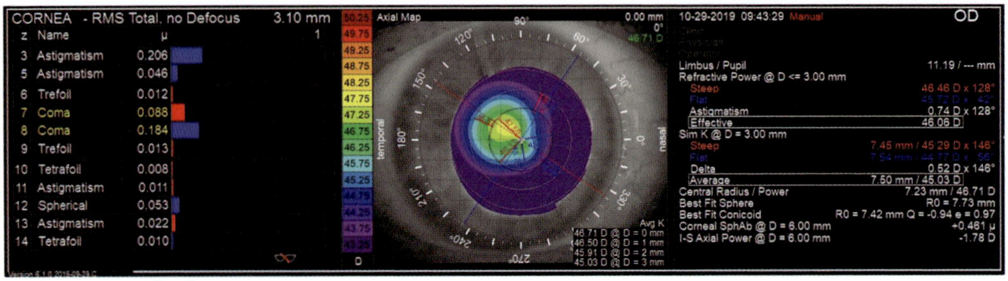

Figure 5-1 This patient has irregular astigmatism with higher-order aberrations, especially coma, after hyperopic LASIK. *(Courtesy of Bryan S. Lee, MD, JD.)*

Tülü Aygün B, Çankaya Kİ, Ağca A, et al. Five-year outcomes of small-incision lenticule extraction vs femtosecond laser–assisted laser in situ keratomileusis: a contralateral eye study. *J Cataract Refract Surg.* 2020;46(3):403–409.

Xia LK, Yu J, Chai GR, Wang D, Li Y. Comparison of the femtosecond laser and mechanical microkeratome for flap cutting in LASIK. *Int J Ophthalmol.* 2015;8(4):784–790.

Central Islands

A central island is a small-diameter (1–3 mm) steepening of at least 1.00 D that causes undesirable visual effects. This steepening is relative to the surrounding paracentral flattening from a myopic treatment (Fig 5-2). Central islands may be associated with decreased visual acuity, monocular diplopia and multiplopia, ghost images, and decreased contrast sensitivity.

The occurrence of central islands has decreased significantly with the use of modern scanning and variable-spot-size lasers and is now rarely encountered. Most central islands diminish over time, especially after surface ablation, although resolution may take 6–12 months. Treatment options such as topography-guided ablations may be helpful in treating persistent central islands.

Decentered Ablations

Accurate centration during the excimer laser procedure is important in optimizing the visual results, especially for hyperopic treatments. A decentered ablation can occur if the patient's head is positioned improperly by the surgeon, if the patient's eye begins to drift and loses fixation, or if the patient's eye is not perpendicular to the laser treatment (Fig 5-3). The incidence of decentration increases with surgeon inexperience, hyperopic ablations, and higher refractive correction because of longer ablation times. Modern tracking systems have reduced the risk of decentration. Treatment of decentration with topography-guided technology may help make the cornea more regular.

Kanellopoulos AJ, Asimellis G. LASIK ablation centration: an objective digitized assessment and comparison between two generations of an excimer laser. *J Refract Surg.* 2015;31(3):164–169.

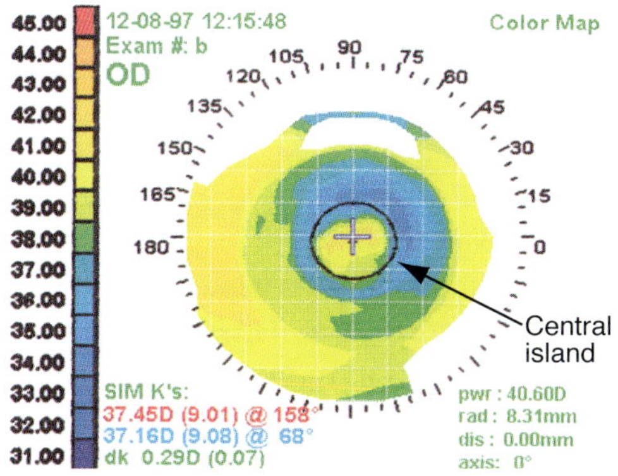

Figure 5-2 Corneal topography findings of a myopic ablation *(blue)* with a central island *(yellow)* in the visual axis. *(Courtesy of Roger F. Steinert, MD.)*

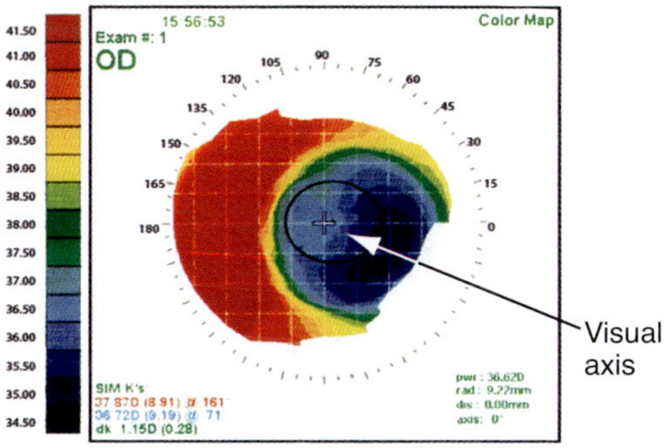

Figure 5-3 Corneal topography findings indicating a decentered ablation. *(Courtesy of Roger F. Steinert, MD.)*

Corticosteroid-Induced Complications

Most cases of postoperative elevation in intraocular pressure (IOP) are associated with prolonged topical corticosteroid therapy after surface ablation. The occurrence of this complication depends not only on the duration of treatment but also on the steroid used. The increase in IOP is usually controlled with topical IOP-lowering medications and typically normalizes after the corticosteroids are decreased or discontinued. It is important to note that refractive surgery can affect the measurement of IOP. For example, Goldmann tonometry readings are less accurate after LVC (see Chapter 7). In addition, fluid may collect in the LASIK flap interface when IOP is elevated and mask dangerously high IOPs. This complication is known as *pressure-induced stromal keratitis (PISK),* and applanation devices will artifactually measure the pressure of the fluid chamber (see the section "Pressure-induced stromal keratopathy" later in this chapter).

Several other corticosteroid-associated complications have been reported after surface ablation. Among them are reactivation of herpes simplex virus keratitis, ptosis, and cataracts.

Shokoohi-Rad S, Daneshvar R, Jafarian-Shahri M, Rajaee P. Comparison between betamethasone, fluorometholone and loteprednol etabonate on intraocular pressure in patients after keratorefractive surgery. *J Curr Ophthalmol.* 2017;30(2):130–135.

Central Toxic Keratopathy

Central toxic keratopathy is a rare, acute, noninflammatory central corneal opacification that can occur within days of uneventful LVC (Fig 5-4). Unlike most other interface entities, this condition has an acute onset without worsening over time. The etiology is unknown, but the resultant stromal thinning may be related to keratinocyte apoptosis.

Confocal microscopy has demonstrated activated keratocytes without inflammatory cells, with initial keratocyte loss from the stromal bed followed by gradual repopulation over time. Central toxic keratopathy has been reported to result in flattening of the anterior corneal curvature without alteration of posterior curvature on anterior segment tomography. However, some cases appear to alter all tomographic parameters, possibly as a measurement artifact.

Marked hyperopic shift is often observed, and it tends to resolve over time. Enhancement can be delayed in these cases until refractive stability is achieved and the clinical findings have resolved. The use of topical hypertonic solutions to treat central toxic keratopathy has been proposed in anecdotal reports.

Moshirfar M, Hazin R, Khalifa YM. Central toxic keratopathy. *Curr Opin Ophthalmol.* 2010;21(4):274–279.

Thornton IL, Foulks GN, Eiferman RA. Confocal microscopy of central toxic keratopathy. *Cornea.* 2012;31(8):934–936.

Sonmez B, Maloney RK. Central toxic keratopathy: description of a syndrome in laser refractive surgery. *Am J Ophthalmol.* 2007;143(3):420–427.

Infectious Keratitis

Infectious keratitis can occur after surface ablation procedures or LASIK, as both types of surgery involve disturbance of the ocular surface (Fig 5-5). Thus, eyelid preparation and

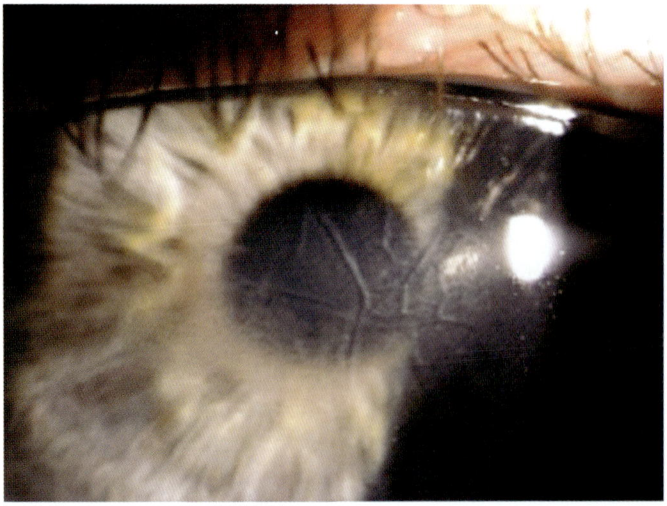

Figure 5-4 Clinical photograph of central toxic keratopathy, a rare, acute, noninflammatory central corneal opacification that can occur within days after uneventful LASIK or photorefractive keratectomy. *(Courtesy of Parag Majmudar, MD.)*

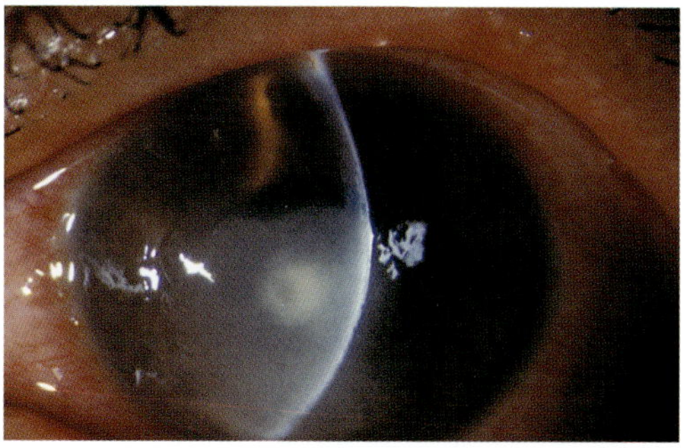

Figure 5-5 Infectious keratitis 1 month after LASIK. *(Courtesy of M. Bowes Hamill, MD.)*

proper draping are recommended. The risk of infection varies depending on the specific technique, with surface ablation conveying a greater risk than LASIK. The most common etiologic agents for these infections are gram-positive organisms, including *Staphylococcus aureus,* methicillin-resistant *Staphylococcus aureus (MRSA), Streptococcus pneumoniae,* and *Streptococcus viridans.* MRSA infections are an increasing cause of keratitis, even in the absence of traditional risk factors such as working in a health care environment. Atypical mycobacteria, *Nocardia asteroides,* and fungi have also been reported to cause infectious keratitis after LVC.

PRK and other surface ablation techniques create an iatrogenic corneal epithelial defect that takes several days to heal. During this time, the risk of postoperative infectious keratitis is highest because of the presence of this defect, use of a bandage contact lens, and administration of topical corticosteroid drops, all of which make it easier for eyelid and conjunctival bacterial flora to gain access to the stroma. Management of postoperative infectious keratitis begins with culturing and sensitivity testing of the contact lens and corneal scrapings, as well as initiation of a broad-spectrum antibiotic, taking into account the higher prevalence of gram-positive organisms. Treatment may require frequent instillation of multiple antimicrobial agents. Because of the risk of fungal keratitis, cultures should include fungal assays, and treatment for keratitis should include antifungal agents in cases that are suspicious or do not respond appropriately to antibacterials (see BCSC Section 8, *External Disease and Cornea*).

During or shortly after LASIK, eyelid and conjunctival flora may enter and remain sequestered under the flap (see the section "LASIK infectious keratitis" later in this chapter). The antimicrobial components in the tears and in topically applied antibiotic drops have difficulty penetrating into the stroma to reach the organisms (Fig 5-6).

Llovet F, de Rojas V, Interlandi E, et al. Infectious keratitis in 204 586 LASIK procedures. *Ophthalmology.* 2010;117(3):232–8.e84.

Mozayan A, Madu A, Channa P. Laser in-situ keratomileusis infection: review and update of current practices. *Curr Opin Ophthalmol.* 2011;22(4):233–237.

Ortega-Usobiaga J, Llovet-Osuna F, Djodeyre MR, Llovet-Rausell A, Beltran J, Baviera J. Incidence of corneal infections after laser in situ keratomileusis and surface ablation when moxifloxacin and tobramycin are used as postoperative treatment. *J Cataract Refract Surg.* 2015;41(6):1210–1216.

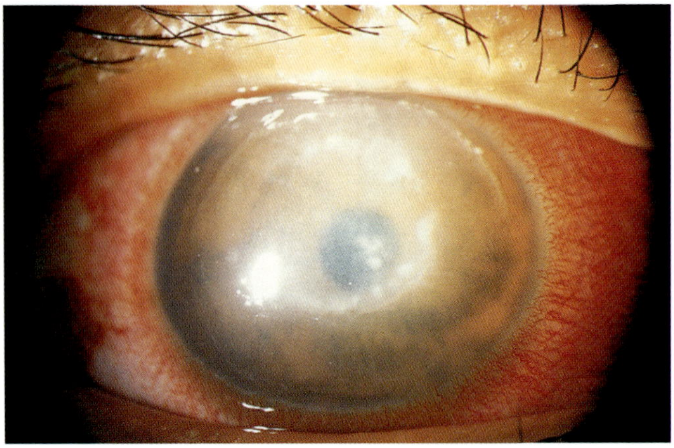

Figure 5-6 Infectious keratitis in a LASIK flap after recurrent epithelial abrasion. *(Courtesy of Jayne S. Weiss, MD.)*

Complications Unique to Surface Ablation

Persistent Epithelial Defects

Usually, the epithelial defect created during surface ablation heals within 3 or 4 days with the aid of a bandage contact lens, although it is sometimes necessary to exchange the bandage contact lens if it is too tight. A frequent cause of delayed re-epithelialization is keratoconjunctivitis sicca or other tear film abnormalities (see Chapter 7). Treatment options include aggressive nonpreserved lubricants, topical cyclosporine, temporary punctal occlusion, amniotic membrane grafting, and autologous serum drops. Patients who have autoimmune connective tissue disease or diabetes mellitus and those who smoke may have poor epithelial healing and thus may not be good candidates for surface ablation. They may require a more aggressive ocular surface regimen before surgery. Topical nonsteroidal anti-inflammatory drugs (NSAIDs) should be discontinued in patients with delayed re-epithelialization.

Oral antibiotics in the tetracycline family may be beneficial for persistent epithelial defects because they inhibit collagenase activity, which in turn improves wound healing. In some cases, epithelial healing may be hindered by the presence of necrotic epithelium on the corneal surface. Gentle debridement of the necrotic epithelial border may help. Patients must be monitored closely until re-epithelialization occurs because a persistent epithelial defect increases the risk of corneal haze, irregular astigmatism, refractive instability, delayed recovery of vision, and infectious keratitis.

Sterile Infiltrates

The use of bandage contact lenses is associated with sterile infiltrates, which may occur more frequently in patients using topical NSAIDs for longer than 24 hours without concomitant topical corticosteroids. The infiltrates, which have been reported in approximately 1 in 300 cases, are secondary to an immune reaction (Fig 5-7). Any infiltrate should first be

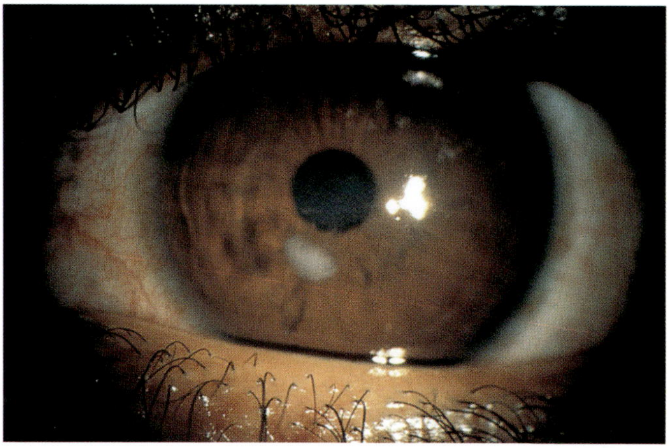

Figure 5-7 Stromal sterile infiltrate after use of a bandage contact lens following photorefractive keratectomy. *(Courtesy of Jayne S. Weiss, MD.)*

presumed to be infectious. Once an infiltrate is determined to be sterile, it is treated with topical corticosteroids, discontinuation of topical NSAIDs, and close follow-up.

Teal P, Breslin C, Arshinoff S, Edmison D. Corneal subepithelial infiltrates following excimer laser photorefractive keratectomy. *J Cataract Refract Surg.* 1995;21(5):516–518.

Corneal Haze

The patient's wound healing after surface ablation is important in determining postoperative topical corticosteroid management. Eyes that have haze or that are undercorrected may benefit from increased corticosteroid use, while those that are overcorrected but clear may benefit from a reduction in topical corticosteroids, which may lead to regression.

If subepithelial corneal haze develops, it typically appears several weeks after surface ablation, peaks in intensity at 1–2 months, and gradually diminishes or disappears over the following 6–12 months (Fig 5-8). *Late-onset corneal haze* may occur several months or more postoperatively after a period in which the cornea was relatively clear. Histologic studies in animals with corneal haze after PRK demonstrate abnormal glycosaminoglycans and/or nonlamellar collagen deposited in the anterior stroma as a consequence of epithelial–stromal wound healing. Most histologic studies from animals and humans show an increase in the number and activity of stromal keratocytes, suggesting that increased keratocyte activity may be the source of the extracellular deposits.

Persistent severe haze is usually associated with greater amounts of correction or smaller ablation zones. Animal studies have demonstrated that ultraviolet B exposure after PRK prolongs stromal healing and increases subepithelial haze. Clinical cases of haze after high ultraviolet exposure, such as at high altitude, corroborate these studies, so surgeons often recommend sunglass wear after surface ablation. Intraoperative mitomycin C reduces the risk of corneal haze.

If clinically unacceptable haze persists, superficial keratectomy or phototherapeutic keratectomy may be performed, often with mitomycin C. Because haze can resolve

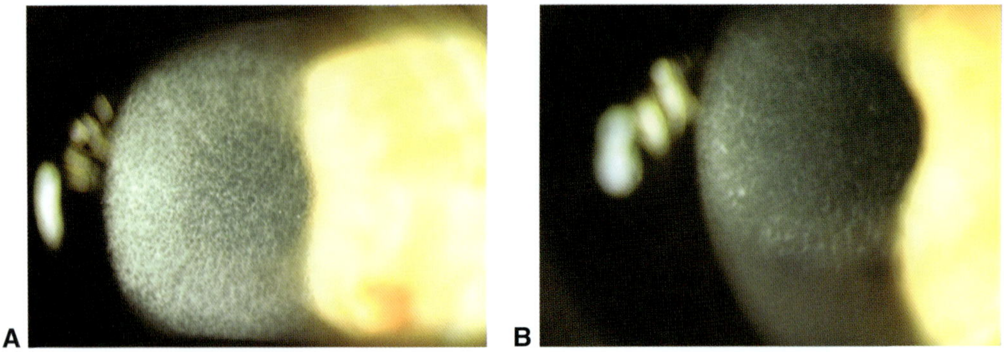

Figure 5-8 Corneal haze after photorefractive keratectomy (PRK). **A,** Severe haze 5 months after PRK. The reticular pattern is characteristic of PRK-induced haze. **B,** Haze has improved to a moderate level by 13 months postoperatively. *(Courtesy of Roger F. Steinert, MD.)*

spontaneously with normal wound remodeling, re-treatment should be delayed for at least 6–12 months. In the presence of haze, refraction is often inaccurate.

Hofmeister EM, Bishop FM, Kaupp SE, Schallhorn SC. Randomized dose-response analysis of mitomycin-C to prevent haze after photorefractive keratectomy for high myopia. *J Cataract Refract Surg.* 2013;39(9):1358–1365.

Kaiserman I, Sadi N, Mimouni M, Sela T, Munzer G, Levartovsky S. Corneal breakthrough haze after photorefractive keratectomy with mitomycin C: incidence and risk factors. *Cornea.* 2017;36(8):961–966.

Majmudar PA, Schallhorn SC, Cason JB, et al. Mitomycin-C in corneal surface excimer laser ablation techniques: a report by the American Academy of Ophthalmology. *Ophthalmology.* 2015;122(6):1085–1095.

Complications Unique to LASIK

The complications associated with LASIK are primarily related to flap creation, postoperative flap positioning, or interface problems.

Microkeratome Complications

In the past, the most severe complications associated with LASIK were related to problems with the manual microkeratome, which caused the planned LASIK procedure to be abandoned in an estimated 0.6%–1.6% of cases. In current practice, advances in microkeratome technology and the advent of femtosecond laser–created flaps have substantially reduced the incidence of severe, sight-threatening complications.

When a manual microkeratome is used, meticulous care must be taken in the cleaning and assembly of the instrument to ensure a smooth, uninterrupted passage. Defects in the blade, poor suction, or uneven progression of the microkeratome across the cornea can produce an irregular, thin, or buttonhole flap (Fig 5-9), which can lead to irregular astigmatism with loss of corrected distance visual acuity (CDVA). Steep corneal curvature

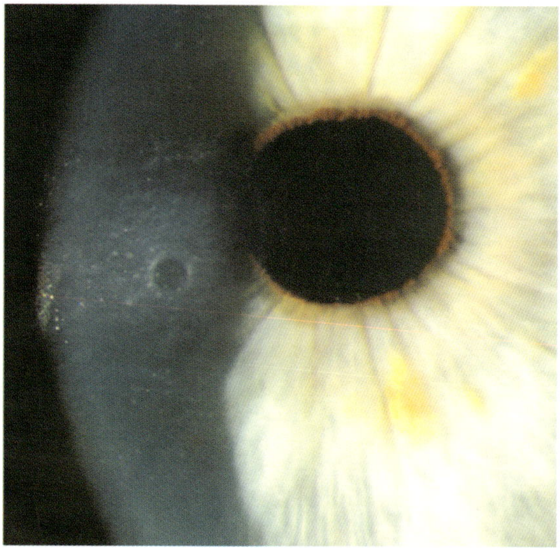

Figure 5-9 LASIK flap with buttonhole. *(Reproduced with permission from Feder RS, Rapuano CJ.* The LASIK Handbook: A Case-Based Approach. *Lippincott Williams & Wilkins; 2007:95. Image courtesy of Christopher J. Rapuano, MD.)*

can result in a nonuniform fit of the keratome suction device or corneal buckling, increasing the risk of thin, irregular, or buttonhole flaps. If a thin or buttonhole flap is created, or if an incomplete flap does not provide sufficient area for the laser ablation, the flap should ideally not be lifted. If the problem was not recognized until the flap was lifted, it should be replaced, a bandage contact lens should be applied, and the ablation should not be performed. Substantial vision loss can be prevented if the flap is allowed to heal before another refractive procedure is attempted. Although a new flap can usually be made safely using a deeper cut after at least 3 months of healing, most surgeons prefer to use a surface ablation technique.

Occasionally, a free cap is created instead of a hinged flap (Fig 5-10). In these cases, if the stromal bed is large enough to accommodate the laser treatment, the corneal cap is placed in a moist chamber while the ablation is performed. It is important to replace the cap with the epithelial side up and to position it properly on a dried stromal bed, using previously placed radial marks—a prudent step to take before microkeratome cases. A temporary 10-0 nylon suture can be placed to create an artificial hinge, but the physiologic dehydration of the stroma by the endothelial pump will generally keep the cap secured in proper position. A bandage contact lens can help protect the cap. A flat corneal curvature (<40.00 D) is a risk factor for creating a free cap because the flap diameter is often smaller than average in flat corneas.

Corneal perforation is a rare but devastating intraoperative complication that can occur if the microkeratome is not properly assembled or the depth plate in older microkeratomes was not properly placed. It is imperative for the surgeon to double-check that the microkeratome has been properly assembled. Modern microkeratomes are constructed with a prefixed depth plate.

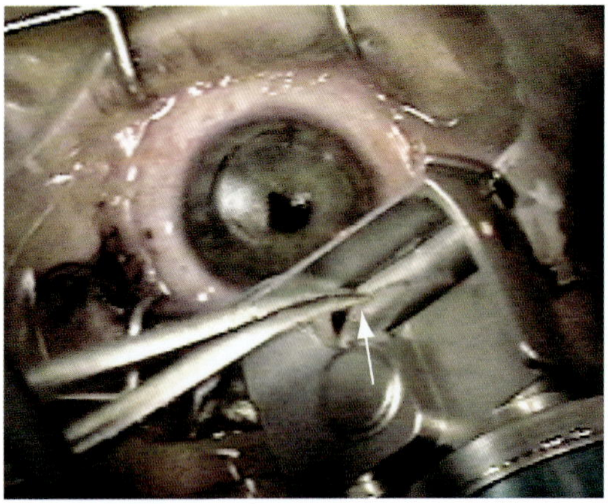

Figure 5-10 Free cap resulting from transection of the hinge. The cap is being lifted from the microkeratome with forceps *(arrow),* and care is being taken to maintain the orientation of the epithelial external layer in order to prevent accidental inversion of the cap when it is replaced. *(Courtesy of Roger F. Steinert, MD.)*

Kahuam-López N, Navas A, Castillo-Salgado C, Graue-Hernandez EO, Jimenez-Corona A, Ibarra A. Laser-assisted in-situ keratomileusis (LASIK) with a mechanical microkeratome compared to LASIK with a femtosecond laser for LASIK in adults with myopia or myopic astigmatism. *Cochrane Database Syst Rev.* 2020;4(4):CD012946.

Epithelial Sloughing or Defects

The friction of microkeratome passage across the pressurized cornea may loosen a sheet of epithelium *(epithelial sloughing)* or cause a frank epithelial defect. Although patients with epithelial basement membrane dystrophy are at particular risk—in which case surface ablation rather than LASIK is advisable—others show no preoperative epithelial abnormalities. The risk of epithelial abnormality during LASIK increases with age. Techniques suggested to decrease the rate of epithelial defects include limiting medications to avoid toxicity, using chilled proparacaine, minimizing topical anesthetic, using nonpreserved drops as much as possible; and, in microkeratome cases, meticulous maintenance of the device and shutting off of suction on the reverse pass. There is a reduced incidence of epithelial defects with femtosecond laser flap creation, which avoids passage of a microkeratome over the cornea.

In cases of significant epithelial defects, a bandage contact lens is often applied immediately postoperatively and retained until stable re-epithelialization occurs, with concomitant intensive lubrication and, often, punctal occlusion. Persistent abnormal epithelium with recurrent erosions or loss of CDVA may require debridement or phototherapeutic keratectomy. Epithelial defects are associated with an increased incidence of postoperative diffuse lamellar keratitis, infectious keratitis, flap striae, and epithelial ingrowth, and surgeons should watch closely for these conditions.

Chen S, Feng Y, Stojanovic A, Jankov MR 2nd, Wang Q. IntraLase femtosecond laser vs mechanical microkeratomes in LASIK for myopia: a systematic review and meta-analysis. *J Refract Surg.* 2012;28(1):15–24.

Moshirfar M, Gardiner JP, Schliesser JA, et al. Laser in situ keratomileusis flap complications using mechanical microkeratome versus femtosecond laser: retrospective comparison. *J Cataract Refract Surg.* 2010;36(11):1925–1933.

Flap Striae

Flap folds, or *striae,* may decrease visual quality or acuity after LASIK. When present, most folds are noted on the first postoperative day, and almost all occur within the first week. Risk factors for development of folds include excessive irrigation under the flap during LASIK, thin flaps, and deep ablations with mismatch of the flap to the new bed. Early recognition and intervention are crucial in treating folds that cause loss of CDVA or visual distortion.

Striae are typically not treated if the patient is asymptomatic and CDVA and UDVA are not affected. Folds are examined with a slit lamp using direct illumination, retroillumination, and fluorescein staining. Circumferential folds may be associated with high myopia and typically resolve with time. Folds that are parallel and emanate from the flap hinge grouped in the same direction indicate flap slippage, which requires prompt intervention. Folds are often categorized as either macrostriae or microstriae, but there is significant overlap clinically (Table 5-1).

Macrostriae

Macrostriae are full-thickness, undulating stromal folds resulting from initial flap malposition or postoperative slippage (Fig 5-11A). Techniques to replace and smooth the flap vary, but after the flap is repositioned, the surgeon should use coaxial and oblique illumination to examine carefully for the presence of striae (Video 5-1). Checking the patient in the early postoperative period is important to detect flap slippage. A protective plastic shield is often used for the first 24 hours to discourage the patient from touching the eyelids and inadvertently disrupting the flap.

VIDEO 5-1 LASIK flap repositioning.
Courtesy of Sarah M. Nehls, MD.

In a large series, striae requiring flap lift were reported in 1.2% of eyes. Careful examination will disclose a wider gutter on the side where the folds are most prominent. Flap slippage should be rectified as soon as it is recognized because the folds rapidly become fixed. The surgeon relifts the flap, copiously irrigates the interface with sterile balanced salt solution, and then stretches the flap perpendicular to the folds. Using hypotonic saline or sterile distilled water swells the flap and may initially reduce the striae; however, such swelling also reduces the flap diameter, which widens the gutter, delays flap adhesion because of prolonged endothelial dehydration time, and may worsen the striae after the flap dehydrates. If the macrostriae have been present for more than 24 hours, reactive epithelial changes tend to fix the folds into position. In addition to refloating the flap, the surgeon may de-epithelialize the central 6 mm of the flap over the macrostriae to remove this impediment to smoothing the wrinkles. A bandage contact lens should be used to stabilize the flap and to protect the surface until full re-epithelialization occurs. In cases of intractable macrostriae, sutures may be placed and retained for several weeks, but irregular astigmatism may still be present after suture removal.

Mimouni M, Vainer I, Assad N, et al. Incidence, indications, and outcomes of eyes needing early flap lifting after LASIK. *Cornea.* 2018;37(9):1118–1123.

Table 5-1 Differentiation Between Macrostriae and Microstriae in LASIK Flaps

Characteristic		Macrostriae	Microstriae
Pathology		Large folds involving entire flap thickness	Fine folds, principally in Bowman layer
Cause		Flap slippage	Mismatch of flap to new bed; contracture of flap
Slit-lamp appearance	Direct illumination	Broad undulations seen as parallel or radial converging lines; widened flap gutter may be present	Fine folds, principally in Bowman layer; gutter usually symmetric
	Retroillumination	Same as above	Folds more obvious on retroillumination
	Fluorescein	Same as above, with negative staining pattern	May show normal fluorescein pattern or negative staining
Analogy		Wrinkles in skewed carpet	Dried, cracked mud
Topography		Possible disruption over striae	Color map may be normal or slightly disrupted; Placido disk mires show fine irregularity
Vision		Decreased CDVA and/or multiplopia if central	Subtly decreased CDVA or multiplopia if clinically significant; microstriae masked by epithelium are universal and asymptomatic
Treatment options	Acute	Refloat/reposition flap immediately	Usually observe; support surface with aggressive lubrication
	Established	Refloat, de-epithelialize over striae, hydrate and stroke, apply traction, or suture Phototherapeutic keratectomy	If visually significant, refloat; try hydration, stroking, suturing Phototherapeutic keratectomy

CDVA = corrected distance visual acuity; LASIK = laser in situ keratomileusis.

Microstriae

Microstriae are fine, hairlike optical irregularities that are best viewed on red reflex retroillumination or by light reflected off the iris (Fig 5-11B). They are very small folds in the Bowman layer, and this anterior location accounts for the reduction of CDVA in some eyes. Computer topographic color maps usually do not show these subtle irregularities. However, disruption of the surface contour may result in irregularity of the Placido disk image. In addition, application of dilute fluorescein often reveals *negative staining,* in which the elevated striae disrupt the tear film, and fluorescence is lost over them.

If optically significant microstriae persist, they can be addressed in the same manner as described earlier for macrostriae. An alternative procedure is phototherapeutic keratectomy. Approximately 200 pulses from a broad-beam laser, set to a maximal diameter of 6.5 mm, are initially applied to penetrate the epithelium. The epithelium acts as a masking

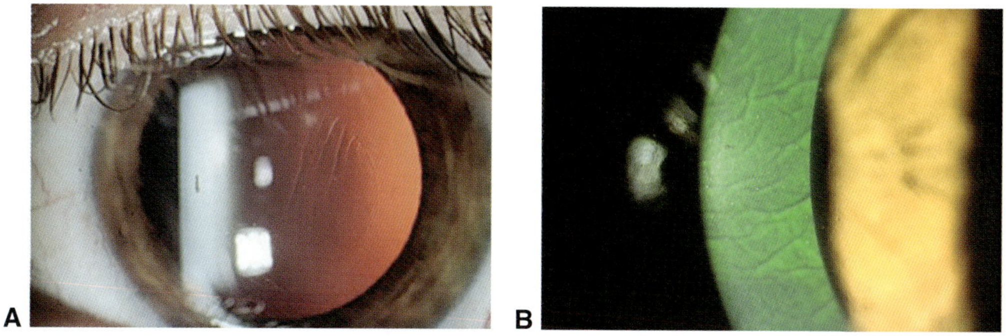

Figure 5-11 Post-LASIK striae. **A,** Retroillumination of multiple horizontal parallel macrostriae in the visual axis from mild flap dislocation. **B,** Numerous randomly directed microstriae on fluorescein staining. These striae resemble dried, cracked mud; are apparent on the first day after LASIK; and usually resolve without intervention. *(Part A courtesy of Parag Majmudar, MD; part B courtesy of Steven C. Schallhorn, MD.)*

agent, exposing the elevated striae before the valleys between the striae. After the transepithelial ablation, additional pulses are applied, and a thin film of medium-viscosity artificial tears is administered every 5–10 pulses, up to a maximum of 100 additional pulses. If these suggestions are followed, little to no haze results, and an average hyperopic shift of less than +1.00 D occurs as a result of the minimal tissue removal.

Ashrafzadeh A, Steinert RF. Results of phototherapeutic keratectomy in the management of flap striae after LASIK before and after developing a standardized protocol: long-term follow-up of an expanded patient population. *Ophthalmology.* 2007;114(6):1118–1123.

Traumatic Flap Dislocation

The rare complication of LASIK flap dislocation most often occurs on the first postoperative day, when dryness and adhesion of the flap to the upper tarsal conjunctiva are sufficient to cause the flap to slip. After the first day, re-epithelialization of the gutter begins to increase flap stability. Within several weeks, keratocytes begin to lay down new collagen at the cut edge of the Bowman layer, and eventually a fine scar is established at the edge of the flap. However, minimal healing occurs across the stromal interface. Late flap dislocation from blunt trauma has been reported many years after LASIK. Flap dislocation requires urgent treatment to replace the flap in its proper anatomical position. To reduce the chance of epithelial ingrowth, the surgeon should make sure that there is no epithelium on the underside of the flap or in the interface.

Ting DSJ, Danjoux JP. Late-onset traumatic dislocation of laser in situ keratomileusis corneal flaps: a case series with many clinical lessons. *Int Ophthalmol.* 2019;39(6):1397–1403.

LASIK Interface Complications

Diffuse lamellar keratitis

The presentation of diffuse lamellar keratitis (DLK; Fig 5-12) can range from asymptomatic interface haze near the edge of the flap to marked central diffuse haze with decreased

A B C

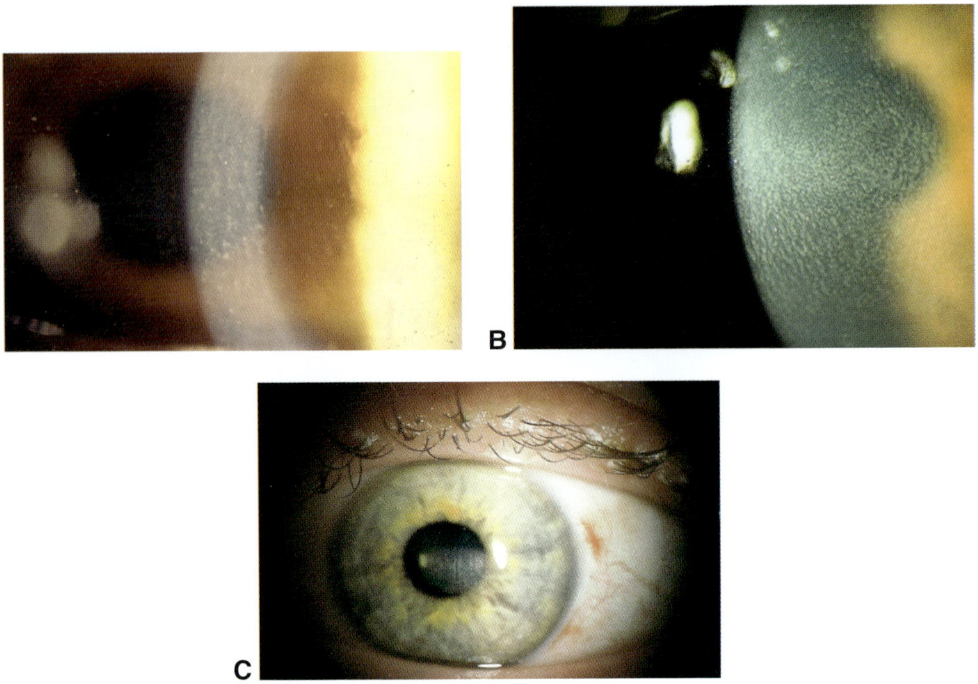

Figure 5-12 Diffuse lamellar keratitis (DLK). **A,** High-magnification image of stage 2 DLK. Note the accumulation of inflammatory cells in the fine ridges created by the oscillating microkeratome blade. **B,** Stage 3 DLK showing dense accumulation of inflammatory cells centrally. **C,** Stage 4 DLK with central scar and folds. *(Parts A and B courtesy of Roger F. Steinert, MD; part C courtesy of Jayne S. Weiss, MD.)*

CDVA. The condition represents a nonspecific sterile inflammatory response to a variety of mechanical and toxic insults. The interface under the flap is a potential space in which any cause of anterior stromal inflammation can trigger the accumulation of white blood cells. DLK has been reported in association with epithelial defects months or even years after LASIK, and the prevalence is higher with a femtosecond flap. Other reported inciting factors include foreign material on the surface of the microkeratome blade or motor, trapped meibomian gland secretions, povidone-iodine solution from the preoperative skin preparation, marking ink, substances produced by laser ablation, contamination of the sterilizer with gram-negative endotoxin, and red blood cells in the interface. The inflammation generally resolves with topical corticosteroid treatment alone without sequelae, but severe cases can lead to scarring or flap melting.

DLK is typically classified by the stages described in Table 5-2. Although stages 1 and 2 usually respond to frequent topical corticosteroid application, stages 3 and 4 usually require lifting of the flap and irrigation, followed by intensive topical corticosteroid treatment. Oral corticosteroids may be used adjunctively in severe cases. Recovery of vision in DLK is usually excellent if the condition is detected and treated promptly.

A surgeon should have a low threshold for lifting or irrigating underneath the flap in suspected cases of severe DLK. Lifting the flap allows removal of inflammatory mediators

Table 5-2 Staging of Diffuse Lamellar Keratitis

Stage	Findings
1	Peripheral faint white blood cells; granular appearance
2	Central scattered white blood cells; granular appearance
3	Central dense white blood cells in visual axis
4	Permanent scarring or stromal melting

from the interface and direct placement of corticosteroids and NSAIDs to suppress inflammation and necrosis. If there is any suspicion that the inflammation is due to infection, the surgeon should consider flap lift and interface culture, with placement of topical antibiotics in the interface. If the presumed DLK does not respond to corticosteroids within 7–10 days of initiation, the diagnosis should be reconsidered, as infectious keratitis or PISK (both discussed in the following sections) can mimic DLK and require corticosteroid cessation.

Holland SP, Mathias RG, Morck DW, Chiu J, Slade SG. Diffuse lamellar keratitis related to endotoxins released from sterilizer reservoir biofilms. *Ophthalmology.* 2000;107(7):1227–1233.

Smith RJ, Maloney RK. Diffuse lamellar keratitis. A new syndrome in lamellar refractive surgery. *Ophthalmology*. 1998;105(9):1721–1726.

Wilson SE, de Oliveira RC. Pathophysiology and treatment of diffuse lamellar keratitis. *J Refract Surg*. 2020;36(2):124–130.

LASIK infectious keratitis

It is important to differentiate sterile interface inflammation from potentially devastating infectious inflammation. Because LASIK patients commonly experience both postoperative discomfort and reduced corneal sensation, pain is not a reliable symptom of infection. Infection after LASIK is usually associated with redness, photophobia, and decreased vision. Several characteristics can help distinguish between DLK and infectious keratitis (Table 5-3). DLK is usually visible with slit-lamp biomicroscopy within 24 hours of surgery and typically begins at the periphery of the flap. There is usually a gradient of inflammation, with the inflammation being most intense at the periphery and diminishing toward the center of the cornea. In general, the inflammatory reaction in DLK is confined to the area of the flap interface and does not extend far beyond the edge of the flap (Fig 5-13). In contrast, post-LASIK infectious keratitis usually begins 2 or 3 days after surgery and involves a more focal inflammatory reaction that is not confined to the lamellar interface. An anterior chamber reaction is more typical of infection, and an infectious inflammatory reaction can extend up into the flap, deeper into the stromal bed, and beyond the confines of the flap.

Infection within the interface can lead to flap melting, severe irregular astigmatism, and corneal scarring that may require corneal transplantation. If infection is suspected, the flap should be lifted and the interface cultured and irrigated with antibiotics. The most common infections are from gram-positive organisms, followed in frequency by those caused by atypical mycobacteria. Mycobacterial infection can be diagnosed more rapidly

Table 5-3 Diffuse Lamellar Keratitis vs Infectious Keratitis After LASIK

Diffuse Lamellar Keratitis	Infectious Keratitis
Usually visible within first 24 hours	Usual onset at least 2–3 days postoperatively
Typically begins at flap periphery	Can occur anywhere under flap
More intense inflammation at periphery decreasing toward center	
Inflammation primarily confined to interface	Inflammation extends above and below interface and beyond flap edge
Diffuse inflammation	Focal inflammation around infection
Minimal to no anterior chamber reaction	Mild to moderate anterior chamber reaction
Flap melts can occur	Flap melts can occur

Modified from Culbertson WW, 2006.

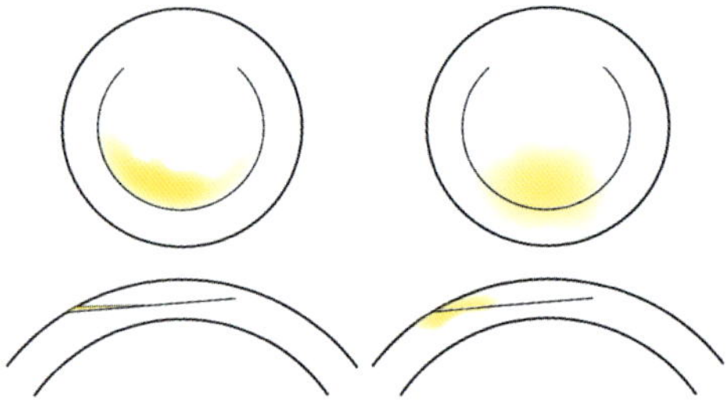

Figure 5-13 DLK is differentiated from infectious keratitis by the confinement of the cells to the flap interface alone in DLK. *(Reproduced from Culbertson WW, 2006.)*

by using acid-fast and fluorochrome stains than by waiting for culture results, which require special media (see Figure 5-5). If there is lack of clinical progress, cultures may need to be repeated, and the flap may need to be amputated to improve antimicrobial penetration.

In general, the timing of the onset of symptoms provides a clue to the etiology of the infection. Infections occurring within 10 days of surgery are typically bacterial (see BCSC Section 8, *External Disease and Cornea*). The fourth-generation fluoroquinolones gatifloxacin and moxifloxacin have excellent efficacy against the most common bacteria that cause post-LASIK infections, including some atypical mycobacteria; however, monotherapy with these drugs may not be sufficient. Late LASIK flap infection may occur after a recurrent erosion (see Figure 5-6).

Bostan C, Slim E, Choremis J, et al. Successful management of severe post-LASIK *Mycobacterium abscessus* keratitis with topical amikacin and linezolid, flap ablation, and topical corticosteroids. *J Cataract Refract Surg.* 2019;45(7):1032–1035.

John T, Velotta E. Nontuberculous (atypical) mycobacterial keratitis after LASIK: current status and clinical implications. *Cornea.* 2005;24(3):245–255.

Pressure-induced stromal keratopathy

A diffuse stromal and interface opacity, PISK has been reported to occur as a result of elevated IOP. It can be mistaken for DLK but is sometimes associated with a visible fluid cleft in the interface (Fig 5-14). The surgeon must be aware of this rare condition

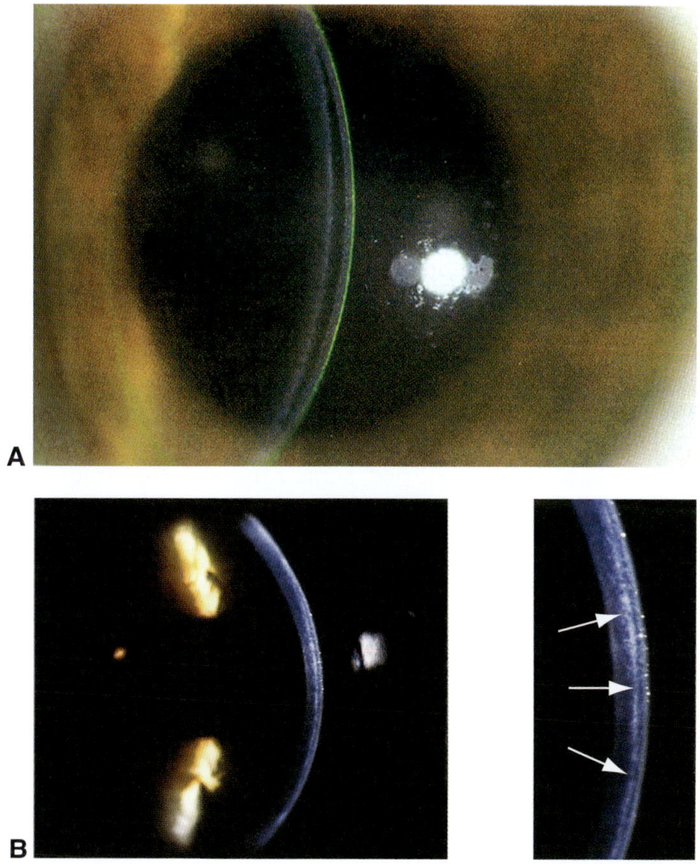

Figure 5-14 Pressure-induced stromal keratopathy (PISK) after LASIK. **A,** An optically clear, fluid-filled space between the flap and stromal bed. This condition is hypothesized to be caused by transudation of fluid across the endothelium as a result of corticosteroid-induced elevation of intraocular pressure (IOP). **B,** PISK without interface gap. A diffuse stromal and interface opacity without an interface fluid cleft can also result from elevated IOP with prolonged corticosteroid use *(left panel)*. Close-up *(right panel, arrows)* further demonstrates the opacification of the stroma and interface. *(Part A reproduced with permission from Hamilton DR, Manche EE, Rich LF, Maloney RK. Steroid-induced glaucoma after laser in situ keratomileusis associated with interface fluid.* Ophthalmology. *2002;109(4):659–665. Part B courtesy of Theofilos Tourtas, MD.)*

because treatment of PISK involves rapid cessation of corticosteroid drops and the use of glaucoma medications to lower IOP. The haze from PISK is associated with prolonged corticosteroid treatment and usually presents after 10 days to 2 weeks. Key differentiators between DLK and PISK are the earlier onset and normal IOP in DLK. Because the fluid cleft may falsely lower Goldmann measurements, IOP should be measured both centrally and peripherally in suspected cases of PISK and with a pneumotonometer, Tono-Pen (Reichert Technologies), or dynamic contour tonometry if available. High-resolution anterior segment optical coherence tomography is helpful for the diagnosis of PISK. Severe glaucomatous vision loss has been reported in cases with delayed diagnosis.

Cabral-Macias J, García-De la Rosa G, Rodríguez-Matilde DF, et al. Pressure-induced stromal keratopathy after laser in situ keratomileusis: acute and late-onset presentations. *J Cataract Refract Surg.* 2018;44(10):1284–1290.

Randleman JB, Lesser GR. Glaucomatous damage from pressure-induced stromal keratopathy after LASIK. *J Refract Surg.* 2012;28(6):378–379.

Epithelial ingrowth

Epithelial ingrowth occurs rarely after primary LASIK, with published prevalence usually less than 3% (Fig 5-15). There is no need to treat isolated nests of epithelial cells in the peripheral lamellar interface that are not advancing and are not affecting vision. However, if the ingrowth is advancing toward the visual axis, is associated with decreased vision from irregular astigmatism identified on topography or tomography (Fig 5-16), or triggers overlying flap melting, it should be removed by lifting the flap, scraping the epithelium from both the underside of the flap and the stromal bed, and then repositioning the flap. After scraping the under-flap surface and stromal bed, some surgeons also remove epithelium from both the periphery of the flap and the bed to allow for flap adherence before the healing

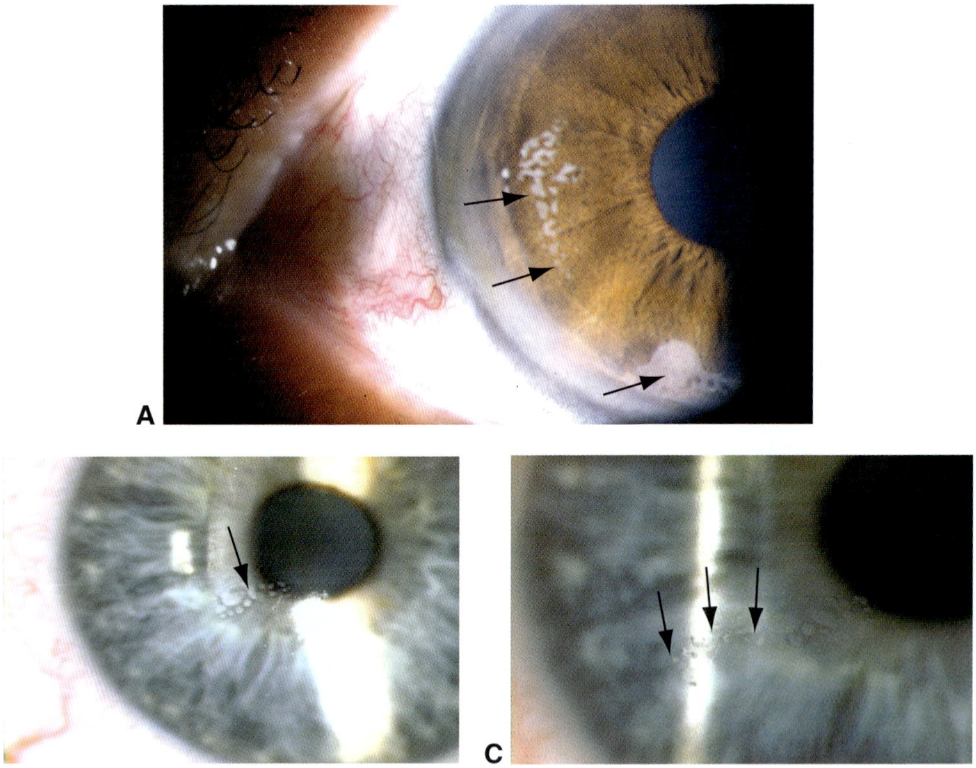

Figure 5-15 Epithelial ingrowth in the interface under a LASIK flap. **A,** Peripheral ingrowth of 1–2 mm *(arrows)* is common and usually inconsequential and does not require intervention unless it induces melting of the overlying flap. **B,** Central nests of epithelial cells *(arrow)* disrupt the patient's vision by elevating and distorting the flap. The flap must be lifted and the epithelium debrided. **C,** Inspection of the midperiphery shows the track followed by the invading epithelium from the periphery toward the center *(arrows)*. *(Courtesy of Roger F. Steinert, MD.)*

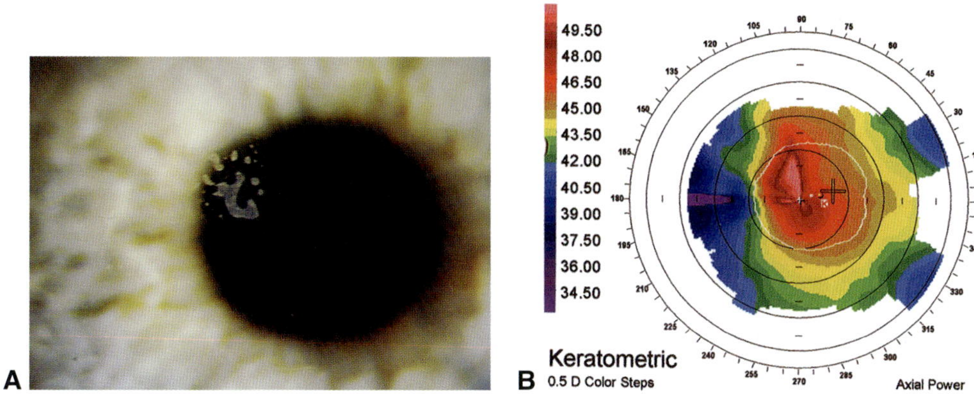

Figure 5-16 Epithelial ingrowth in the visual axis. **A,** Clinical appearance. **B,** Corresponding topographic steepening and irregularity. *(Courtesy of J. Bradley Randleman, MD.)*

epithelium reaches the flap edge. Additional techniques include flap suturing or fibrin glue at the flap edge. Some surgeons treat the undersurface of the flap with absolute alcohol to remove any residual epithelium. Nd:YAG laser has also been described to treat early epithelial ingrowth in lieu of flap lift.

The incidence of epithelial ingrowth is higher in eyes that develop an epithelial defect at the time of the procedure, undergo a re-treatment with lifting of a preexisting flap, or have traumatic flap dehiscence. In such cases, special care should be taken to ensure that no epithelium is caught under the edge of the flap when it is repositioned. Placement of a bandage contact lens at the conclusion of the procedure may decrease the incidence of epithelial ingrowth.

Ayala MJ, Alió JL, Mulet ME, De La Hoz F. Treatment of laser in situ keratomileusis interface epithelial ingrowth with neodymium:yttrium-aluminum-garnet laser. *Am J Ophthalmol.* 2008;145(4):630–634.

Friehmann A, Mimouni M, Nemet AY, Sela T, Munzer G, Kaiserman I. Risk factors for epithelial ingrowth following microkeratome-assisted LASIK. *J Refract Surg.* 2018;34(2):100–105.

Yesilirmak N, Chhadva P, Cabot F, Galor A, Yoo SH. Post–laser in situ keratomileusis epithelial ingrowth: treatment, recurrence, and long-term results. *Cornea.* 2018; 37(12):1517–1521.

Interface debris

The principal indication for lifting the flap and irrigating for debris is an inflammatory reaction elicited by the foreign material, as small amounts of lint, nondescript particles, or tiny metal particles from stainless steel surgical instruments are usually well tolerated. A small amount of blood that has oozed into the interface from transected peripheral vessels may also be tolerated and typically resolves spontaneously with time. However, significant amounts can elicit an inflammatory cell response and should be irrigated from the interface at the time of LASIK (Fig 5-17). Although use of a topical vasoconstrictor such as epinephrine reduces this problem, it can also cause pupillary dilation, making it harder for patients to fixate or for the surgeon to engage pupil tracking.

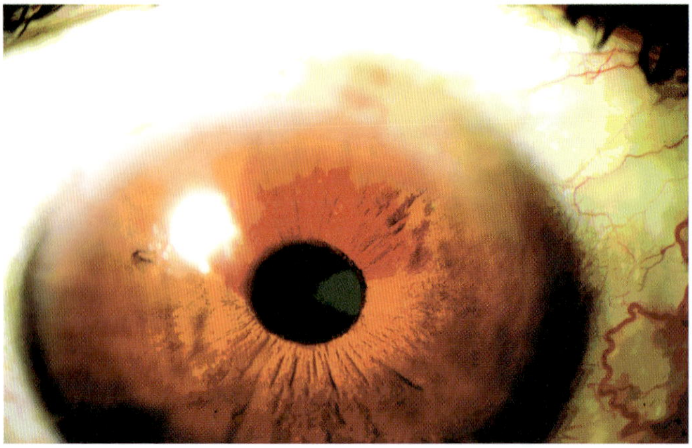

Figure 5-17 Blood in the LASIK interface. *(Courtesy of Jayne S. Weiss, MD.)*

Complications Related to Femtosecond Laser–Assisted LASIK Flaps

Opaque bubble layer and gas breakthrough

One of the most common adverse effects of the intrastromal photodisruption procedure is the generation of an *opaque bubble layer* (*OBL;* Fig 5-18). This bubble layer is composed of carbon dioxide and water. Laser tracking systems can be significantly impaired by an OBL. Time and/or mechanical massage will allow the OBL to dissipate. Newer-generation femtosecond lasers with higher repetition rates tend to create less OBL.

Epithelial gas breakthrough is a rare but serious complication of OBL production, and the presence of a corneal scar is a contraindication to a femtosecond flap. As in the case of a buttonhole from a mechanical keratome, the flap should not be lifted if the problem is identified in time. After the breach is healed, surface ablation may be performed.

In rare cases, gas liberated from the plasma cavitation bubbles can travel into the anterior chamber, potentially interfering with the laser tracking systems. If this occurs, the surgeon can wait a few hours for the bubbles to resolve. In addition, instillation of a mydriatic drop may cause the pupil to dilate around the bubbles, allowing laser recognition and capture to proceed.

Farjo AA, Sugar A, Schallhorn SC, et al. Femtosecond lasers for LASIK flap creation: a report by the American Academy of Ophthalmology. *Ophthalmology*. 2013;120(3):e5–e20.

Transient light sensitivity

After femtosecond LASIK, some patients experience acute onset of pain and light sensitivity in an otherwise white and quiet eye with excellent UDVA. The cornea and flap interface appear normal. It has been speculated that an acute onset of ocular inflammation or dry eye is somehow related to use of the femtosecond laser. Treatment consists of frequent administration of topical corticosteroids and topical cyclosporine. Almost all cases respond to treatment and resolve in weeks to months.

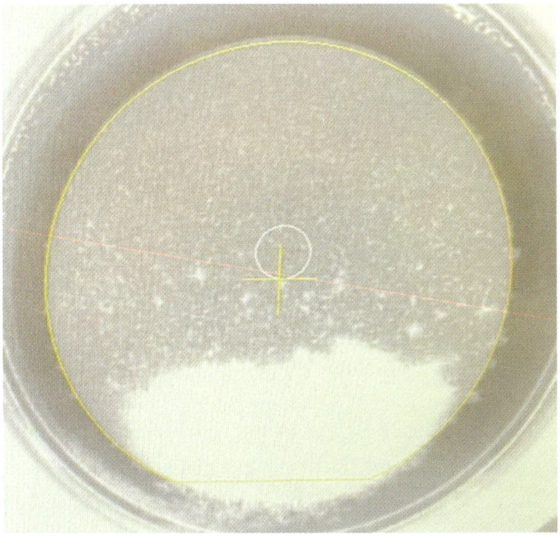

Figure 5-18 Opaque bubble layer after femtosecond laser–assisted LASIK flap creation. *(Courtesy of George O. Waring IV, MD.)*

Rainbow glare

Rainbow glare, an optical adverse effect of treatment with the femtosecond laser, is described as bands of color around white lights at night. This complication may be related to higher raster energy levels and increased length of time between service calls for the laser as well as the laser model and settings. One report described improvement with treatment of the stromal side of the flap, although rainbow glare tends to resolve with time.

Gatinel D, Saad A, Guilbert E, Rouger H. Simultaneous correction of unilateral rainbow glare and residual astigmatism by undersurface flap photoablation after femtosecond laser-assisted LASIK. *J Refract Surg.* 2015;31(6):406–410.

Zhang Y, Chen YG. High incidence of rainbow glare after femtosecond laser assisted-LASIK using the upgraded FS200 femtosecond laser. *BMC Ophthalmol.* 2018;18(1):71.

Ectasia

Corneal ectasia develops after excimer laser ablation when the corneal biomechanical integrity is reduced beyond its functional threshold. This complication results from performing surgery in patients who either are predisposed to developing corneal ectatic disorders or have a significantly reduced postablation residual stromal bed (see Chapter 2). Ectasia has been reported far more frequently after LASIK than after surface ablation. One large retrospective study estimated the post-LASIK ectasia rate at 0.033% in 2018, suggesting that improvements in screening have resulted in significant reduction compared to the 0.66% rate published by Pallikaris in 2001.

Retrospective analysis has found that ectasia is usually associated with LASIK performed in patients who had preoperative topographic abnormalities. Other risk factors include younger patient age, thinner corneas, and higher myopic corrections. In a series of patients who developed ectasia despite normal preoperative topography, the most significant factor was 40% or more tissue altered (see the sidebar Risk Factors for Ectasia in

Chapter 2). However, ectasia without any demonstrable risk factors has also been reported. Additional technologies being evaluated to reduce ectasia prevalence include corneal biomechanical analysis and use of artificial intelligence to evaluate preoperative topography.

Corneal crosslinking is the first-line treatment to stabilize the cornea. Often, functional visual acuity can be restored with rigid gas-permeable or hybrid contact lenses. The implantation of symmetric or asymmetric intrastromal ring segments to reduce the irregular astigmatism can help in selected cases. Crosslinking has been combined with simultaneous or sequential excimer laser treatment to reduce astigmatism. In extreme cases, corneal transplantation may be required. Treatment for unstable corneas is discussed in further detail in BCSC Section 8, *External Disease and Cornea,* Chapter 9.

American Academy of Ophthalmology Cornea/External Disease Panel. Preferred Practice Pattern Guidelines. *Corneal Ectasia.* American Academy of Ophthalmology; 2018. www.aao.org/ppp

Bohac M, Koncarevic M, Pasalic A, et al. Incidence and clinical characteristics of post LASIK ectasia: a review of over 30,000 LASIK cases. *Semin Ophthalmol.* 2018;33(7–8):867–877.

Randleman JB, Woodward M, Lynn MJ, Stulting RD. Risk assessment for ectasia after corneal refractive surgery. *Ophthalmology.* 2008;115(1):37–50.

Richoz O, Mavrakanas N, Pajic B, Hafezi F. Corneal collagen cross-linking for ectasia after LASIK and photorefractive keratectomy: long-term results. *Ophthalmology.* 2013;120(7):1354–1359.

Santhiago MR, Smadja D, Gomes BF, et al. Association between the percent tissue altered and post–laser in situ keratomileusis ectasia in eyes with normal preoperative topography. *Am J Ophthalmol.* 2014;158(1):87–95.e1.

Seiler T, Koufala K, Richter G. Iatrogenic keratectasia after laser in situ keratomileusis. *J Refract Surg.* 1998;14(3):312–317.

Rare Complications

Rare and sometimes coincidental complications of LASIK include optic nerve ischemia, premacular subhyaloid hemorrhage, macular hemorrhage associated with preexisting lacquer cracks or choroidal neovascularization, choroidal infarcts, postoperative corneal edema associated with preoperative cornea guttae, and ring scotoma. Binocular diplopia may occur in patients whose refractive error has been corrected and who have iatrogenic monovision, improper control of accommodation, or decompensated phorias.

Gimbel HV, Penno EE, van Westenbrugge JA, Ferensowicz M, Furlong MT. Incidence and management of intraoperative and early postoperative complications in 1000 consecutive laser in situ keratomileusis cases. *Ophthalmology.* 1998;105(10):1839–1848.

Mehta A, Reed D, Miller KE. Diplopia and strabismus after corneal refractive surgery. *Mil Med.* 2020;185(5–6):e755–e758.

CHAPTER 6

Femtosecond Lenticule Extraction

This chapter includes a related video. Go to www.aao.org/bcscvideo_section13 or scan the QR code in the text to access this content.

Highlights

- Small-incision lenticule extraction (SMILE) offers an alternative to surface ablation or laser in situ keratomileusis (LASIK) refractive surgery.
- SMILE uses a femtosecond laser to remove a refractive lenticule to treat myopia and astigmatism.
- Clinical outcomes of SMILE are comparable to those of photorefractive keratectomy or LASIK at 6 months.

Refractive Lenticule Extraction

In 1996, investigators first described the use of a picosecond laser to generate an intrastromal lenticule that was removed manually after the flap was lifted. The main drawbacks of this procedure, which was a precursor to modern refractive lenticule extraction (commonly referred to as *ReLEx*), were the relatively low precision and accuracy of the laser. In 1998, the first studies involving this technology were performed in rabbit eyes and in partially sighted eyes.

Following the debut of the VisuMax femtosecond laser (Carl Zeiss Meditec) in 2007, the intrastromal lenticule method was reintroduced in a procedure named *femtosecond lenticule extraction* (commonly referred to as *FLEx*). This procedure involved intrastromal dissection of a refractive lenticule as well as creation of a corneal flap and was performed entirely with a femtosecond laser. The refractive results were similar to those observed with laser in situ keratomileusis (LASIK), but the visual recovery time was longer.

More recently, a method called *small-incision lenticule extraction (SMILE)* was developed. This technique employs a 1043-nm laser that fires at 500 kHz with a pulse duration of 220–580 fs. Although SMILE is a form of lenticule extraction, it has the advantage of being performed entirely within a pocket, obviating the need for a flap. SMILE obtained Conformité Européenne marking in 2009 and received US Food and Drug Administration approval in September 2016.

Krueger RR, Juhasz T, Gualano A, Marchi V. The picosecond laser for nonmechanical laser in situ keratomileusis. *J Refract Surg.* 1998;14(4):467–469.

Reinstein DZ, Archer TJ, Carp GI. *The Surgeon's Guide to SMILE (Small Incision Lenticule Extraction).* Slack Inc; 2018.

Sekundo W, Kunert KS, Blum M. Small incision corneal refractive surgery using the small incision lenticule extraction (SMILE) procedure for the correction of myopia and myopic astigmatism: results of a 6-month prospective study. *Br J Ophthalmol.* 2011;95(3):335–339.

Shah R, Shah S. Effect of scanning patterns on the results of femtosecond laser lenticule extraction refractive surgery. *J Cataract Refract Surg.* 2011;37(9):1636–1647.

US Food and Drug Administration. Summary of Safety and Effectiveness Data. VisuMax Femtosecond Laser System for Refractive Correction. September 13, 2016. Accessed October 6, 2021. https://www.accessdata.fda.gov/cdrh_docs/pdf15/P150040B.pdf

Vestergaard A, Ivarsen A, Asp S, Hjortdal JØ. Femtosecond (FS) laser vision correction procedure for moderate to high myopia: a prospective study of ReLEx(®) FLEx and comparison with a retrospective study of FS-laser in situ keratomileusis. *Acta Ophthalmol.* 2013;91(4):355–362.

Indications and Preoperative Evaluation

The SMILE procedure is currently approved for the treatment of myopia with or without astigmatism from −1.00 D to −10.00 D sphere, and −0.75 D to −3.00 D cylinder with a manifest refraction spherical equivalent greater than −10.00 D in the eye to be treated in patients aged 22 years or older who have documentation of stable manifest refraction over the past year. Clinical trials are under way investigating the use of SMILE to treat hyperopia. Preoperative evaluation is similar to that for patients undergoing photoablative procedures such as LASIK or photorefractive keratectomy (PRK). (See Chapter 2 for additional details.) As in all refractive procedures involving tissue removal, a primary goal of evaluation is to exclude patients with corneal ectatic diseases or susceptibility to postoperative ectasia. Table 6-1 reviews relative contraindications for SMILE.

Table 6-1 Relative Contraindications to SMILE

Insufficient corneal tissue thickness for the amount of correction needed
Abnormal findings on topography/tomography
Unstable refraction
Irregular astigmatism
Severe or untreated dry eye
Active eye infection or inflammation
Active or prior herpetic keratitis or neurotrophic keratitis
Autoimmune or connective tissue disease (eg, rheumatoid arthritis, systemic lupus erythematosus)
Uncontrolled glaucoma
Uncontrolled diabetes
Pregnancy or lactation
Unrealistic patient expectations
Hyperopic treatments (studies currently under way)

SMILE = small-incision lenticule extraction.

Ambrósio R Jr, Ramos I, Lopes B, et al. Ectasia susceptibility before laser vision correction. *J Cataract Refract Surg.* 2015;41(6):1335–1336.

US Food and Drug Administration. VisuMax Femtosecond Laser. Approval for expanded indications. October 4, 2018. Accessed October 6, 2021. https://www.accessdata.fda.gov/cdrh_docs/pdf15/p150040s003a.pdf

Use of the VisuMax Femtosecond Laser Lenticule Removal Procedure for the Correction of Hyperopia (V1601CI). Accessed October 6, 2021. https://clinicaltrials.gov/ct2/show/NCT03431571

Advantages of SMILE

As the popularity of SMILE increases, its theoretical advantages in comparison to PRK and LASIK are becoming better understood. For example, no flap is created in SMILE, resulting in a potentially more biomechanically stable cornea (preservation of stronger anterior corneal lamellae compared with LASIK) and less disruption of anterior corneal innervation (reduced dry eye symptoms). The procedure may be particularly appropriate for patients who are involved in contact sports or high-risk professions. In addition, environmental factors such as ambient air quality, temperature, and humidity have less impact on refractive outcomes of SMILE compared with LASIK; and the excimer lasers used in LASIK and PRK have more stringent specifications with respect to these factors, which can affect treatment predictability.

Guo H, Hosseini-Moghaddam SM, Hodge W. Corneal biomechanical properties after SMILE versus FLEX, LASIK, LASEK, or PRK: a systematic review and meta-analysis. *BMC Ophthalmol.* 2019;19(1):167.

Walter KA, Stevenson AW. Effect of environmental factors on myopic LASIK enhancement rates. *J Cataract Refract Surg.* 2004;30(4):798–803.

Wong AHY, Cheung RKY, Kua WN, Shih KC, Chan TCY, Wan KH. Dry eyes after SMILE. *Asia Pac J Ophthalmol (Phila).* 2019;8(5):397–405.

Disadvantages of SMILE

Compared with LASIK, the potential drawbacks of SMILE include a smaller therapeutic range (no hyperopic treatments, limited astigmatic treatment), slower visual recovery, longer procedure time, lack of automated cyclotorsion compensation for astigmatism correction, and the inability to perform wavefront-guided or topography-guided treatments. In addition, SMILE enhancements are generally performed with PRK, and although there are claims for stronger biomechanics, corneal ectasia is still possible. Many of these drawbacks may be eliminated or improved by further development and innovations in the hardware and software delivering SMILE treatments.

Surgical Technique

SMILE is generally performed as an office-based procedure under topical anesthesia. A curved interface is placed on the eye to dock with the femtosecond laser. Centration is achieved by having the patient look at a fixation light and confirming fixation with an infrared light. During SMILE, the femtosecond laser first creates the lower interface of the intrastromal lenticule (using an *out-to-in* direction to minimize the time that the patient's

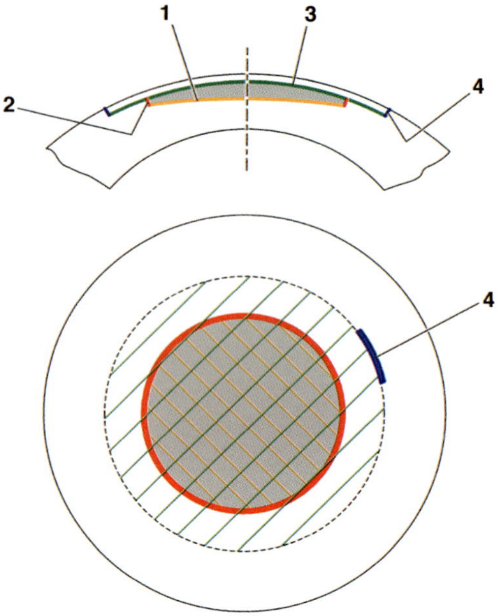

Figure 6-1 Incisional geometry of the SMILE procedure. *1,* Lenticule cut (under side of lenticule). *2,* Lenticule side cut. *3,* Cap cut (concurrently upper side of lenticule). *4,* Cap opening incision. *(Reproduced from Reinstein DZ, Archer TJ, Gobbe M. Small incision lenticule extraction (SMILE) history, fundamentals of a new refractive surgery technique and clinical outcomes.* Eye Vis (Lond). *2014;1:3.)*

central vision is blurred) and then the upper interface of the lenticule (using an *in-to-out* direction). The laser then makes a side cut to allow access to the newly created refractive lenticule (Fig 6-1). The total time to complete the incisions is between 20 and 35 seconds, regardless of the magnitude of the refractive error.

A spatula is then inserted through the tunnel incision to separate residual lenticular attachments, first within the anterior lamella and then within the posterior plane. After both planes have been separated, microforceps are used to extract the intrastromal lenticule (Fig 6-2). The corneal pocket is hydrated with balanced salt solution, and the corneal epithelial surface is gently squeegeed with a moist surgical sponge. Topical antibiotics, anti-inflammatories, and lubricants are placed. The treatment is repeated on the fellow eye if indicated (Video 6-1).

VIDEO 6-1 Small-incision lenticule extraction procedure.
Courtesy of William F. Wiley, MD.

Moshirfar M, McCaughey MV, Reinstein DZ, Shah R, Santiago-Caban L, Fenzl CR. Small-incision lenticule extraction. *J Cataract Refract Surg.* 2015;41(3):652–665.

Reinstein DZ, Archer TJ, Gobbe M. Small incision lenticule extraction (SMILE) history, fundamentals of a new refractive surgery technique and clinical outcomes. *Eye Vis (Lond).* 2014;1:3. Published 2014 Oct 16.

Outcomes

Several studies have compared refractive outcomes of SMILE with those of LASIK. Overall, studies have shown that SMILE results are nearly identical to those of femtosecond laser–assisted LASIK (FS-LASIK). Currently, the disadvantage of SMILE is its slightly

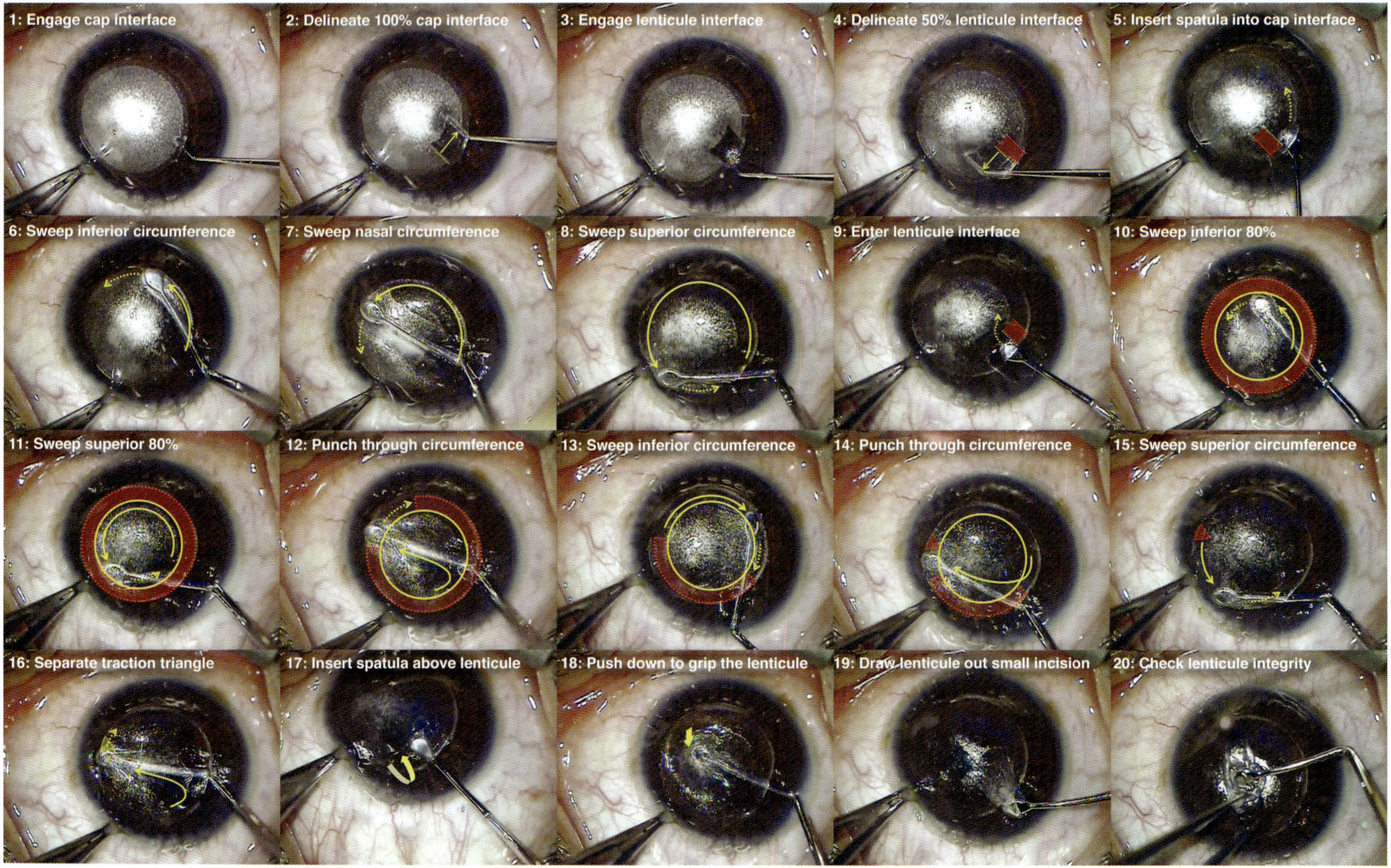

Figure 6-2 Series of still images showing standard lenticule removal technique. *(Used with permission from Reinstein D, Archer J.* The Surgeon's Guide to SMILE: Small Incision Lenticule Extraction. *SLACK Incorporated; 2018.)*

slower visual recovery on postoperative day 1 (Fig 6-3). In a study comparing SMILE with FS-LASIK, the uncorrected distance visual acuity (UDVA) in the LASIK group was at first statistically better than in the SMILE group, but at 6 months, no difference in vision was observed between the 2 groups. In addition, spherical aberration was lower in the SMILE group. Another study reported that 84% of eyes in each group achieved a UDVA of 20/20; however, 12% in the SMILE group and 4% in the LASIK group achieved a UDVA of 20/15. Higher-order aberrations, postoperative dry eye, and glare were significantly more common in the LASIK group. A recent study reported similar outcomes as in prior studies, although a higher—but not statistically significant—percentage of patients in the SMILE group (80%) than in the FS-LASIK group (65%) were within ±0.5 D of the attempted spherical equivalent at 3 years. Another study showed no statistical difference in refractive outcomes in a contralateral eye study comparing SMILE with FS-LASIK at 5 years.

Ganesh S, Gupta R. Comparison of visual and refractive outcomes following femtosecond laser–assisted LASIK with SMILE in patients with myopia or myopic astigmatism. *J Refract Surg.* 2014;30(9):590–596.

Han T, Xu Y, Han X, et al. Three-year outcomes of small incision lenticule extraction (SMILE) and femtosecond laser–assisted laser in situ keratomileusis (FS-LASIK) for myopia and myopic astigmatism. *Br J Ophthalmol.* 2019;103(4):565–568.

Liu M, Chen Y, Wang D, et al. Clinical outcomes after SMILE and femtosecond laser–assisted LASIK for myopia and myopic astigmatism: a prospective randomized comparative study. *Cornea.* 2016;35(2):210–216.

Tülü Aygün B, Çankaya Kİ, Ağca A, et al. Five-year outcomes of small-incision lenticule extraction vs femtosecond laser–assisted laser in situ keratomileusis: a contralateral eye study. *J Cataract Refract Surg.* 2020;46(3):403–409.

Complications

Studies have reported a low incidence of complications related to SMILE. Because the procedure can be technically challenging, most of the complications described in the literature occurred early in the surgeon's learning curve. In a study that enrolled 1800 eyes treated with

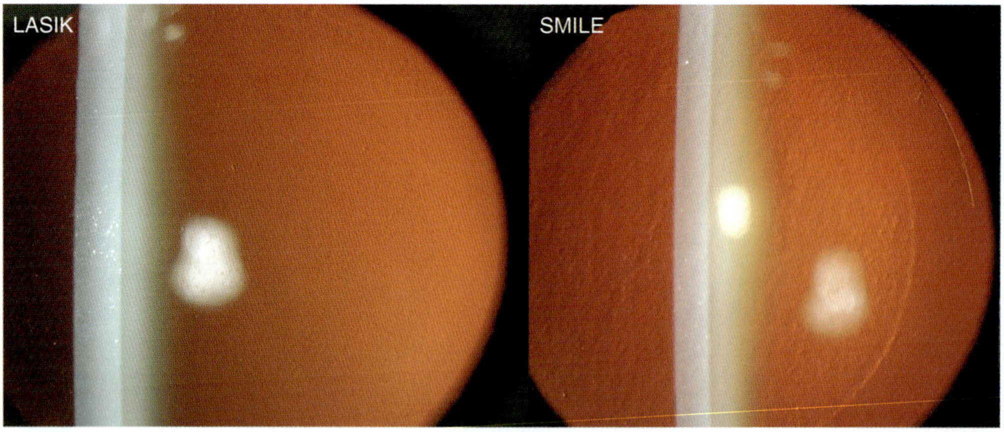

Figure 6-3 Slit-lamp retroillumination photograph at the 1-day postoperative visit comparing LASIK and SMILE. *(Used with permission from Reinstein D, Archer J.* The Surgeon's Guide to SMILE: Small Incision Lenticule Extraction. *SLACK Incorporated; 2018.)*

SMILE, perioperative complications included epithelial abrasions (6.0% of eyes), difficult lenticule extraction (1.9%), small tears in the cornea at the incision (1.8%), and cap perforation (0.22%); a major tear occurred in 1 eye (0.06%) (Fig 6-4). However, none of these patients reported late visual symptoms. Postoperative complications included trace haze (8.0%), epithelial dryness on postoperative day 1 (5.0%), interface inflammation secondary to central abrasion (0.3%), and minor interface infiltrates (0.3%). Topographic irregular astigmatism was described in 1.0% of eyes, resulting in reduced 3-month corrected distance visual acuity or ghost images. A complication unique to SMILE is the presence of a lenticule remnant in the interface. Diffuse lamellar keratitis and postoperative ectasia have also been reported.

Dong Z, Zhou X. Irregular astigmatism after femtosecond laser refractive lenticule extraction. *J Cataract Refract Surg.* 2013;39(6):952–954.

Ivarsen A, Asp S, Hjortdal J. Safety and complications of more than 1500 small-incision lenticule extraction procedures. *Ophthalmology.* 2014;121(4):822–828.

Moshirfar M, Albarracin JC, Desautels JD, Birdsong OC, Linn SH, Hoopes PC Sr. Ectasia following small-incision lenticule extraction (SMILE): a review of the literature. *Clin Ophthalmol.* 2017;11:1683–1688.

Zhao J, He L, Yao P, et al. Diffuse lamellar keratitis after small-incision lenticule extraction. *J Cataract Refract Surg.* 2015;41(2):400–407.

Re-treatment After SMILE

Surgeons have different options for re-treatment to improve refractive outcomes after SMILE, and the choice is often dictated by the primary cap thickness and the availability of the technology. The cap may be converted into a flap, and a thin-flap LASIK procedure may be performed. PRK may also be used to re-treat SMILE patients. However, a primary SMILE cannot be enhanced with an additional SMILE procedure.

In a retrospective study of surface ablation enhancement after SMILE, PRK was performed on 43 of 1963 eyes treated with SMILE (≈2%). The spherical equivalent was −6.35 ± 1.31 D before SMILE and −0.86 ± 0.43 D before the PRK. Surface ablation was performed after a mean of 9.82 ± 5.27 months and resulted in a spherical equivalent of 0.03 ± 0.57 D at 3 months ($P < .0001$). The number of patients within ±0.5 and ±1.0 D of their target refraction increased, respectively, from 23% to 80% and from 73% to 93%. In these 43 PRK-enhanced eyes, mean uncorrected distance acuity improved from 0.23 ± 0.20 logMAR (a little worse than 20/32) to 0.08 ± 0.15 logMAR (about 20/20; $P < .0001$).

Riau AK, Ang HP, Lwin NC, Chaurasia SS, Tan DT, Mehta JS. Comparison of four different VisuMax circle patterns for flap creation after small incision lenticule extraction. *J Refract Surg.* 2013;29(4):236–244.

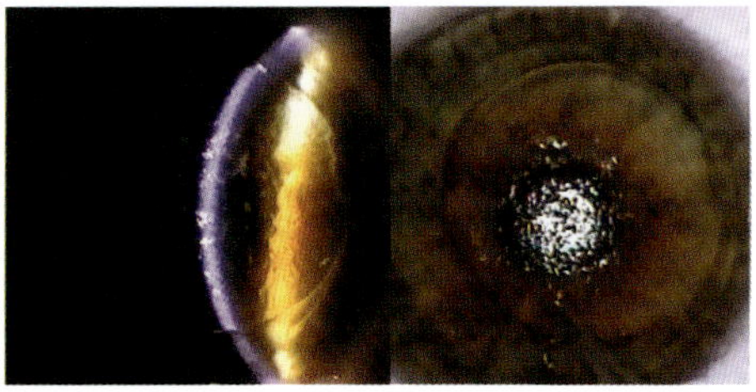

Figure 6-4 Intraoperative photograph of an extracted lenticule placed on the cornea at the end of a case. There is a small sliver of tissue missing at 2 o'clock. *(Used with permission from Reinstein D, Archer J.* The Surgeon's Guide to SMILE: Small Incision Lenticule Extraction. *SLACK Incorporated; 2018.)*

Siedlecki J, Luft N, Kook D, et al. Enhancement after myopic small incision lenticule extraction (SMILE) using surface ablation. *J Refract Surg.* 2017;33(8):513–518.
Zhao J, Yao P, Chen Z, et al. Enhancement of femtosecond lenticule extraction for visual symptomatic eye after myopia correction. *BMC Ophthalmol.* 2014;14:68.

Emerging Technologies

Currently, several manufacturers are developing SMILE platforms. Technique and treatment algorithms continue to evolve, which should lead to enhanced outcomes. Indications continue to expand, with current studies under way for hyperopic treatment profiles.

CHAPTER 7

Refractive Surgery in Ocular and Systemic Disease

Highlights

- Patients should be screened for ocular surface disease, which can negatively affect refractive outcomes.
- Keratoconus is a contraindication to refractive surgery, and patients should be screened with topography or tomography to assess risk of corneal ectatic disease before surgery.
- Myopic patients undergoing excimer laser refractive surgery do not have a higher risk of retinal detachment than the general population of myopes.
- Refractive surgery can be beneficial in certain patients with anisometropic amblyopia or accommodative burden.
- Corneal diseases such as endothelial dysfunction and prior herpes simplex virus or other types of infectious keratitis are relative contraindications to refractive surgery.
- Systemic autoimmune disease may lead to complications after refractive surgery, so patients with such diseases warrant special evaluation and coordination with other providers preoperatively.

Introduction

Over the past decades, refractive surgery has evolved into a subspecialty with increasingly precise laser-assisted procedures that play an important role in the surgical armamentarium of today's ophthalmologists. As the cumulative number of patients who have undergone refractive surgery has grown, so has the prevalence of patients with concomitant known ocular or systemic diseases who wish to undergo these procedures.

Many patients who would have been excluded from the original US Food and Drug Administration (FDA) clinical trials have since been successfully treated with refractive surgery, and some formerly absolute contraindications are now considered to be relative contraindications. With increased experience, surgeons have performed laser in situ keratomileusis (LASIK) and photorefractive keratectomy (PRK) safely and effectively in patients with concomitant ocular or systemic diseases. However, laser vision correction (LVC) procedures in these patients are considered off-label. Performing off-label surgery is permissible if the surgeon judges that the benefit of a procedure outweighs the potential risk. In these cases, it is the surgeon's ethical, legal, and medical responsibility to explain the concept of off-label surgery to the patient, to determine whether the procedure meets the standard of care in the community, and to candidly discuss the potential risks and benefits with the patient. In the era of collaborative care, the surgeon may find that consultation with the patient's primary physician or rheumatologist provides important information about the patient's systemic health and may allow optimization of underlying chronic disease.

American Academy of Ophthalmology Refractive Management/Intervention Panel. Preferred Practice Pattern Guidelines. *Refractive Errors & Refractive Surgery.* American Academy of Ophthalmology; 2017. www.aao.org/ppp

Bower KS, Woreta F. Update on contraindications for laser-assisted in situ keratomileusis and photorefractive keratectomy. *Curr Opin Ophthalmol.* 2014;25(4):251–257.

Ocular Conditions

Ocular Surface Disease

Because ocular surface disease (OSD) can affect the outcome of keratorefractive procedures, the surgeon should identify and address OSD as needed before performing surgery. Dry eye after LASIK is the most common and anticipated consequence of LVC, although symptoms are typically self-limited. Many patients seeking refractive surgery have preexisting dry eye disease that caused them to become intolerant of contact lenses; thus, a history of contact lens intolerance should suggest the possibility of underlying dry eye. During the informed consent discussion, patients should be cautioned that their dry eye condition could worsen postoperatively or later in life, possibly leading to additional discomfort or decreased vision that could be permanent.

A preoperative screening algorithm suggests that all refractive patients should be assessed for signs and symptoms of OSD. Questionnaires and modern point-of-care testing—such as tear film osmolarity and matrix metalloproteinase (MMP)-9 assays—allow clinicians to diagnose OSD in potential refractive surgery patients at an earlier stage than with traditional approaches such as reliance on examination findings or patient-reported symptoms alone. Hyperosmolarity has been associated with increased variance in refractive measurements, and elevated MMP-9 levels have been found in patients with abnormal corneal epithelial function.

External examination should include evaluation of eyelid anatomy and function for conditions, including incomplete blink, lagophthalmos, entropion, ectropion, and eyelid notching. The conjunctiva should be examined for the presence of conjunctival chalasis, subconjunctival fibrosis, or symblepharon. Meibomian gland dysfunction has a high prevalence, and oil flow and gland architecture should be assessed in addition to tear film quantity and quality. Commonly performed tear film parameter tests include osmolarity; MMP-9; tear breakup time; and staining with fluorescein, lissamine green, or rose bengal. Imaging the tear lipid layer and performing meibography are also valuable screening tools. Corneal topography should be reviewed for evidence of irregularity or poor image quality, which often indicates an unstable tear film or epithelial basement membrane dystrophy.

In addition to OSD assessment, screening questions should include a review of any history of connective tissue diseases or conjunctival cicatrizing disorders. These conditions are relative contraindications to refractive procedures and should be addressed prior to any surgical consideration (see Chapter 2).

Optimizing the ocular surface

The clinician's goal should be to improve the quality of the tear film, clear the cornea of any punctate erosions, and resolve OSD symptoms before surgery. In addition to typical symptoms of OSD, such as foreign body sensation, fluctuating vision between blinks may occur, so optimization of the ocular surface is necessary to achieve optimal visual quality. A delay in surgery may be necessary to allow time for treatment response.

Treatment of OSD may include topical tear replacement; punctal occlusion; use of topical anti-inflammatory drugs such as corticosteroids, cyclosporine, or lifitegrast (see BCSC Section 8, *External Disease and Cornea*); and meibomian gland therapeutic procedures. Often, combination therapy is instituted. Dietary supplements containing omega fatty acids, such as from flaxseed or fish oil, have been shown to improve OSD symptoms in some studies. Meibomian gland inflammation may also benefit from oral or topical macrolides such as doxycycline or azithromycin.

Postoperative ocular surface disease

In LVC, the severing of corneal nerves during flap creation or ablation of corneal tissue may cause corneal anesthesia. Although most patients have temporary anesthesia lasting 3–6 months, others may have persistent dysfunction. After LVC, patients may develop punctate epithelial erosions, decreased tear production, reduced tear breakup time, and related symptoms as a result of the temporary neurotrophic state of the cornea. In a review of patients who had undergone LASIK, dry eye symptoms and blepharitis were the most common diagnoses among patients dissatisfied with the procedure, even those who had obtained good postoperative visual outcomes. In the great majority of these patients, symptoms resolved 3–6 months after surgery, but those whose symptoms persisted were among the least satisfied in this series.

American Academy of Ophthalmology Cornea/External Disease Panel. Preferred Practice Pattern Guidelines. *Blepharitis.* American Academy of Ophthalmology; 2018. www.aao.org/ppp

American Academy of Ophthalmology Cornea/External Disease Panel. Preferred Practice Pattern Guidelines. *Dry Eye Syndrome.* American Academy of Ophthalmology; 2018. www.aao.org/ppp

Bower KS, Sia RK, Ryan DS, Mines MJ, Dartt DA. Chronic dry eye in photorefractive keratectomy and laser in situ keratomileusis: manifestations, incidence, and predictive factors. *J Cataract Refract Surg.* 2015;41(12):2624–2634.

Levinson BA, Rapuano CJ, Cohen EJ, Hammersmith KM, Ayres BD, Laibson PR. Referrals to the Wills Eye Institute Cornea Service after laser in situ keratomileusis: reasons for patient dissatisfaction. *J Cataract Refract Surg.* 2008;34(1):32–39.

Salib GM, McDonald MB, Smolek M. Safety and efficacy of cyclosporine 0.05% drops versus unpreserved artificial tears in dry-eye patients having laser in situ keratomileusis. *J Cataract Refract Surg.* 2006;32(5):772–778.

Starr CE, Gupta PK, Farid M, et al. An algorithm for the preoperative diagnosis and treatment of ocular surface disorders. *J Cataract Refract Surg.* 2019;45(5):669–684.

Herpes Simplex and Herpes Zoster Virus Infection

Many surgeons avoid LVC in patients with a history of herpes simplex virus (HSV) keratitis because trauma from the lamellar dissection or exposure to the excimer laser may reactivate the virus and cause recurrent HSV keratitis. However, some authors have concluded that such recurrence reflects the natural course of the disease rather than reactivation due to excimer laser ablation.

The role of excimer laser ablation in inciting recurrence of HSV keratitis has been investigated in the laboratory. Rabbits infected with HSV type 1 demonstrated viral reactivation after exposure of the corneal stroma to 193-nm ultraviolet radiation during PRK and LASIK. The use of systemic valacyclovir before the laser treatment decreased the rate of recurrence in the rabbit model. In another rabbit study, systemic valacyclovir reduced ocular shedding of HSV after LASIK.

Reactivation of HSV keratitis has been reported in humans after radial keratotomy (RK), phototherapeutic keratectomy (PTK), PRK, and LASIK. Fagerholm and colleagues reported a 25% incidence of postoperative HSV keratitis in the 17 months after excimer laser compared with a 45% recurrence rate in an equivalent period before the laser. The authors concluded that the procedure does not seem to significantly increase the incidence of recurrences.

A retrospective review of 13,200 PRK-treated eyes with no history of corneal HSV revealed a 0.14% incidence of HSV keratitis. Of these cases, 16.5% occurred within 10 days of the procedure; the authors postulated that this finding may indicate a direct effect of the excimer ultraviolet laser. In 78% of cases, HSV keratitis occurred within 15 weeks, which could be related to the corticosteroid therapy.

Cases of reactivation of herpes zoster ophthalmicus after LASIK have also been reported, with some authors suggesting the benefit of topical and oral antiviral treatment. There are anecdotal reports of flap interface inflammation resembling diffuse lamellar keratitis after LASIK in patients with herpes simplex or herpes zoster keratitis. In these cases, topical corticosteroids may also be required.

Because of the potential for vision loss from recurrence of HSV keratitis, some refractive surgeons consider prior herpetic keratitis a contraindication to refractive surgery. Others may consider performing PRK, PTK, or LASIK in patients with a history of HSV keratitis who have not had any recent recurrences and who have good corneal sensation, minimal or no corneal vascularization or scarring, and normal corrected distance visual acuity (CDVA). Preoperative and postoperative prophylaxis with systemic antiviral drugs should be strongly considered in these patients. Results of the Herpetic Eye Disease Study (HEDS) showed a 50% reduction in the risk of recurrence with a prophylactic dose of oral acyclovir over the course of 1 year in patients with latent HSV with no inciting factors, such as treatment with an excimer laser. Patients with pronounced corneal hypoesthesia or anesthesia, vascularization, thinning and scarring, or recent herpetic attacks should not be considered candidates for refractive surgery. Any patient with a history of herpes simplex or herpes zoster keratitis should be counseled about the continued risk of recurrence and its potential to cause vision loss after excimer LVC.

Asbell PA. Valacyclovir for the prevention of recurrent herpes simplex virus eye disease after excimer laser photokeratectomy. *Trans Am Ophthalmol Soc.* 2000;98:285–303.

de Rojas Silva V, Rodriguez-Conde R, Cobo-Soriano R, Beltrán J, Llovet F, Baviera J. Laser in situ keratomileusis in patients with a history of ocular herpes. *J Cataract Refract Surg.* 2007;33(11):1855–1859.

Fagerholm P, Ohman L, Orndahl M. Phototherapeutic keratectomy in herpes simplex keratitis. Clinical results in 20 patients. *Acta Ophthalmol (Copenh).* 1994;72(4):457–460.

Jain V, Pineda R. Reactivated herpetic keratitis following laser in situ keratomileusis. *J Cataract Refract Surg.* 2009;35(5):946–948.

Levy J, Lapid-Gortzak R, Klemperer I, Lifshitz T. Herpes simplex virus keratitis after laser in situ keratomileusis. *J Refract Surg.* 2005;21(4):400–402.

Nagy ZZ, Keleman E, Kovács A. Herpes simplex keratitis after photorefractive keratectomy. *J Cataract Refract Surg.* 2003;29(1):222–223.

Keratoconus

Keratoconus is considered a contraindication to LASIK or surface ablation. Creating the LASIK flap weakens the cornea, resulting in a loss of structural integrity along with excimer removal of tissue. Therefore, LVC may significantly increase the risk of exacerbating the ectasia. Although advanced stages of keratoconus can be diagnosed by slit-lamp examination, more sensitive analyses using corneal topography, tomography, and pachymetry can reveal findings early in the disease process. There is no consensus on a specific test or measurement that is diagnostic of a corneal ectatic disorder, but corneal topography/tomography and corneal pachymetry should be part of the evaluation. Subtle corneal thinning, curvature, or elevation changes can be overlooked on slit-lamp evaluation.

In cases of forme fruste keratoconus where the fellow eye appears normal, studies have suggested several risk factors for progression to keratoconus in either eye or post-LASIK ectasia in the operated eye. These include interocular asymmetry of inferior corneal steepening or asymmetric bow-tie topographic patterns with skewed steep radial axes above and below the horizontal meridian (Fig 7-1). Patients with suspected keratoconus have

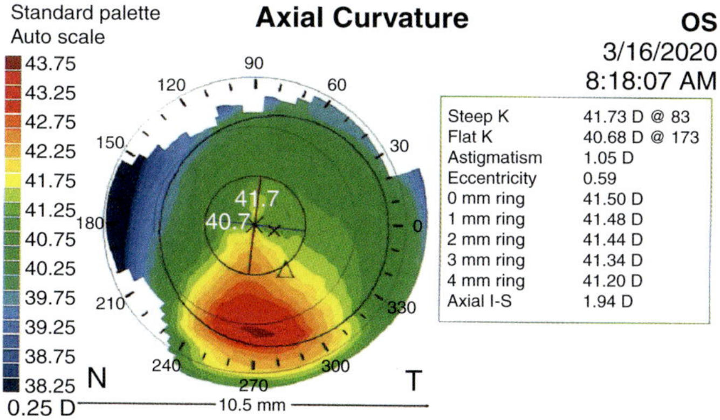

Figure 7-1 Corneal topographic map indicating keratoconus with asymmetric irregular steepening. *(Courtesy of Preeya K. Gupta, MD.)*

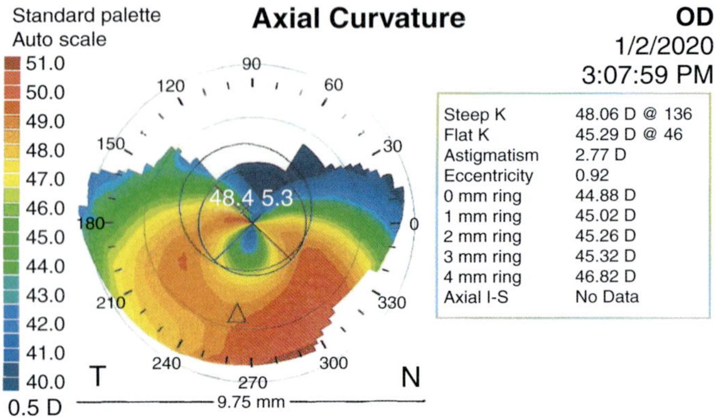

Figure 7-2 Topography of pellucid marginal degeneration showing the "crab-claw" pattern. N = nasal; T = temporal. *(Courtesy of Preeya K. Gupta, MD.)*

the aforementioned features in either or both eyes, and LVC should not be considered for them. Patients with an inferior "crab-claw" pattern accompanied by central flattening are at risk of developing pellucid marginal degeneration (Fig 7-2) or a "low-sagging cone" variety of keratoconus, even in the absence of clinical signs. This pattern may be designated "pellucid suspect," and LVC should be avoided in these eyes.

Global pachymetry measurements may help rule out forme fruste keratoconus. Posterior curvature evaluation with newer corneal imaging technology may also detect subtle disease (Fig 7-3). Often, the refractive surgeon is the first physician to detect and inform a patient of the presence of corneal ectasia. The patient may have excellent vision with glasses or contact lenses and may be seeking the convenience of a more permanent correction through LASIK. It is important for the ophthalmologist to clearly convey that although forme fruste keratoconus does not necessarily indicate the presence of a progressive disease, refractive surgery should not be performed because of the potential for unpredictable results and progressive vision loss. The patient should also be informed about the importance of follow-up examinations to monitor for any signs of progression. Corneal crosslinking with riboflavin administration and ultraviolet-A exposure can be used to slow or halt corneal ectasia. In addition, intrastromal corneal ring segments are FDA approved for use in keratoconus. (See BCSC Section 8, *External Disease and Cornea,* for further detail on these therapies.)

Alessio G, L'Abbate M, Sborgia C, La Tegola MG. Photorefractive keratectomy followed by cross-linking versus cross-linking alone for management of progressive keratoconus: two-year follow-up. *Am J Ophthalmol.* 2013;155(1):54–65.

Ambrósio R Jr, Alonso RS, Luz A, Coca Velarde LG. Corneal-thickness spatial profile and corneal-volume distribution: tomographic indices to detect keratoconus. *J Cataract Refract Surg.* 2006;32(11):1851–1859.

Belin MW, Asota IM, Ambrósio R, Khachikian SS. What's in a name: keratoconus, pellucid marginal degeneration, and related thinning disorders. *Am J Ophthalmol.* 2011;152(2):157–162.

Binder PS, Lindstrom RL, Stulting RD, et al. Keratoconus and corneal ectasia after LASIK. *J Cataract Refract Surg.* 2005;31(11):2035–2038.

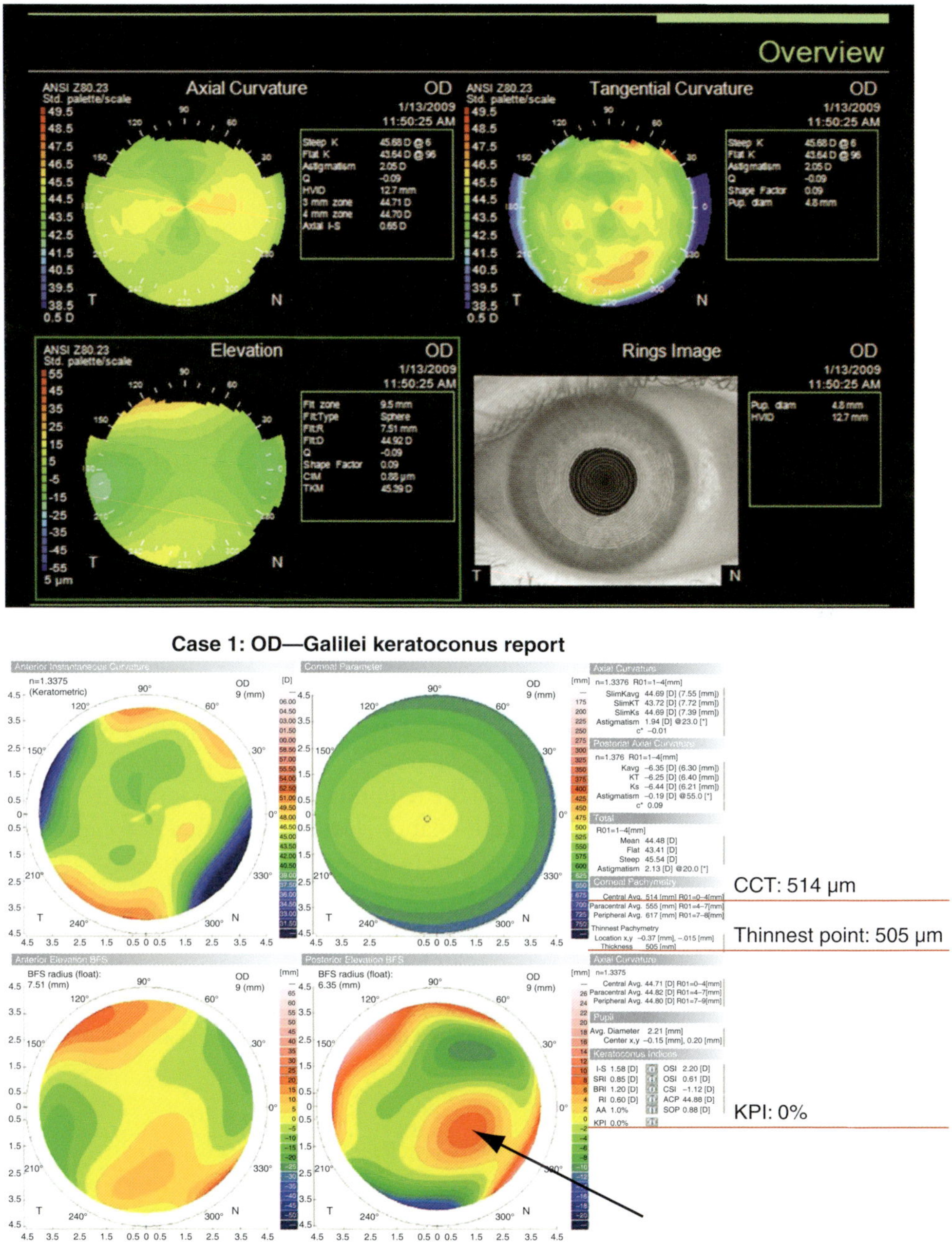

A

B

Figure 7-3 A 40-year-old man wishes to correct his myopia and high astigmatism. He does not wear contact lenses. His manifest refraction is –4.00 +3.00 × 4 OD and –3.75 +3.00 × 168 OS; corrected distance visual acuity is 20/20 OU. Both eyes appear normal on slit-lamp examination. **A,** Although the topographic examination appears normal on first glance, there is subtle inferior steepening that requires close inspection to appreciate. **B,** A clearly abnormal hot spot *(arrow)* is apparent on the dual Scheimpflug analyzer posterior elevation map, which is concerning for keratoconus. Technologies that evaluate regional corneal thickness and posterior corneal elevation in addition to anterior curvature may improve the identification of patients with early keratoconus. CCT = central corneal thickness; KPI = keratoconus prediction index. *(Courtesy of Douglas D. Koch, MD.)*

Randleman JB, Russell B, Ward MA, Thompson KP, Stulting RD. Risk factors and prognosis for corneal ectasia after LASIK. *Ophthalmology.* 2003;110(2):267–275.

Saad A, Gatinel D. Topographic and tomographic properties of forme fruste keratoconus corneas. *Invest Ophthalmol Vis Sci.* 2010;51(11):5546–5555.

Corneal Dystrophies

Epithelial basement membrane dystrophy (also called *map-dot-fingerprint dystrophy*) is a common corneal dystrophy that can be an incidental finding in many asymptomatic patients. In determining the safety of refractive surgery in these eyes, the surgeon must ensure that the irregularity in the epithelium is not affecting the refractive error. Generally, centrally located corneal irregularities should be considered visually significant. In cases of limited or isolated peripheral basement membrane dystrophy deemed stable enough to proceed with refractive surgery, surface ablation may be the preferred approach, as epithelial sloughing may occur more frequently with LASIK and lead to inflammation or epithelial ingrowth. In addition, surface ablation may help reduce irregular astigmatism and recurrent erosions, which are frequent in these patients.

Published reports on refractive surgery in patients with Fuchs endothelial dystrophy are limited. Among the small number of patients with mild guttae and a family history of Fuchs dystrophy who have been reported on after LASIK, the majority developed progressive corneal edema, loss of endothelial cells, and loss of CDVA. The progressive nature of this disease and the fluctuations in corneal refractive power due to variable edema make these eyes difficult to stabilize for accurate measurements and postoperative management. Patients who have guttae without edema or a family history of Fuchs may be better candidates for surface ablation in order to avoid the flap interface created in LASIK. The flap interface can act as a reservoir for fluid accumulation, leading to further decompensation of the cornea, and the flap may be more likely to be dislodged.

Moshirfar M, Feiz V, Feilmeier MR, Kang PC. Laser in situ keratomileusis in patients with corneal guttata and family history of Fuchs' endothelial dystrophy. *J Cataract Refract Surg.* 2005;31(12):2281–2286.

Vroman DT, Solomon KD, Holzer MP, Peng Q, Apple DJ, Bowie EM. Endothelial decompensation after laser in situ keratomileusis. *J Cataract Refract Surg.* 2002;28(11):2045–2049.

Post–Penetrating Keratoplasty

Refractive error after penetrating keratoplasty (PKP) is extremely common owing to the inherent imprecision of the operation, with many series documenting a mean postoperative astigmatism of 4.00–5.00 D. In many cases, these refractive errors are not amenable to spectacle correction and may require rigid gas-permeable contact lens correction to achieve good vision. However, contact lens fitting may not be successful in post-PKP patients because of abnormal corneal curvature or the patient's inability to tolerate or manipulate a contact lens.

Given the success of the excimer laser in treating myopia and astigmatism, PRK has been studied and used to treat post-PKP refractive errors. PRK has the disadvantages associated with epithelial removal in a corneal transplant and may lead to corneal haze when high refractive errors are treated. The use of prophylactic topical mitomycin C has made PRK a more acceptable treatment option after PKP. Although the refractive results are often good, surface ablation in patients who have had PKP is generally less predictable and less effective than it is for those with naturally occurring astigmatism and myopia.

Optimal timing of refractive surgery after PKP is controversial. All sutures should be removed, and the refraction should be stable. To avoid wound dehiscence, many surgeons wait at least 1 year after PKP, and an additional 4 months after all sutures are removed, before performing the refractive surgery. An interval of at least 18–24 months after PKP provides sufficient wound healing in most cases. No matter how much time has elapsed since the PKP surgery, the entirety of the graft–host wound should be carefully inspected to identify areas of variability in coaptation of the graft–host junction. Refraction and corneal topography should be stable, as documented by 2 consecutive readings on separate visits at least 1 month apart. Refractive surgery should be avoided if the corneal graft shows evidence of inflammation, diffuse vascularization, ectasia, inadequate healing of the graft–host interface, or refractive instability, or if there are signs of rejection or endothelial decompensation. Corneal graft rejection has been described after PRK; thus, higher and more prolonged dosing with topical corticosteroids should be considered for post-PKP refractive surgery patients to decrease this risk.

Fares U, Sarhan AR, Dua HS. Management of post-keratoplasty astigmatism. *J Cataract Refract Surg.* 2012;38(11):2029–2039.

Hardten DR, Chittcharus A, Lindstrom RL. Long term analysis of LASIK for the correction of refractive errors after penetrating keratoplasty. *Cornea.* 2004;23(5):479–489.

Huang PY, Huang PT, Astle WF, et al. Laser-assisted subepithelial keratectomy and photorefractive keratectomy for post-penetrating keratoplasty myopia and astigmatism in adults. *J Cataract Refract Surg.* 2011;37(2):335–340.

Ocular Hypertension and Glaucoma

Of particular concern in patients with ocular hypertension or primary open-angle glaucoma (POAG) is the effect of the acute rise in intraocular pressure (IOP) to more than 65 mm Hg when suction is applied during the creation of the stromal flap for LASIK or the epithelial flap for epi-LASIK. There have been reports of new visual field defects arising immediately after LASIK that are attributed to mechanical compression or ischemia of the optic nerve head from the temporary increase in IOP.

Evaluation of a patient with ocular hypertension or POAG includes a complete history and ocular examination with peripheral visual field testing and corneal pachymetry. A history of poor IOP control, nonadherence to treatment, maximal medical therapy, or prior surgical interventions may suggest progressive disease, which may be a contraindication for refractive surgery. The surgeon should also note the status of the angle, the presence and amount of optic nerve cupping, and the degree of visual field loss, especially if split fixation is present.

Several reports have confirmed that central corneal thickness affects Goldmann applanation tonometry (GAT) and Tono-Pen (Reichert Technologies) measurement of IOP (see the section Glaucoma After Refractive Surgery in Chapter 8). Studies have demonstrated that thinner-than-normal corneas give falsely low IOP readings, whereas thicker corneas give falsely high readings. Although all reports agree that central corneal thickness affects GAT IOP measurement, there is no consensus on a specific formula to compensate for this effect in clinical practice.

Myopic LVC removes tissue to reduce the steepness of the cornea; this sculpting process results in a thinner central cornea, which leads to artifactually lower IOP measurements postoperatively. Such inaccurately low measurements on central applanation tonometry hinder the diagnosis of corticosteroid-induced glaucoma after keratorefractive procedures, which can lead to optic nerve cupping, visual field loss, and decreased vision (Fig 7-4).

Because PRK and LASIK interfere with accurate measurement of IOP, these refractive procedures should not be considered for a patient whose IOP is poorly controlled. Furthermore, patients should be advised of the effect of refractive surgery on their IOP measurements and urged to inform future ophthalmologists about their surgery. Patients should be referred to a glaucoma specialist when indicated.

Patients with ocular hypertension often can safely undergo refractive surgery. Such patients should be counseled preoperatively that refractive surgery treats only the refractive error and not the natural history of the ocular hypertension, which sometimes progresses to glaucoma, accompanied by optic nerve cupping and visual field loss. The ophthalmologist should pay particular attention to the risk factors for progression to glaucoma, including older age, reduced corneal thickness, increased cup–disc ratio, family history of glaucoma, and elevated IOP. All patients with ocular hypertension should be informed of the greater difficulty in assessing IOP after excimer laser ablation.

The decision about whether to perform refractive surgery in a patient with glaucoma is controversial, although LASIK is contraindicated in any patient with marked optic nerve cupping, visual field loss, or visual acuity loss. There are no long-term studies of

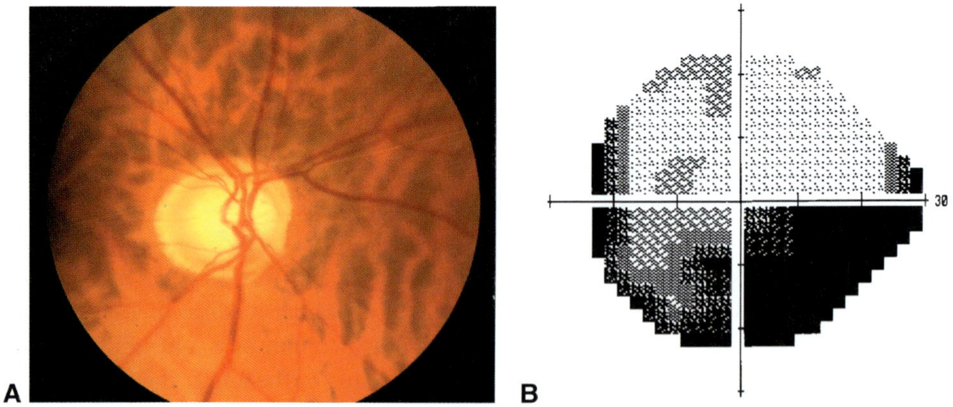

Figure 7-4 Glaucomatous optic nerve atrophy in a patient with "normal" intraocular pressure (IOP) after laser in situ keratomileusis (LASIK). **A,** Fundus photograph demonstrates increased cup–disc ratio in a patient who received a diagnosis of glaucoma 1 year after LASIK. The patient had decreased vision, with corrected distance visual acuity of 20/40 and IOP of 21 mm Hg. **B,** Humphrey 24-2 visual field with extensive inferior arcuate visual field loss corresponding to thinning of the superior optic nerve rim. *(Parts A and B courtesy of Jayne S. Weiss, MD.)*

refractive surgery in this population. The refractive surgeon may consider use of an ancillary informed consent that documents the patient's understanding that POAG may cause progressive vision loss independent of any refractive surgery and that IOP elevation during a LASIK or an epi-LASIK procedure or following LASIK or surface ablation (often due to a corticosteroid response) can cause glaucoma progression.

The surgeon should be aware that placement of a suction ring may not be possible if there is a functioning filtering bleb or a tube shunt. In rare cases in which both filtering surgery and LASIK are being planned, it is preferable to perform LASIK before the filter is placed, although the glaucoma surgery may induce astigmatism. Suction time should be minimized to decrease the chance of optic nerve damage from the transient increase in IOP. Alternatively, surface ablation may be preferable to avoid the IOP rise associated with LASIK flap creation. The surgeon must exercise caution when using postoperative corticosteroids because of their potential for elevating IOP. The patient should be informed as to when to resume postoperative topical medications for glaucoma. Finally, to avoid trauma to the flap, the surgeon generally should not check IOP for at least 72 hours after LASIK or until reepithelialization has occurred and bandage contact lenses have been removed after PRK.

Bashford KP, Shafranov G, Tauber S, Shields MB. Considerations of glaucoma in patients undergoing corneal refractive surgery. *Surv Ophthalmol.* 2005;50(3):245–251.

Hamilton DR, Manche EE, Rich LF, Maloney RK. Steroid-induced glaucoma after laser in situ keratomileusis associated with interface fluid. *Ophthalmology.* 2002;109(4):659–665.

Pepose JS, Feigenbaum SK, Qazi MA, Sanderson JP, Roberts CJ. Changes in corneal biomechanics and intraocular pressure following LASIK using static, dynamic, and noncontact tonometry. *Am J Ophthalmol.* 2007;143(1):39–47.

Schallhorn JM, Schallhorn SC, Ou Y. Factors that influence intraocular pressure changes after myopic and hyperopic LASIK and photorefractive keratectomy: a large population study. *Ophthalmology.* 2014;122(3):471–479.

Shaikh NM, Shaikh S, Singh K, Manche E. Progression to end-stage glaucoma after laser in situ keratomileusis. *J Cataract Refract Surg.* 2002;28(2):356–359.

Sharma N, Sony P, Gupta A, Vajpayee RB. Effect of laser in situ keratomileusis and laser-assisted subepithelial keratectomy on retinal nerve fiber layer thickness. *J Cataract Refract Surg.* 2006;32(3):446–450.

Yang CC, Wang IJ, Chang YC, Lin LL, Chen TH. A predictive model for postoperative intraocular pressure among patients undergoing laser in situ keratomileusis (LASIK). *Am J Ophthalmol.* 2006;141(3):530–536.

Retinal Disease

High myopia

Patients with high myopia are at increased risk of retinal tears and detachment. A thorough dilated retinal examination (including scleral depression, if indicated) should be performed on all patients with high myopia, and referral to a retina specialist should be considered for patients with predisposing retinal pathology. One study of 4800 consecutive patients in a private refractive surgery practice found that 52 (1.1%) had posterior segment pathology that required intervention. Another study of 29,916 myopic and hyperopic eyes undergoing LASIK demonstrated that 1.5% of patients required preoperative treatment of retinal pathology.

Brady J, O'Keefe M, Kilmartin D. Importance of fundoscopy in refractive surgery. *J Cataract Refract Surg.* 2007;33(9):1602–1607.

Retinal detachment

Patients with high myopia should be counseled that refractive surgery corrects only the refractive aspect of the myopia and not the natural history of the highly myopic eye and its known complications. Such patients remain at risk of retinal tears and detachment throughout their lives.

Although no causal link has been established between retinal detachment and excimer laser refractive surgery, the potential adverse effects should be considered. The rapid increase and then decrease in IOP could theoretically stretch the vitreous base, and the acoustic shock waves from the laser could play a role in the development of a posterior vitreous detachment. Although the actual risk to eyes with high myopia or preexisting retinal pathology has not been determined through well-controlled, long-term studies, current data suggest that LVC does not increase the incidence of retinal detachment. In a series of 1554 eyes that underwent LASIK for myopia with a mean refractive error of -13.52 ± 3.38 D, retinal detachments developed in 4 eyes (0.25%) at 11.25 ± 8.53 months after the procedure. Three of the eyes had retinal flap tears, and 1 eye had an atrophic hole. There was no statistically significant difference in CDVA before and after conventional retinal reattachment surgery, although a myopic shift was caused by the scleral buckle.

In a study of 38,823 eyes with mean myopia of –6.00 D, the frequency of rhegmatogenous retinal detachments at a mean of 16.3 months after LASIK was 0.8%. The eyes that developed retinal detachments had a mean preoperative myopia of –8.75 D. In a retrospective review, Blumenkranz reported that the frequency of retinal detachment after excimer laser treatment was similar to the frequency in the general population, averaging 0.034% over 2 years. Another study examined the frequency of rhegmatogenous retinal detachment over 10 years after LASIK in 11,594 patients with myopia. The frequency of detachment was 0.05% at 1 year, 0.15% at 5 years, and 0.19% at 10 years. All patients in this study had a preoperative retinal examination, and any predisposing retinal findings were treated before LASIK surgery.

The retinal detachment rate has been reported to be higher with intraocular procedures such as refractive lens exchange or phakic intraocular lens (IOL) implantation than with excimer laser treatment. Highly myopic eyes undergoing phakic IOL procedures are at risk of retinal detachment from the underlying high myopia as well as from the intraocular surgery. In a recent study of 1248 eyes receiving a phakic IOL, the yearly incidence of retinal detachment was 0.0013%, 0.029%, 0%, 0.011%, and 0.015%, respectively, for years 1 through 5 postoperatively.

Arevalo JF. Posterior segment complications after laser-assisted in situ keratomileusis. *Curr Opin Ophthalmol.* 2008;19(3):177–184.

Arevalo JF, Lasave AF, Torres F, Suarez E. Rhegmatogenous retinal detachment after LASIK for myopia of up to –10 diopters: 10 years of follow-up. *Graefes Arch Clin Exp Ophthalmol.* 2012;250(7):963–970.

Blumenkranz MS. LASIK and retinal detachment: should we be concerned? [editorial]. *Retina.* 2000;20(5):578–579.

Kanclerz P, Grzybowski A. Does corneal refractive surgery increase the risk of retinal detachment? A literature review and statistical analysis. *J Refract Surg.* 2019;35(8):517–524.

Rishi P, Attiku Y, Agarwal M, et al. Retinal detachment after phakic intraocular lens implantation: a 10-year multicenter study. *Ophthalmology.* 2019;126(8):1198–1200.

Previous retinal detachment surgery

Patients who have had prior scleral buckle surgery or vitrectomy may seek refractive surgery because of their myopia. A buckle can result in a myopic shift because of axial elongation of the eye. Refractive surgery can be considered in selected cases that have symptomatic ametropia with good CDVA. The surgeon should determine whether the scleral buckle or conjunctival scarring will interfere with placement of the suction ring in preparation for creation of the LASIK flap. If these conditions are thought to interfere, a surface ablation procedure may be preferable to LASIK. Preoperative informed consent is critical, as patients may not understand that CDVA will be limited by post-detachment retinal dysfunction despite anatomical repair. Both the patient and the surgeon should realize that the final visual results may not be as predictable as after refractive surgery in patients with normal anatomy. Patients should also be aware that if the scleral buckle needs to be removed, the refractive status could change dramatically. Unexpected corneal steepening has been reported in patients undergoing LASIK with previously placed scleral buckles.

Barequet IS, Levy J, Klemperer I, et al. Laser in situ keratomileusis for correction of myopia in eyes after retinal detachment surgery. *J Refract Surg.* 2005;21(2):191–193.

Amblyopia and Strabismus in Adults and Children

Amblyopia and anisometropic amblyopia

Amblyopia is defined as a decrease in visual acuity without evidence of organic eye disease, typically resulting from unequal visual stimulation during visual development. The prevalence of amblyopia is 2%–4% in the United States; up to half of these cases represent anisometropic amblyopia. Patients with anisometropia greater than 3.00 D between the 2 eyes are likely to develop amblyopia that may be more resistant to traditional amblyopia therapy, such as glasses, contact lenses, patching, or atropine penalization therapy, partly because of the significant amount of aniseikonia.

Evaluation of a patient with amblyopia should include a thorough medical history to identify any known cause of amblyopia, a history of ocular disease or surgery, assessment of ocular alignment and motility, and a comprehensive anterior segment and retinal examination. Patients should be referred to a strabismus specialist when indicated. Preoperative counseling of a patient with amblyopia should inform the patient that even after refractive surgery, the vision in the amblyopic eye will not be as good as that in the nonamblyopic eye. The patient should also understand that CDVA will likely be the same or similar, with or without refractive surgery, although in some cases there is improvement in CDVA.

Typically, refractive surgery is performed in this group of patients to treat high anisometropia or astigmatism in 1 eye or high refractive error in both eyes. LVC and phakic IOL implantation have been successfully performed in the more myopic, amblyopic eye in adult patients with anisometropic amblyopia. Some studies suggest that postoperative CDVA may even improve modestly compared with preoperative levels in a subset of adults who undergo refractive surgery. In a study of 327 amblyopic patients undergoing LASIK or PRK, CDVA improved more than 1 line in 45%, 2 lines in 22.9%, and 3 lines in 9.8% of patients. In a study of phakic IOL implantation in patients with greater than 3.00 D of anisometropia, there was an average gain of 3 lines of vision; 91% of eyes gained more than 1 line, and no eyes lost CDVA. This improvement in vision was attributed to an increase in magnification and a decrease in optical aberrations rather than an actual improvement in the amblyopia.

However, performing refractive surgery in the normal eye of an adult patient with amblyopia requires additional consideration. The decision depends on many factors, including the level of CDVA in the amblyopic eye and the normal eye as well as the ocular alignment. To increase safety, unilateral surgery in the amblyopic eye followed by surgery in the nonamblyopic eye may be considered. However, deviation in ocular alignment has been reported after unilateral LASIK for high myopia as a result of focus disparity causing esodeviation and impairment of fusion. In some cases, a preoperative contact lens trial may be helpful in assessing this potential risk. If CDVA in the amblyopic eye is 20/200 or worse, the patient would be considered legally blind if he or she were to lose significant vision after refractive surgery in the normal eye. In such cases, refractive surgery in the amblyopic eye may or may not offer much benefit, and proceeding with surgery in the nonamblyopic eye should be very carefully considered.

Alió JL, Ortiz D, Abdelrahman A, de Luca A. Optical analysis of visual improvement after correction of anisometropic amblyopia with a phakic intraocular lens in adult patients. *Ophthalmology.* 2007;114(4):643–647.

Kim SK, Lee JB, Han SH, Kim EK. Ocular deviation after unilateral laser in situ keratomileusis. *Yonsei Med J.* 2000;41(3):404–406.

CLINICAL EXAMPLE

Consider a patient with anisometropic amblyopia whose vision is corrected to 20/40 with −7.00 D in the right eye and to 20/20 with −1.00 D in the left eye. This patient may be an excellent candidate for refractive surgery in the amblyopic right eye because he or she probably cannot tolerate glasses to correct the anisometropic amblyopia and may not tolerate contact lenses. Even if the post-LASIK uncorrected distance visual acuity (UDVA) were worse than 20/40 in the amblyopic eye, it would be better than the pre-LASIK UDVA of counting fingers.

If the postoperative UDVA in the amblyopic right eye improved to 20/40, the patient could be considered for LVC of −1.00 D in the left eye. However, if the patient has presbyopia, some surgeons would discourage further intervention and discuss the potential advantages of the low myopia. In a younger patient with accommodation, some surgeons would inform the patient of the potential risks associated with treating the better eye but would perform the LVC.

Sakatani K, Jabbur NS, O'Brien TP. Improvement in best corrected visual acuity in amblyopic adult eyes after laser in situ keratomileusis. *J Cataract Refract Surg.* 2004;30(12):2517–2521.
Sorkin N, Varssano D, Smadja D, Klein A, Mimouni M, Rosenblatt A. Visual outcomes of laser vision correction in eyes with preoperative amblyopia. *J Cataract Refract Surg.* 2017;43(3):383–388.

Refractive surgery in children

Pediatric refractive surgery is more challenging because children's eyes and refractive status continue to change over time. Additional studies on the growing eye and the long-term effect of excimer laser treatment and phakic IOLs on the corneal endothelium and crystalline lens are needed to better assess the outcomes. Consequently, these procedures are off-label and are typically regarded as investigational.

However, some authors have reported the successful performance of LVC and phakic IOL implantation in children, mostly 8 years and older, when conventional therapies have failed. Most of these children were treated for anisometropic amblyopia in the more myopic eye. In these studies, refractive error was decreased and visual acuity was maintained or improved in moderately amblyopic eyes. Refractive surgery did not improve CDVA or stereopsis in children older than 8 years with densely amblyopic eyes because of their age. In a study of 40 children aged 1–6 years, PRK was performed (under general anesthesia) because they were unable to wear glasses or contact lenses for high myopia or anisometropic amblyopia from myopia. Patients were treated for existing amblyopia, and mean CDVA improved from 20/70 to 20/40. The study found that corneal haze developed postoperatively in 60% of the eyes. Most patients demonstrated increasing corneal clarity within 1 year, although 2 of 27 patients required PTK for the corneal haze. Regression of effect was attributed to a vigorous healing response and the axial myopic shift associated with growth.

Several studies have reported successful implantation of phakic IOLs in children with high anisometropia and amblyopia. This technique eliminates corneal wound-healing problems associated with keratorefractive procedures and may be considered in patients with high refractive error in whom the traditional methods of amblyopia therapy have failed. However, other potentially serious complications may ensue, depending on the type of phakic IOL. Such complications include progressive corneal endothelial cell loss, cataract formation, pupillary block glaucoma, and persistent inflammation, as well as the usual risks associated with intraocular surgery. Larger clinical trials are necessary to adequately evaluate the safety and efficacy of phakic IOLs in this age group. Furthermore, these patients should be monitored for endothelial cell loss and cataract.

Alió JL, Wolter NV, Piñero DP, et al. Pediatric refractive surgery and its role in the treatment of amblyopia: meta-analysis of the peer-reviewed literature. *J Refract Surg.* 2011;27(5):364–374.
Astle WF, Huang PT, Ells AL, Cox RG, Deschenes MC, Vibert HM. Photorefractive keratectomy in children. *J Cataract Refract Surg.* 2002;28(6):932–941.
Astle WF, Huang PT, Ereifej I, Paszuk A. Laser-assisted subepithelial keratectomy for bilateral hyperopia and hyperopic anisometropic amblyopia in children: one-year outcomes. *J Cataract Refract Surg.* 2010;36(2):260–267.
Lesueur LC, Arne JL. Phakic intraocular lens to correct high myopic amblyopia in children. *J Refract Surg.* 2002;18(5):519–523.

Paysse EA, Coats DK, Hussein MA, Hamill MB, Koch DD. Long-term outcomes of photorefractive keratectomy for anisometropic amblyopia in children. *Ophthalmology.* 2006;113(2):169–176.

Tychsen L, Packwood E, Berdy G. Correction of large amblyopiogenic refractive errors in children using the excimer laser. *J AAPOS.* 2005;9(3):224–233.

Accommodative esotropia

Uncorrected hyperopia can stimulate an increase in accommodation, leading to accommodative convergence. Esotropia arises from insufficient fusional divergence. Traditional treatment includes correction of hyperopia with glasses or contact lenses and muscle surgery for any residual esotropia. As a child ages, the hyperopia typically decreases, often with concomitant resolution of the accommodative esotropia. If significant hyperopia persists, glasses or contact lenses will continue to be needed to control the esotropia.

Before refractive surgery, it is important to perform an adequate cycloplegic refraction (using cyclopentolate 1%) on patients younger than 35 years who have intermittent strabismus or phoria. Accurate refraction is necessary to avoid residual postoperative hyperopia. Otherwise, the postoperative hyperopia may result in a new onset of esotropia with an accommodative element. Several studies performed outside the United States have reported on the use of PRK or LASIK for adults with accommodative esotropia. In one of the studies, orthophoria or microesotropia was achieved after LASIK for hyperopia with accommodative esotropia in a series of 9 patients older than 18 years. A second study demonstrated a reduction in the mean esotropia of 21 prism diopters (Δ) prior to LASIK to 3.7Δ after surgery. However, another study of LASIK in accommodative esotropia in patients aged 10–52 years found that 42% of these patients had no reduction in their esotropia.

Brugnoli de Pagano OM, Pagano GL. Laser in situ keratomileusis for the treatment of refractive accommodative esotropia. *Ophthalmology.* 2012;119(1):159–163.

Hoyos JE, Cigales M, Hoyos-Chacón J, Ferrer J, Maldonado-Bas A. Hyperopic laser in situ keratomileusis for refractive accommodative esotropia. *J Cataract Refract Surg.* 2002;28(9):1522–1529.

Systemic Conditions

Human Immunodeficiency Virus Infection

According to the FDA, patients with an immunodeficiency disease should not undergo LASIK, regardless of the excimer platform, because the risk outweighs the benefit. In a survey of members of the International Society of Refractive Surgery, 51% of respondents considered HIV-seropositive patients who did not have definite acquired immunodeficiency syndrome (AIDS) to be acceptable refractive surgery candidates. Only 13% of respondents thought that patients with definite AIDS were candidates for refractive surgery, while 44% believed that AIDS was an absolute contraindication to refractive surgery. Some surgeons advise patients with AIDS against undergoing refractive surgery because of concerns about postoperative complications, including the increased risk of infection associated with immunosuppression. Infections have been reported among HIV-positive patients who underwent LASIK or PRK. For example, in the US Military HIV Natural History Study, 79 of 2073 patients had LASIK, PRK, or RK, and 6 infections were reported: 5 in the PRK group and 1 in the RK group. This study suggests that HIV-positive patients may be at higher risk for complications with PRK, and a history of AIDS was also identified as a risk factor for complications.

An additional concern is the potential for aerosolizing live virus during laser ablation, which could pose a risk to laser-suite personnel. Because refractive surgeons may operate on patients who do not know they are infected with viruses such as HIV or one of the hepatitis viruses, universal precautions must be followed with all patients. Inhaled particles 5 μm or larger in diameter are deposited in the bronchial, tracheal, nasopharyngeal, and nasal walls; and particles less than 2 μm in diameter are deposited in the bronchioles and alveoli. Even if viral particles are not viable, the excimer laser plume produces particles with a mean diameter of 0.22 μm. Although the health effects of inhaled particles from the plume have not yet been determined, there have been anecdotal reports of respiratory ailments such as chronic bronchitis in high-volume excimer laser refractive surgeons. Evacuation of the laser plume potentially decreases the amount of debris that is inhaled.

If a surgeon is considering performing excimer laser ablation in an HIV-infected patient who is not immunocompromised and has normal results on eye examination, extra precautions are warranted. The surgeon should counsel the patient about the visual risks of HIV infection and the lack of long-term follow-up results for refractive surgery in this population. The surgeon may also consider consulting with the physicians managing the patient's underlying condition, including specialists in infectious diseases. The surgeon may choose to treat 1 eye at a time on separate days and schedule the patient as the last patient of the day. In addition, the surgeon may consider implementing additional precautions for the operating room staff, such as wearing filtering masks during the procedure and evacuating the laser plume.

Aref AA, Scott IU, Zerfoss EL, Kunselman AR. Refractive surgical practices in persons with human immunodeficiency virus positivity or acquired immune deficiency syndrome. *J Cataract Refract Surg.* 2010;36(1):153–160.

Hagen KB, Kettering JD, Aprecio RM, Beltran F, Maloney RK. Lack of virus transmission by the excimer laser plume. *Am J Ophthalmol.* 1997;124(2):206–211.

Tisdale CS, Justin GA, Wang X, et al; Infectious Disease Clinical Research Program HIV Working Group. Refractive surgery in the HIV-positive U.S. Military Natural History Study Cohort: complications and risk factors. *J Cataract Refract Surg.* 2019;45(11):1612–1618.

Diabetes Mellitus

A patient with diabetes mellitus who is considering LVC should have a thorough preoperative history and examination, and the surgeon should pay special attention to the presence of active diabetic ocular disease. The blood glucose of a diabetic patient should be well controlled to ensure an accurate refraction at the time of examination and postoperative stability. A history of treatment for proliferative diabetic retinopathy or cystoid macular edema indicates visually significant diabetic complications that typically preclude refractive surgery.

The ophthalmic examination should include inspection of the corneal epithelium to check the health of the ocular surface, identification of cataract if present, and detailed retinal examination. Preoperative corneal sensation should be assessed because corneal anesthesia can impede epithelial healing. Special consideration should be given to ruling out the presence of diabetic keratopathy by assessing corneal sensitivity and performing a detailed slit-lamp examination specifically looking for irregularities in the epithelium. Diabetic keratopathy can cause delayed epithelial healing, epithelial fragility, persistent defects, or superficial keratitis. In one study, diabetic keratopathy was present in 84% of patients with a diagnosis of diabetic retinopathy, compared with 41% of those without retinal complications. These findings suggest that refractive surgery should be reserved only for those patients with tightly controlled blood glucose and no signs of retinopathy or keratopathy.

A retrospective review performed 6 months after LASIK in 30 eyes of patients with diabetes mellitus reported a complication rate of 47%, compared with a complication rate of 6.9% in the control group. The most common problems in this study were related to epithelial healing and included epithelial loosening and defects. A loss of 2 or more lines of CDVA was reported in less than 1% of both the diabetes mellitus and control groups. However, 6 of the 30 eyes in the diabetes mellitus group required a mean of 4.3 months to heal because of persistent epithelial defects. The authors concluded that the high complication rate in these patients was explained by unmasking subclinical diabetic keratopathy.

Another retrospective review of 24 patients with diabetes mellitus who underwent LASIK demonstrated that 63% achieved UDVA of 20/25 or better. Three of the 24 eyes had an epithelial defect after surgery, and epithelial ingrowth developed in 2 of these eyes. No eye lost CDVA. In contrast, Cobo-Soriano and colleagues evaluated 44 diabetic patients (both insulin dependent and non–insulin dependent) who underwent LASIK in a retrospective observational case-control study. The investigators found no significant differences between diabetic patients and control subjects in perioperative and postoperative complications, including epithelial defects, epithelial ingrowth, and flap complications.

Given these contradictory reports, surgeons should exercise caution in the selection of patients with diabetes mellitus for refractive surgery. Intraoperative technique can be adjusted to ensure maximal epithelial health. To reduce corneal toxicity, the surgeon should use the minimal amount of topical anesthetic (preferably in the form of nonpreserved drops) immediately before performing the procedure. Patients with diabetes mellitus should be counseled preoperatively about the increased risk of postoperative complications and the possibility of prolonged healing time after LASIK. They should also be informed that the procedure treats only the refractive error and not the natural history of the diabetes mellitus, which can lead to future ocular complications and associated vision loss.

Cobo-Soriano R, Beltrán J, Baviera J. LASIK outcomes in patients with underlying systemic contraindications: a preliminary study. *Ophthalmology.* 2006;113(7):1118.e1–e8.

Fraunfelder FW, Rich LF. Laser-assisted in situ keratomileusis complications in diabetes mellitus. *Cornea.* 2002;21(3):246–248.

Halkiadakis I, Belfair N, Gimbel HV. Laser in situ keratomileusis in patients with diabetes. *J Cataract Refract Surg.* 2005;31(10):1895–1898.

Jabbur NS, Chicani CF, Kuo IC, O'Brien TP. Risk factors in interface epithelialization after laser in situ keratomileusis. *J Refract Surg.* 2004;20(4):343–348.

Saini JS, Khandalavla B. Corneal epithelial fragility in diabetes mellitus. *Can J Ophthalmol.* 1995;30(3):142–146.

Simpson RG, Moshirfar M, Edmonds JN, Christiansen SM. Laser in-situ keratomileusis in patients with diabetes mellitus: a review of the literature. *Clin Ophthalmol.* 2012;6:1665–1674.

Connective Tissue and Autoimmune Diseases

Most surgeons consider active, uncontrolled connective tissue diseases, such as rheumatoid arthritis, systemic lupus erythematosus, and polyarteritis nodosa, to be contraindications to refractive surgery. Reports in the literature have discussed corneal melting and perforation following cataract extraction in patients with these conditions, as well as corneal scarring after PRK in a patient with systemic lupus erythematosus.

However, a large retrospective series of 1224 eyes in patients with rheumatoid arthritis, systemic lupus erythematosus, psoriatic arthritis, sarcoidosis, ankylosing spondylitis, multiple sclerosis, or scleroderma undergoing LASIK or PRK suggests that refractive surgery may be considered in patients with well-controlled connective tissue or autoimmune disease. In this study, there were 3 cases of anterior uveitis, 9 cases of epitheliopathy that led to 2 lines of loss in CDVA, and 1 flap melt that was resolved with topical treatment. Another retrospective study of 62 eyes of patients with autoimmune or connective tissue disorders who had undergone LASIK reported that these eyes had a somewhat worse refractive outcome than control eyes but did not sustain any severe complications such as corneal melting, laceration, or interface alterations.

Because the risk from an underlying disease cannot be quantified, increased caution should be exercised if refractive surgery is considered in patients with well-controlled autoimmune or connective tissue disease. It should be emphasized to the patient that ocular manifestations such as OSD and dry eye may not present for many years. Consultation with the treating physician, surgery on 1 eye at a time, and ancillary informed consent should be considered.

Alió JL, Artola A, Belda JI, et al. LASIK in patients with rheumatic diseases: a pilot study. *Ophthalmology.* 2005;112(11):1948–1954.

Schallhorn JM, Schallhorn SC, Hettinger KA, et al. Outcomes and complications of excimer laser surgery in patients with collagen vascular and other immune-mediated inflammatory diseases. *J Cataract Refract Surg.* 2016;42(12):1742–1752.

Simpson RG, Moshirfar M, Edmonds JN, Christiansen SM, Behunin N. Laser in situ keratomileusis in patients with collagen vascular disease: a review of the literature. *Clin Ophthalmol.* 2012;6:1827–1837.

CHAPTER 8

Considerations After Refractive Surgery

This chapter includes a related video. Go to www.aao.org/bcscvideo_section13 or scan the QR code in the text to access this content.

Highlights

- Intraocular lens calculations are affected by both incisional and excimer laser refractive surgery.
- If a patient who has undergone laser vision correction subsequently requires retinal detachment repair, special consideration should be given to maintaining corneal integrity and protecting the LASIK flap.
- Contact lenses can be used after refractive surgery, but irregular astigmatism or severe flattening or steepening of the cornea can make fitting challenging.
- Laser vision correction has an impact on intraocular pressure measurements.

Introduction

The number of patients who have had refractive surgery continues to grow, and ophthalmologists are increasingly confronted with the management of post–refractive surgery patients with other ocular conditions, such as cataract, glaucoma, retinal detachment, corneal opacities, and irregular astigmatism. Calculation of the intraocular lens (IOL) power for cataract surgery presents a particular challenge in this population.

Intraocular Lens Calculations After Refractive Surgery

Numerous formulas have been developed to calculate IOL power for eyes that have undergone refractive surgery, but none is infallible, and these cases are still prone to refractive "surprises." Although the measurement of axial length should remain accurate after refractive surgery, determining the keratometric power of the post–refractive surgery cornea is problematic. The difficulty arises from several factors. Small effective central optical zones after refractive surgery (especially after radial keratotomy [RK]) can lead to inaccurate measurements because keratometers and Placido disk–based corneal topography devices measure the corneal curvature several millimeters away from the center of the cornea and possibly outside the modified treated zone. In addition, the relationship between the anterior and posterior corneal curvatures may be considerably altered after refractive surgery, especially after laser ablative procedures. Generally, if standard keratometry readings are used to calculate IOL power for a previously myopic, post–refractive surgery eye, the refractive error will be hyperopic after cataract surgery because the keratometry readings are erroneously steeper than the true central corneal power (ie, myopic ablations result in flatter-than-measured corneas).

A variety of methods have been developed to better estimate the central corneal power after refractive surgery. None is perfectly accurate, and different methods can lead to disparate values. Intraoperative wavefront aberrometry systems have been shown to decrease residual refractive error after cataract surgery in post–refractive surgery eyes, but there is debate about their utility compared with use of fourth-generation IOL formulas. These devices use Talbot-Moiré–based interferometry to obtain real-time aphakic IOL calculations (Video 8-1). In addition, intraoperative aberrometry can be used to refine astigmatism management with toric lenses. Another novel approach to aid in the management of refractive error is to adjust the IOL after implantation through application of light. Currently, the Light Adjustable Lens (RxSight), approved by the US Food and Drug Administration (FDA) to reduce residual refractive error after cataract surgery (see Chapter 9), is being investigated in the post–refractive surgery population.

VIDEO 8-1 Intraoperative aberrometry in a post–myopic LASIK patient.
Courtesy of Karolinne Maia Rocha, MD, PhD.

At the time of cataract surgery evaluation, patients need to be informed that IOL power calculations are less accurate when performed after refractive surgery. Despite maximum preoperative effort by the surgeon, additional surgery, such as laser vision correction (LVC), IOL exchange, or implantation of a piggyback IOL, may be required in order to attain a better refractive result if the patient is unwilling to wear glasses or contact lenses. Cataract surgery after RK frequently induces short-term corneal swelling, with flattening and a hyperopic shift. For this reason, in the event of a refractive surprise, an IOL exchange should not be performed in post-RK eyes until the cornea and refraction stabilize, which may take several weeks to months. Corneal curvature generally does not change so much when cataract surgery is performed after photorefractive keratectomy (PRK) or LASIK; thus, it may be possible to plan and perform an IOL exchange or refractive surgical procedures earlier in these patients.

In the evaluation of a post–refractive surgery patient for cataract surgery, it is important to perform biometry, assess topography to evaluate the cornea, and know what type of refractive procedure was performed. A myopic ablation induces central flattening, whereas a hyperopic ablation induces central steepening. RK incisions often lead to irregular astigmatism and flattening that will be apparent on topography. Slit-lamp examination may reveal what type of surgery a patient has undergone, as old LASIK flaps and RK incisions are visible. It may be difficult to discern whether a patient has had PRK, as there are often no signs other than topographic changes. In addition, some patients have combinations of LASIK, PRK, and RK. It is also important to look at the centration of the excimer ablation. Patients with a decentered ablation often have irregular astigmatism, which may alter treatment options offered to the patient and limit corrected distance visual acuity (CDVA) after cataract surgery. When possible, pre–refractive surgery information should be kept by both the patient and the refractive surgeon, as it can help the cataract surgeon understand what changes were induced by the refractive surgery. To assist in retaining these data, the American Academy of Ophthalmology and the International Society of Refractive Surgery have codeveloped the K-Card, available in PDF form on the Academy website (www.aao.org/patient-safety-statement/kcard).

Chen X, Yuan F, Wu L. Metaanalysis of intraocular lens power calculation after laser refractive surgery in myopic eyes. *J Cataract Refract Surg.* 2016;42(1):163–170.

Hill WE, Byrne SF. Complex axial length measurements and unusual IOL power calculations. *Focal Points: Clinical Modules for Ophthalmologists.* American Academy of Ophthalmology; 2004, module 9.

Raufi N, James C, Kuo A, Vann R. Intraoperative aberrometry vs modern preoperative formulas in predicting intraocular lens power. *J Cataract Refract Surg.* 2020;46(6):857–861.

Shammas HJ. Intraocular lens power calculation in patients with prior refractive surgery. *Focal Points: Clinical Modules for Ophthalmologists.* American Academy of Ophthalmology; 2013, module 6.

Eyes With Known Pre– and Post–Refractive Surgery Data

One method for calculating IOL power after refractive surgery is the *clinical history method,* in which pre- and post–refractive surgery refraction and keratometry values, if available, are used to approximate the true previous keratometry values for the central cornea. Unfortunately, even with these measurements, this approach has not proved to be accurate in the setting of excimer laser refractive surgery. Moreover, it can be difficult to obtain a post–refractive surgery refraction that is stable; that is, obtained several months after the refractive surgery but before the onset of a myopic shift induced by a developing nuclear sclerotic cataract. In post-RK patients, however, the post-RK refraction and the refractive history were identified as the most important parameters in a recent study assessing IOL power calculation methods. Some authors have also suggested that when no refractive history is available—which is often the case, given the time interval since RK was commonly performed—the Barrett True K and Haigis formulas both performed well.

Chen M. An evaluation of the accuracy of the ORange (Gen II) by comparing it to the IOLMaster in the prediction of postoperative refraction. *Clin Ophthalmol.* 2012;6:397–401.

Fram NR, Masket S, Wang L. Comparison of intraoperative aberrometry, OCT-based IOL formula, Haigis-L, and Masket formulae for IOL power calculations after laser vision correction. *Ophthalmology.* 2015;122(6):1096–1101.

Masket S, Masket SE. Simple regression formula for intraocular lens power adjustment in eyes requiring cataract surgery after excimer laser photoablation. *J Cataract Refract Surg.* 2006;32(3):430–434.

Turnbull AMJ, Crawford GJ, Barrett GD. Methods for intraocular lens power calculation in cataract surgery after radial keratotomy. *Ophthalmology.* 2020;127(1):45–51.

Eyes Without Preoperative Information

If no preoperative information is available, the *hard contact lens method* can be used to calculate corneal power. However, this method is often cumbersome in clinical practice. The CDVA needs to be at least 20/80 in order for this approach to work. First, a baseline manifest refraction is performed; a plano hard contact lens of known base curve (power) is then placed on the eye, and another manifest refraction is performed. If the manifest refraction does not change, the cornea has the same power as the contact lens. If the refraction is more myopic, the contact lens is steeper (more powerful) than the cornea by the amount of change in the refraction; the reverse holds true if the refraction is more hyperopic. For example:

Current spherical equivalent manifest refraction: −1.00 diopter (D)
A hard contact lens of known base curve (8.7 mm) and power (37.00 D) is placed
Overrefraction: +2.00 D
Change in refraction: +2.00 D − (−1.00 D) = +3.00 D
Calculation of corneal power: 37.00 D + 3.00 D = 40.00 D

The ASCRS Online Post-Refractive Intraocular Lens Power Calculator

An online tool for calculating IOL power in a post–refractive surgery patient was developed by Warren Hill, MD; Li Wang, MD, PhD; and Douglas D. Koch, MD. It is available on the website of the American Society of Cataract and Refractive Surgery (ASCRS; www.ascrs.org) and directly at http://iolcalc.ascrs.org.

To use this IOL calculator, the surgeon selects the appropriate prior refractive surgical procedure and enters the patient's biometric data, topography data (from selected devices), and prior data, if known (Fig 8-1). The IOL power is calculated by a variety of formulas and displayed at the bottom of the form, and the surgeon can compare the range of results to select the best IOL power for the individual situation. This online tool is updated regularly with new formulas and information as they become available and, at this time, probably represents the best option for preoperative calculation of IOL powers in post–refractive surgery patients.

Wang L, Hill WE, Koch DD. Evaluation of intraocular lens power prediction methods using the American Society of Cataract and Refractive Surgeons Post-Keratorefractive Intraocular Lens Power Calculator. *J Cataract Refract Surg.* 2010;36(9):1466–1473.

Retinal Detachment Repair After Laser Vision Correction

Even if the eyes of patients with high myopia become emmetropic as a result of refractive surgery, these eyes remain at increased risk of retinal detachment. For this reason, symptoms such as floaters or photopsias warrant a thorough retinal evaluation to ensure that there are no peripheral retinal tears or holes. In addition, if vitreoretinal surgery or laser is deemed necessary, the vitreoretinal surgeon should ask about prior refractive surgery. Eyes undergoing retinal detachment repair after LASIK are prone to flap problems, including flap dehiscence, microstriae, and macrostriae. The surgeon may find it helpful to mark the edge

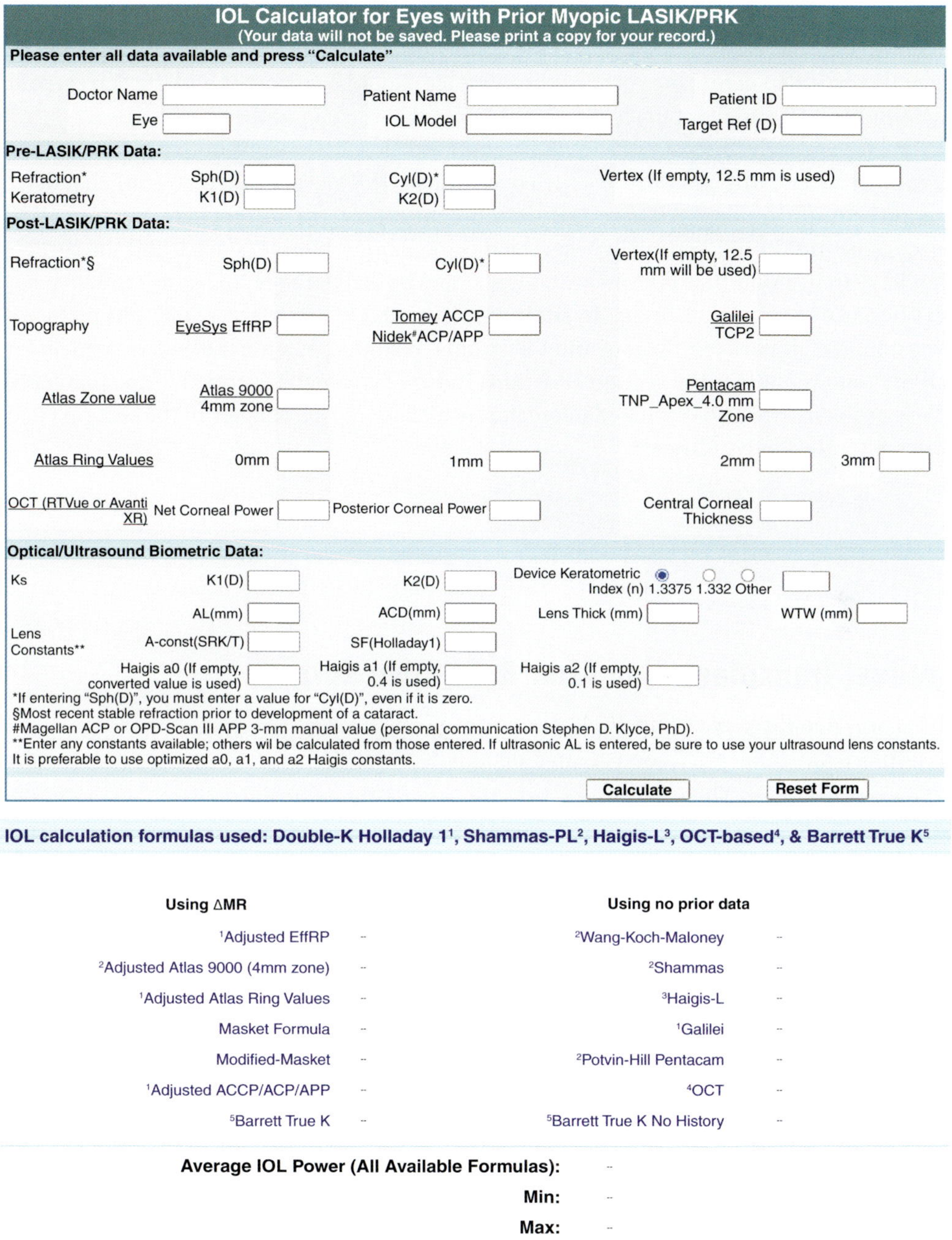

IOL Calculator for Eyes with Prior Myopic LASIK/PRK
(Your data will not be saved. Please print a copy for your record.)
Please enter all data available and press "Calculate"

Doctor Name | Patient Name | Patient ID
Eye | IOL Model | Target Ref (D)

Pre-LASIK/PRK Data:

Refraction* — Sph(D) — Cyl(D)* — Vertex (If empty, 12.5 mm is used)
Keratometry — K1(D) — K2(D)

Post-LASIK/PRK Data:

Refraction*§ — Sph(D) — Cyl(D)* — Vertex(If empty, 12.5 mm will be used)
Topography — EyeSys EffRP — Tomey ACCP Nidek#ACP/APP — Galilei TCP2
Atlas Zone value — Atlas 9000 4mm zone — Pentacam TNP_Apex_4.0 mm Zone
Atlas Ring Values — 0mm — 1mm — 2mm — 3mm
OCT (RTVue or Avanti XR) — Net Corneal Power — Posterior Corneal Power — Central Corneal Thickness

Optical/Ultrasound Biometric Data:

Ks — K1(D) — K2(D) — Device Keratometric Index (n) 1.3375 1.332 Other
AL(mm) — ACD(mm) — Lens Thick (mm) — WTW (mm)
Lens Constants** — A-const(SRK/T) — SF(Holladay1)
Haigis a0 (If empty, converted value is used) — Haigis a1 (If empty, 0.4 is used) — Haigis a2 (If empty, 0.1 is used)

*If entering "Sph(D)", you must enter a value for "Cyl(D)", even if it is zero.
§Most recent stable refraction prior to development of a cataract.
#Magellan ACP or OPD-Scan III APP 3-mm manual value (personal communication Stephen D. Klyce, PhD).
**Enter any constants available; others wil be calculated from those entered. If ultrasonic AL is entered, be sure to use your ultrasound lens constants. It is preferable to use optimized a0, a1, and a2 Haigis constants.

Calculate | Reset Form

IOL calculation formulas used: Double-K Holladay 1[1], Shammas-PL[2], Haigis-L[3], OCT-based[4], & Barrett True K[5]

Using ΔMR		Using no prior data	
[1]Adjusted EffRP	--	[2]Wang-Koch-Maloney	--
[2]Adjusted Atlas 9000 (4mm zone)	--	[2]Shammas	--
[1]Adjusted Atlas Ring Values	--	[3]Haigis-L	--
Masket Formula	--	[1]Galilei	--
Modified-Masket	--	[2]Potvin-Hill Pentacam	--
[1]Adjusted ACCP/ACP/APP	--	[4]OCT	--
[5]Barrett True K	--	[5]Barrett True K No History	--

Average IOL Power (All Available Formulas): --
Min: --
Max: --

Figure 8-1 The American Society of Cataract and Refractive Surgery (ASCRS) post-refractive intraocular lens (IOL) power calculator (available at http://iolcalc.ascrs.org). The cataract surgeon enters the patient's pre–refractive surgery data (if known) and current data into the form. After the "calculate" button at the bottom of the form is clicked, the IOL power calculated by a variety of formulas is displayed. *(Used with permission from the American Society of Cataract and Refractive Surgery.)*

of the flap prior to surgery to aid in flap replacement in case the flap is dislodged. The risk of flap problems increases dramatically if the epithelium is debrided during the retinal detachment repair. If flap dehiscence occurs, the interface should be irrigated and the flap carefully repositioned. A bandage contact lens may be placed at the end of the procedure.

Postoperatively, the patient should be observed closely for signs of flap problems such as epithelial ingrowth and diffuse lamellar keratitis (DLK), especially if an epithelial defect was present on the flap. After retinal detachment repair, the intraocular pressure (IOP) needs to be monitored, especially when an intraocular gas bubble is used, and the surgeon should keep in mind that IOP measurements may be artifactually low after refractive surgery because of corneal thinning. In addition, elevated IOP can cause a DLK-like picture or even a fluid cleft between the flap and the stroma, resulting in a misleading, extremely low IOP measurement (see the section "Pressure-induced stromal keratopathy" in Chapter 5). These problems are also discussed in greater detail later in this chapter in the section Glaucoma After Refractive Surgery.

Qin B, Huang L, Zeng J, Hu J. Retinal detachment after laser in situ keratomileusis in myopic eyes. *Am J Ophthalmol.* 2007;144(6):921–923.

Wirbelauer C, Pham DT. Imaging interface fluid after laser in situ keratomileusis with corneal optical coherence tomography. *J Cataract Refract Surg.* 2005;31(4):853–856.

Corneal Transplantation After Refractive Surgery

Corneal transplantation is occasionally required after refractive surgery for indications including significant scarring, irregular astigmatism, ectasia, and edema. Issues unrelated to refractive surgery, such as trauma, infectious keratitis, or corneal edema after cataract surgery, can also necessitate corneal transplantation. Each type of refractive surgical procedure is unique in the reasons a graft may be required and in ways to avoid problems with the corneal transplant. Indications and techniques for corneal transplantation are discussed in greater detail in BCSC Section 8, *External Disease and Cornea.*

After RK, a graft may be required because of trauma resulting in incisional rupture, central scarring not responsive to phototherapeutic keratectomy, irregular astigmatism, excessive flattening of the central cornea, contact lens intolerance, or progressive hyperopia. The RK incisions can gape or dehisce during penetrating keratoplasty trephination, preventing creation of a uniform and deep trephination. One method for avoiding RK wound gape or dehiscence during keratoplasty is to mark the cornea with the trephine and then reinforce the RK incisions with interrupted sutures outside the trephine mark prior to trephination. If the RK incisions open during the corneal transplant surgery, then X, mattress, or lasso sutures may be required to close these stellate wounds.

After LASIK, corneal transplantation may be required to treat central scarring (eg, after infection or with a buttonhole) or corneal ectasia. A significant challenge in this scenario is that most LASIK flaps are larger than a typical trephine size (8 mm). Trephination through the flap increases the risk that the flap peripheral to the corneal transplant wound may separate. This complication may be avoidable through careful trephination and use of a gentle suturing technique that incorporates the LASIK flap under the corneal transplant suture.

Corneal transplantation is occasionally required in a patient with intrastromal corneal ring segments. The polymethyl methacrylate ring segments may be removed prior to grafting; or, if they lie centrally enough, they may be left in place and removed in toto with the host tissue or removed at the time of trephination.

Contact Lens Use After Refractive Surgery

Indications

Contact lenses can be used before and after refractive surgery to obtain valuable clinical information. For example, a patient with presbyopia can use a temporary trial with soft contact lenses to experience monovision before undergoing surgery, thus reducing the risk of postoperative dissatisfaction. Contact lenses can also be used preoperatively in a patient with a motility abnormality (eg, esotropia or exotropia) to simulate expected vision after refractive surgery and to ensure that diplopia does not become manifest.

In the perioperative period, hydrophilic soft contact lenses can help promote epithelial healing or prevent flap-related complications. Rigid gas-permeable (RGP) or scleral contact lenses are more effective than soft lenses in correcting reduced vision or irregular astigmatism after RK and LVC. Night-vision problems caused by a persistent, uncorrected refractive error or irregular astigmatism may also be reduced by using contact lenses. However, if the symptoms are related to higher-order aberrations, they may persist despite contact lens use. Contact lenses for refractive purposes should not be fitted until surgical wounds and serial refractions are stable.

Contact Lenses After Radial Keratotomy

Centration is a challenge in fitting contact lenses after RK, in part because the corneal apex is displaced to the midperiphery and radial incisions can induce excessive flattening of the central cornea (Fig 8-2). Frequently used fitting techniques involve referring to the preoperative keratometry readings and basing the initial lens trial on the average keratometry values. Contact lens stability is achieved by adjusting the lens diameter. In general, larger-diameter lenses take advantage of the eyelid to achieve stability. However, they also increase the effective steepness of the lens owing to the increased sagittal depth. If the preoperative

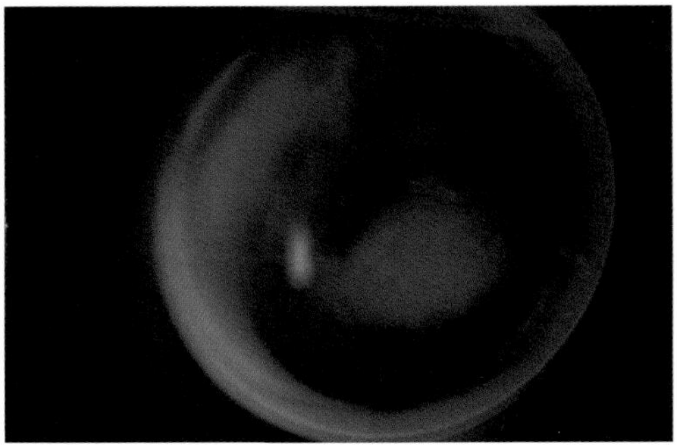

Figure 8-2 Fluorescein staining pattern in a contact lens patient who had undergone radial keratotomy and LASIK shows pooling centrally and touch in the midperiphery. This pattern is the result of central corneal flattening and steepening in the midperiphery. *(Courtesy of Robert S. Feder, MD.)*

keratometry reading is not available, the ophthalmologist can use a paracentral or midperipheral curve, as measured with postoperative corneal topography, as a starting point. When a successful fit cannot be obtained with a standard RGP lens, a reverse-geometry lens can be used. The secondary curves can be designed to be as steep as necessary to achieve a stable fit. The larger the optical zone, the flatter the fit.

Hydrophilic soft lenses and scleral lenses can also be used after RK. Toric soft lenses can be helpful when regular astigmatism is present. Soft lenses are less helpful in eyes with irregular astigmatism because they are less able to mask an irregular surface. Specialized lens designs may be helpful for patients with significant irregular astigmatism who are intolerant of conventional RGP lenses. Such designs include hybrid contact lenses, which consist of an RGP center surrounded by a soft contact lens skirt, and scleral RGP lenses, which vault the cornea and rest on the perilimbal conjunctiva/sclera. Whenever contact lenses are prescribed for post-RK eyes, as in the preceding scenarios, the ophthalmologist should continue to monitor the cornea for possible neovascularization of the wounds. If neovascularization occurs, contact lens wear should cease. Once the vessels have regressed, refitting can commence.

Contact Lenses After Surface Ablation and LASIK

Immediately after surface ablation, a soft contact lens is placed on the cornea as a bandage to help promote epithelialization and reduce discomfort. The lens is worn until the corneal epithelium has healed. Healing time depends on the size of the epithelial defect but generally takes between 4 and 7 days. A tight-fitting lens should be removed or replaced if there is evidence of corneal hypoxia (eg, corneal edema, folds in the Descemet membrane, or iritis).

The indications for contact lens fitting after LASIK are similar to those following other types of refractive surgery. The corneal contour is usually stable by 3 months after LASIK for myopia; however, it may take up to 6 months for the cornea to stabilize after LASIK for hyperopia. A soft contact lens may be used immediately after LASIK surgery when the epithelium is disrupted to promote epithelialization and to prevent epithelial ingrowth. When needed, it is generally used for a few days on an extended-wear basis until epithelial defects are resolved and then removed by the surgeon. Daily-wear contact lenses for refractive purposes should not be considered until the surgeon believes the risk of flap displacement is low.

Glaucoma After Refractive Surgery

Corneal thickness, geometry, and hysteresis are all altered by refractive surgery, and these 3 factors have a significant impact on the accuracy of IOP measurement. When measured with Goldmann applanation tonometry, IOP is artifactually reduced after surface ablation and LASIK for myopia, both of which decrease central corneal thickness and hysteresis. Similar inaccuracies in IOP measurement can occur after LVC for hyperopia. After excimer laser refractive surgery, the mean reduction in IOP measurement is 0.63 mm Hg per diopter of correction, with a wide standard deviation. In general, the reduction of measured IOP is greater after LASIK than after surface ablation. Surface ablation patients with a preoperative refractive error of less than 5.00 D may have a negligible decrease in IOP measurements. Adjusting IOP measurements for corneal hysteresis has been shown to be less dependent upon central corneal thickness measurements and thus may represent a more accurate IOP after corneal refractive surgery.

The topical corticosteroids used after refractive surgery pose a serious risk of corticosteroid-induced IOP elevation, particularly because an accurate IOP measurement is difficult to obtain. By 3 months postoperatively, up to 15% of surface ablation patients may have IOP higher than 22 mm Hg. If the elevated IOP is not recognized early enough, optic nerve damage and visual field loss can occur. When topical corticosteroids are used postoperatively for an extended time, periodic, careful disc evaluation is essential. Optic nerve and nerve fiber layer imaging may facilitate the evaluation. Periodic visual field assessment may be more effective than IOP measurement for identifying at-risk patients before severe visual field loss occurs (see Chapter 7, Figure 7-4).

Chang DH, Stulting RD. Change in intraocular pressure measurements after LASIK: the effect of refractive correction and the lamellar flap. *Ophthalmology.* 2005;112(6):1009–1016.

Hamilton DR, Manche EE, Rich LF, Maloney RK. Steroid-induced glaucoma after laser in situ keratomileusis associated with interface fluid. *Ophthalmology.* 2002;109(4):659–665.

Kaufmann C, Bachmann LM, Thiel MA. Comparison of dynamic contour tonometry with Goldmann applanation tonometry. *Invest Ophthalmol Vis Sci.* 2004;45(9):3118–3121.

Yang CC, Wang IJ, Chang YC, Lin LL, Chen TH. A predictive model for postoperative intraocular pressure among patients undergoing laser in situ keratomileusis (LASIK). *Am J Ophthalmol.* 2006;141(3):530–536.

Zhang H, Sun Z, Li L, Sun R, Zhang H. Comparison of intraocular pressure measured by ocular response analyzer and Goldmann applanation tonometer after corneal refractive surgery: a systematic review and meta-analysis. *BMC Ophthalmol.* 2020;20(1):23.

CHAPTER 9

Intraocular Refractive Surgery

This chapter includes related videos. Go to www.aao.org/bcscvideo_section13 or scan the QR codes in the text to access this content.

Highlights

- Phakic intraocular lens implantation allows for the treatment of high levels of myopia and myopic astigmatism while maintaining the eye's ability to accommodate.
- Refractive lens exchange is typically used for the correction of refractive errors and presbyopia in presbyopic or peripresbyopic patients. It is important to manage patient expectations if any natural accommodative ability remains and will be lost in the procedure.
- Bioptics is the planned combination of phakic intraocular lens implantation or refractive lens exchange with subsequent corneal laser vision correction to correct high refractive errors.

Intraocular Refractive Procedures

In its early history, *refractive surgery* was synonymous with *corneal refractive (keratorefractive)* surgery. In recent years, however, the scope of refractive surgery has expanded to include lens-based intraocular surgical techniques for achieving refractive outcomes.

In crystalline lens–sparing procedures, termed *phakic intraocular lens implantation,* the implantation of a phakic intraocular lens (PIOL) allows treatment of more extreme refractive errors, especially high myopia. Available PIOLs in the United States include iris-fixated and posterior chamber (sulcus) lenses for myopia and myopic astigmatism. Outside the United States, iris-fixated and posterior chamber lenses are available for hyperopia and myopia, as well as hyperopic and myopic astigmatism.

In crystalline lens–extraction procedures, termed *refractive lens exchange (RLE),* the patient's lens is removed and replaced with a prosthetic lens to address refractive errors of the eye. Advances in cataract surgical technique and technologies and expanded choices of IOLs have afforded more accurate and predictable refractive outcomes, allowing the elective correction of spherical, astigmatic, and presbyopic refractive errors.

The combination of corneal and intraocular refractive surgery, termed *bioptics,* allows patients at the extremes of refractive error, both spherical (myopia, hyperopia) and cylindrical (astigmatism), to attain good, predictable outcomes. These outcomes are achieved by combining the advantages of intraocular refractive surgery in treating large corrections with the adjustability of keratorefractive techniques. In addition, the optical quality may be improved by dividing the refractive correction between the two surgical procedures.

This chapter discusses the intraocular surgical techniques that are now, or are soon expected to be, available to the refractive surgeon.

Phakic Intraocular Lenses

Background

Use of the PIOL in correcting refractive error began in Europe in the 1950s, but limitations in manufacturing quality precluded these IOLs from achieving widespread adoption until the 1990s. Refinements in IOL design have reduced the incidence of complications and consequently increased the use of these PIOLs both within and outside the United States. Within the United States, 4 PIOLs are currently approved by the US Food and Drug Administration (FDA) for myopia: 2 nonfoldable polymethyl methacrylate (PMMA) iris-fixated PIOLs, and 2 foldable collamer posterior chamber PIOLs. The 2 nonfoldable PMMA lenses have an identical design but different dioptric ranges. Outside the United States, available models include foldable versions of the PIOLs and hyperopic and toric versions of all of these PIOLs. Representative lenses in each category (Table 9-1) are discussed in the following sections.

Alshamrani AA, Alharbi SS. Phakic intraocular lens implantation for the correction of hyperopia. *J Cataract Refract Surg.* 2019;45(10):1503–1511.

Pineda R 2nd, Chauhan T. Phakic intraocular lenses and their special indications. *J Ophthalmic Vis Res.* 2016;11(4):422–428.

Advantages

Phakic intraocular lenses provide the advantage of allowing for treatment of a much wider range of refractive errors than can be treated safely and effectively through corneal refractive surgery. The skills required for insertion are, with a few exceptions, similar to those used in cataract surgery. The equipment needed for IOL implantation is substantially less expensive than an excimer laser and similar to the equipment used for cataract surgery. In addition, the PIOL is removable; therefore, the refractive effect is theoretically reversible. However, any intervening change caused by the PIOL implantation is often permanent. Compared with refractive lens exchange (discussed later in this chapter), PIOL implantation has the advantage of preserving natural accommodation; it also has lower risks of endophthalmitis and postoperative retinal detachment because the crystalline lens barrier is preserved and vitreous destabilization is minimal.

Disadvantages

Phakic intraocular lens insertion is an intraocular procedure, carrying all the potential risks associated with intraocular surgery. In addition, each PIOL style has its own set of associated risks. Lenses currently available in the United States with PMMA optics are

Table 9-1 Phakic Intraocular Lenses

Position	Model	Available Power (Diopters)	Optic Size/Effective Diameter (mm)	Length (mm)	Material	Manufacturer	FDA Approval
Iris-supported	Verisyse model[a] VRSM5US	–5.00 to –20.00	5.0	8.5	PMMA	Johnson & Johnson Vision	Approved
	Verisyse model[a] VRSM6US	–5.00 to –15.00	6.0	8.5	PMMA	Johnson & Johnson Vision	Approved
	Artisan model 203	+3.00 to +12.00	5.0 or 6.0	8.5	PMMA	Ophtec	
	Artisan toric IOL	Custom	5.0 or 6.0	8.5	PMMA	Ophtec	
	Artiflex/Veriflex	–3.00 to –23.50	5.0 or 6.0	8.5	Polysiloxane	Ophtec	
Sulcus-supported	Visian ICL[b]	–3.00 to –20.00	4.9–5.8	12.1–13.7	Collamer	STAAR Surgical	Approved
	Visian ICL	+3.00 to +12.00		11.5–13.2	Collamer	STAAR Surgical	
	Visian Toric ICL	–3.00 to –16.00 myopia and 1.00 to 4.00 cylinder	4.9–5.8	12.1–13.7	Collamer	STAAR Surgical	Approved
	EVO/EVO+ Visian ICL[c]	–3.00 to –18.00 myopia and 1.00 to 6.00 cylinder	4.9–5.8 (EVO) 4.9–6.1 (EVO+)	11.5–13.2	Collamer	STAAR Surgical	

FDA = US Food and Drug Administration; ICL = implantable collamer lens; IOL = intraocular lens; PMMA = polymethyl methacrylate.

[a] The Artisan lens (Ophtec), marketed in the United States as the Verisyse lens (Johnson & Johnson Vision), is FDA approved for use in the lens power range of –5.00 to –20.00 D.

[b] The Visian ICL (STAAR Surgical) posterior chamber phakic IOL is FDA approved to correct myopia in the range of –3.00 to –20.00 D.

[c] The EVO Visian ICL (STAAR Surgical) has a 360-µm pore in the center of its optic to allow aqueous flow, eliminating the need for peripheral iridotomies. The EVO+ model is available in optic diameters up to 6.1 mm for larger pupil sizes but is otherwise identical to the EVO model.

not foldable, so their insertion requires creation of a relatively large wound, which may result in postoperative astigmatism. Posterior chamber PIOLs have a higher incidence of cataract formation. For patients with PIOLs in whom a visually significant cataract eventually develops, the PIOL will have to be explanted at the time of cataract surgery, possibly through a larger-than-usual wound. Although PIOLs to correct hyperopia are available outside the United States, indications for their implantation are narrower because the anterior chamber tends to be shallower than in patients with myopia, causing the IOL to sit too close to the corneal endothelium and resulting in increased endothelial cell loss.

Patient Selection

Indications

Phakic intraocular lenses can be offered as the primary surgical option for anyone who has refractive errors within the available treatment range and meets other screening criteria (discussed later). However, most surgeons reserve PIOL use for patients whose refractive limits are near or beyond the FDA-approved limits for laser vision correction, or who are otherwise not good candidates for keratorefractive surgery. Although excimer lasers can be used to treat high degrees of myopia, many surgeons have reduced the upper limits for laser in situ keratomileusis (LASIK) and surface ablation in their refractive practices because of the decreased predictability, high rate of regression, large amount of stromal tissue removed, increased incidence of microstriae, and night-vision problems that can occur with treatment of a patient with high myopia. Similarly, LASIK and surface ablation for correction of hyperopia greater than +4.00 diopters (D) and astigmatism greater than 4.00 D of cylinder are less accurate than for lower corrections. If surgeons become comfortable with the use of PIOLs, they may also choose to implant them for refractive powers significantly lower than the maximal limits for programmable excimer laser treatments. In addition, owing to the rapid visual recovery and low complication rate associated with currently available PIOLs, increasing numbers of surgeons are implanting these lenses bilaterally on the same day, providing a patient experience similar to bilateral same-day LASIK. The Ophthalmic Mutual Insurance Company (OMIC) has evaluated this practice.

PIOLs are available in the United States in powers between −3.00 D and −20.00 D, and for 1.00–4.00 D of astigmatism at the spectacle plane (see Table 9-1). Outside the United States, PIOLs are available for correcting hyperopia up to +12.00 D. PIOLs may be considered off-label treatment for eyes with irregular topographies from forme fruste or frank keratoconus.

Ophthalmic Mutual Insurance Company (OMIC). [OMIC website]. Am I covered for performing bilateral same-day RLE or bilateral same-day phakic implant procedures? Updated Oct. 2, 2019. Accessed October 6, 2021. https://goo.gl/bb9IcI

Contraindications

Phakic intraocular lenses have specific contraindications, which include preexisting intraocular disease such as a compromised corneal endothelium, iritis, significant iris abnormality, rubeosis iridis, cataract, or glaucoma. The anterior chamber diameter, anterior chamber depth, and pupil size must be appropriate for the specific PIOL being considered.

Patient evaluation

A thorough preoperative evaluation is necessary, as detailed in Chapter 2. Although PIOLs are FDA approved in the United States for patients 21 years or older, they are sometimes used off-label on younger patients with extreme refractive errors.

Tychsen L, Faron N, Hoekel J. Phakic intraocular collamer lens (Visian ICL) implantation for correction of myopia in spectacle-aversive special needs children. *Am J Ophthalmol.* 2017;175:77–86.

Informed consent

As with any refractive procedure, an informed consent specifically for this procedure should be obtained before surgery. The patient should be informed of the potential short-term and long-term risks of the procedure and of available alternatives; he or she should also be counseled about the importance of long-term follow-up because of the potential for endothelial cell loss over time. It is also important for the surgeon to ensure that the patient has realistic expectations about the visual outcomes of the procedure.

Ancillary tests

Specular microscopy or confocal microscopy is performed preoperatively to confirm that endothelial cell count and morphology are adequate. Anterior chamber depth must also be assessed because adequate depth is required for safe implantation of a PIOL. If the anterior chamber depth is less than 3.2 mm, the risk of endothelial and iris or angle trauma from placement of an anterior chamber, iris-fixated, or posterior chamber PIOL is increased. Anterior chamber depth can be measured by ultrasound biomicroscopy, anterior segment optical coherence tomography (OCT), partial coherence interferometry, slit-beam topography, or Scheimpflug imaging. In the United States, PIOL implantation is contraindicated in individuals who do not meet the minimum endothelial cell count specified for each PIOL and do not have a minimum internal anterior chamber depth (measured from the endothelium to the anterior capsule) of 3.0 mm. Methods for IOL power selection are specific to each PIOL and manufacturer; some manufacturers provide software for use in IOL power calculation.

Surgical Technique

Topical anesthesia with an intracameral supplement is appropriate if the patient can cooperate and the PIOL can be inserted through a small incision. If the patient cannot cooperate in the use of topical anesthesia or if a large incision is required, peribulbar or general anesthesia is preferable. Retrobulbar anesthesia should be used with caution in patients whose eyes have a high axial length because of the increased risk of globe perforation.

A peripheral iridotomy is performed for implantation of all currently FDA-approved PIOLs to reduce the risk of pupillary block and angle closure. One or more laser iridotomies can be performed before the PIOL surgery, or an iridectomy can be performed as part of the implant procedure. Meticulous removal of viscoelastic material at the conclusion of surgery lowers the risk of postoperative elevation of intraocular pressure (IOP).

Iris-fixated phakic intraocular lens

Most surgeons induce pupillary miosis before they initiate iris-fixated PIOL implantation, both to protect the crystalline lens and to make the iris easier to manipulate. The lens is generally inserted through a superior limbal incision but can be implanted with the wound placed at the steep meridian to minimize postoperative astigmatism. The long axis of the PIOL is ultimately oriented perpendicular to the axis of the incision. A side port incision is made approximately 2–3 clock-hours on either side of the center of the incision; thus, a 12 o'clock incision requires side port incisions near the 10 and 2 o'clock meridians. The "claw" haptics are fixated to the iris in a process called *enclavation.*

After the PIOL has been carefully centered over the pupil, it is stabilized with forceps while a specially designed enclavation needle is introduced through 1 of the side port incisions, and a small amount of iris is brought up into the claw haptic. This procedure is repeated on the other side. If adjustment of the PIOL position becomes necessary after fixation, the iris must be released before the PIOL is moved. Careful wound closure helps minimize surgically induced astigmatism. PMMA PIOLs require a 6-mm wound and thus generally require sutures for proper closure, whereas iris-fixated PIOLs made of flexible materials can be inserted through a small, self-sealing wound of approximately 3 mm. Video 9-1 demonstrates implantation of an iris-fixated PIOL.

VIDEO 9-1 Implantation of an iris-fixated phakic IOL.
Courtesy of David R. Hardten, MD.

Sizing the iris-fixated phakic intraocular lens Because this type of PIOL is fixated to the midperipheral iris, not to the angle or sulcus, it has the advantage of having a "one-size-fits-all" length. The PIOL is 8.5 mm long in total, including the 5.0- or 6.0-mm-long PMMA optic (Fig 9-1).

Posterior chamber phakic intraocular lens

Posterior chamber PIOLs require pupillary dilation before implantation. These PIOLs are made of a flexible collamer material and are implanted through a small wound approximately 3 mm long (Fig 9-2). The optic of the PIOL is vaulted to avoid contact with the crystalline lens and to allow aqueous to flow over the crystalline lens. This vaulting can be viewed at the slit lamp as well as with ultrasound biomicroscopy or Scheimpflug imaging (Fig 9-3). The lens manufacturers suggest that an acceptable amount of vaulting of the lens optic over the crystalline lens is 1.0 ± 0.5 corneal thicknesses. Using the appropriate vault is crucial for reducing complications (discussed later in the chapter).

For lens implantation, following pupil dilation, a 3.0- to 3.2-mm temporal clear corneal incision is made, and 1–2 additional paracentesis incisions are created, usually superiorly and inferiorly, to facilitate lens positioning. The lens is inserted using a cohesive viscoelastic material; after the lens unfolds, the footplates are positioned under the iris (Fig 9-4). The leading footplate is marked for identification to allow confirmation of correct orientation of the lens as it is injected. The surgeon should avoid contact with the central 6.0 mm of the lens, as any contact might damage the thin lens optic. Care should also be taken to avoid touching the crystalline lens with the PIOL to minimize the risk

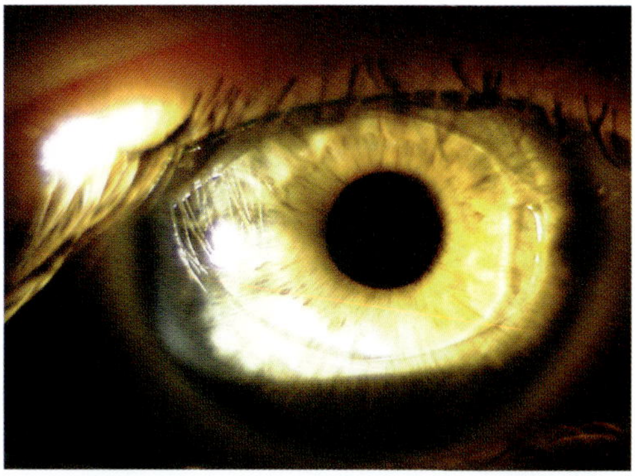

Figure 9-1 An iris-fixated phakic intraocular lens (PIOL) for myopic correction. The iris clip portion of the lens is visible on the right side of the image. *(Courtesy of Sherman W. Reeves, MD, MPH.)*

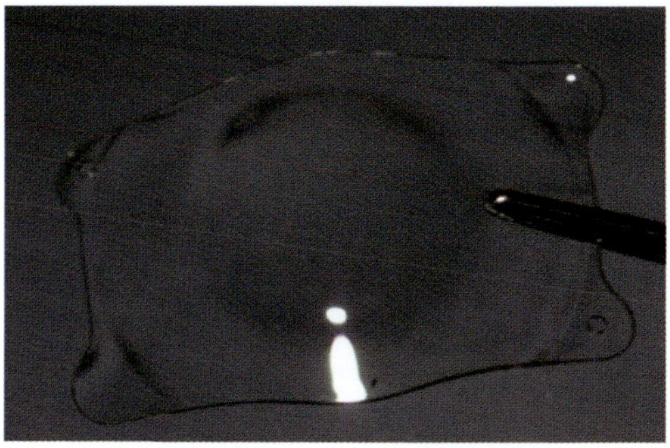

Figure 9-2 An implantable collamer posterior chamber PIOL. *(Courtesy of John B. Cason, MD.)*

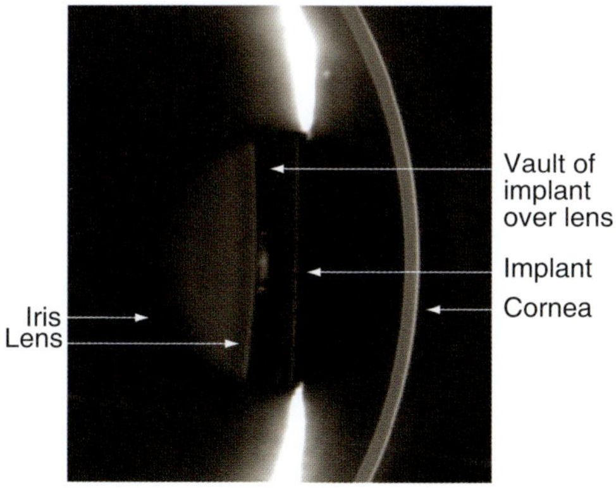

Figure 9-3 Scheimpflug image of a posterior chamber PIOL in place within the ciliary sulcus. The clear space between the implant and the native lens of the eye is termed the *vault* of the implant. *(Courtesy of Sherman W. Reeves, MD, MPH.)*

of cataract formation. Positioning instruments should be inserted through the paracenteses and kept peripheral to this central area. The pupil is then constricted. It is crucial to remove all viscoelastic material at the conclusion of the procedure to reduce the risk of a postoperative spike in IOP. Video 9-2 shows implantation of a posterior chamber PIOL.

VIDEO 9-2 Implantation of a posterior chamber phakic IOL.
Courtesy of George O. Waring IV, MD.

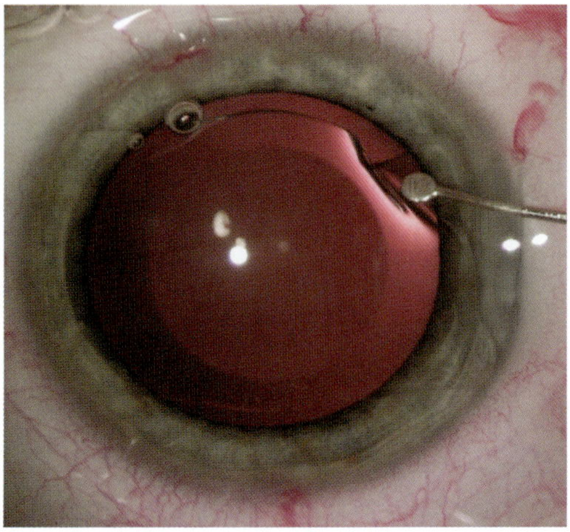

Figure 9-4 The footplate of a collamer posterior chamber PIOL is manipulated into position behind the iris. *(Courtesy of John B. Cason, MD.)*

Sizing the posterior chamber phakic intraocular lens The correct IOL length is selected by using the white-to-white measurement between the 3 and 9 o'clock meridians or by direct sulcus measurements made by a variety of techniques, including high-frequency ultrasound, anterior segment OCT, slit-beam or Scheimpflug imaging, and laser interferometry. Although the FDA-approved technique for measurement remains white-to-white measurement, there is growing evidence that direct sulcus measurement using any of these methods is superior and minimizes the risk of incorrect PIOL sizing. For more information on PIOLs, please refer to the FDA website.

Dougherty PJ, Rivera RP, Schneider D, Lane SS, Brown D, Vukich J. Improving accuracy of phakic intraocular lens sizing using high-frequency ultrasound biomicroscopy. *J Cataract Refract Surg.* 2011;37(1):13–18.

US Food and Drug Administration. [Medical devices website]. Phakic intraocular lenses. Updated March 26, 2018. Accessed October 6, 2021. https://goo.gl/aRyPgK

Angle-supported phakic intraocular lens

No angle-supported PIOLs are currently approved by the FDA. Previously, a flexible acrylic, angle-fixated PIOL was available outside the United States but was later removed from the market because of high rates of endothelial cell loss.

Outcomes

With better methods for determining PIOL power, outcomes have steadily improved. The significant postoperative gains over preoperative values in lines of corrected distance visual acuity (CDVA) are likely the result of a reduction in the image minification present with spectacle correction of high myopia. Loss of CDVA is rare. Moreover, the loss of contrast sensitivity noted after LASIK for high myopia does not occur after PIOL surgery. In fact, in all spatial frequencies, contrast sensitivity increases from preoperative levels with best spectacle correction.

Chen H, Liu Y, Niu G, Ma J. Excimer laser versus phakic intraocular lenses for myopia and astigmatism: a meta-analysis of randomized controlled trials. *Eye Contact Lens.* 2018;44(3):137–143.

Pérez-Cambrodí RJ, Piñero DP, Ferrer-Blasco T, Cerviño A, Brautaset R. The posterior chamber phakic refractive lens (PRL): a review. *Eye (Lond).* 2013;27(1):14–21.
US Food and Drug Administration. [FDA website]. Summary of safety and effectiveness data. Artisan phakic lens. PMA No. P030028. Accessed October 6, 2021. https://goo.gl/nTYyG2
US Food and Drug Administration. [FDA website]. Summary of safety and effectiveness data. STAAR Visian Toric ICL (Implantable Collamer Lens). PMA No. P030016/S001. Accessed October 6, 2021. https://www.accessdata.fda.gov/cdrh_docs/pdf3/P030016S001b.pdf

Complications

Phakic intraocular lens surgery shares the same possible risks and complications as other forms of IOL surgery. However, the most relevant potential complications include raised IOP, persistent anterior chamber inflammation, traumatic PIOL dislocation, cataract formation, and endothelial cell loss. Some of these complications do not manifest for years, thus requiring long-term follow-up.

Iris-fixated phakic intraocular lens

At 1-year follow-up in an FDA clinical trial of 662 patients who had an iris-fixated PIOL implanted for myopia, 1 patient had a hyphema, 5 had IOL dislocations, and 3 had iritis. Night-vision concerns about glare, starbursts, and halos were reported in 13.5%, 11.8%, and 18.2%, respectively, in patients who did not have these symptoms preoperatively. However, improvement in symptoms of 12.9%, 9.7%, and 9.8%, respectively, occurred in patients after PIOL implantation. In general, nighttime symptoms were worse in patients with larger pupil diameters.

Stulting and colleagues reported a 3-year follow-up study on 232 eyes of the 662 eyes enrolled in the FDA study. A total of 5 lenses dislocated and required reattachment, and an additional 20 lenses required surgery for insufficient lens fixation. No eyes required IOP-lowering medications after the first month. The mean decrease in endothelial cell density from baseline to 3 years was 4.8%. Six eyes required retinal detachment repair (rate, 0.3% per year), and 3 eyes underwent cataract surgery. Iris deformation, though rare, can also occur with iris-fixated PIOLs.

Pop M, Payette Y. Initial results of endothelial cell counts after Artisan lens for phakic eyes: an evaluation of the United States Food and Drug Administration Ophtec Study. *Ophthalmology.* 2004;111(2):309–317.
Stulting RD, John ME, Maloney RK, Assil KK, Arrowsmith PN, Thompson VM; U.S. Verisyse Study Group. Three-year results of Artisan/Verisyse phakic intraocular lens implantation. Results of the United States Food and Drug Administration clinical trial. *Ophthalmology.* 2008;115(3):464–472.

Posterior chamber phakic intraocular lens

In addition to the potential risks associated with implantation of other types of PIOLs, implantation of posterior chamber PIOLs increases the risk of cataract formation, pupillary block ocular hypertension, and pigmentary dispersion. If the posterior chamber PIOL is too large, vaulting increases, and if the peripheral iridotomies are not patent or blocked, pupillary block ocular hypertension can occur, or more chronically, iris chafing with pigmentary dispersion could result. If the PIOL is too small, the vaulting is reduced, decreasing the chance of chafing but increasing the risk of cataract. Incorrect PIOL vault can necessitate enlarging the peripheral iridotomies or exchange of the implanted lens for one with a better fit. Creation of the peripheral iridotomy may also lead to iris bleeding, focal cataract, synechia, or visual symptoms such as monocular diplopia or glare.

In an FDA clinical trial for 1 posterior chamber PIOL model, the incidence of nighttime visual symptoms was approximately 10%, but a similar percentage showed improvement in these symptoms after surgery. The incidence of visually significant cataract development in the FDA clinical trial as reported by Sanders and colleagues was 0.4% for anterior subcapsular cataracts and 1% for nuclear sclerotic cataracts.

Kamiya and colleagues reported 4-year follow-up results for 56 eyes of 34 patients with implanted posterior chamber PIOLs. No eyes developed pupillary block or a significant increase in IOP. The mean central endothelial cell loss was 3.7%. Symptomatic cataracts requiring surgery developed in 2 eyes, and asymptomatic anterior subcapsular cataracts developed in 6 other eyes. In a study of more than 500 eyes monitored for an average of 4.7 years, Sanders reported that anterior subcapsular opacities developed in 6%–7% of eyes, and visually significant cataracts developed in 1%–2% of eyes.

The incidence of retinal detachment after posterior chamber PIOL insertion is very low. In a series of 418 eyes that underwent a posterior chamber PIOL procedure, rhegmatogenous retinal detachment developed in 3 eyes (0.7%) at a mean of 19.8 months postoperatively, a rate comparable to the expected natural history of detachment in eyes with similar degrees of myopia.

Al-Abdullah AA, Al-Falah MA, Al-Rasheed SA, Khandekar R, Suarez E, Arevalo JF. Retinal complications after anterior versus posterior chamber phakic intraocular lens implantation in a myopic cohort. *J Refract Surg.* 2015;31(12):814–819.

Kamiya K, Shimizu K, Igarashi A, Hikita F, Komatsu M. Four-year follow-up of posterior chamber phakic intraocular lens implantation for moderate to high myopia. *Arch Ophthalmol.* 2009;127(7):845–850.

Sanders DR. Anterior subcapsular opacities and cataracts 5 years after surgery in the Visian Implantable Collamer Lens FDA trial. *J Refract Surg.* 2008;24(6):566–570.

Sanders DR, Vukich JA, Doney K, Gaston M; Implantable Contact Lens in Treatment of Myopia Study Group. U.S. Food and Drug Administration clinical trial of the Implantable Contact Lens for moderate to high myopia. *Ophthalmology.* 2003;110(2):255–266.

Angle-supported phakic intraocular lens

Previously, several angle-supported PIOLS were used internationally, but all were subsequently withdrawn from the market because of unacceptably high complication rates. The complications reported most frequently for angle-supported PIOLs are nighttime glare and halos, pupil ovalization, and endothelial cell loss.

Although glare and halos are the most commonly reported symptoms after angle-supported PIOL insertion, occurring in 18.8%–20.0% of patients, these symptoms appear to decrease by as much as 50% over a postoperative period of 7 years. The degree of endothelial cell loss occurring 1–7 years after insertion ranges from 4.6% to 8.4%. Pupil ovalization can occur because of iris tuck during insertion, or it can occur over time as a result of chronic inflammation and fibrosis around the haptics within the anterior chamber angle. The incidence of pupil ovalization ranges from 5.9% to 27.5% and is directly related to the postoperative interval studied. Ovalization is more likely when the implant is too large. In contrast, endothelial damage and decentration are most often associated with movement of a lens that is too small.

Alió JL, Toffaha BT, Peña-Garcia P, Sádaba LM, Barraquer RI. Phakic intraocular lens explantation: causes in 240 cases. *J Refract Surg.* 2015;31(1):30–35.

Refractive Lens Exchange

Advantages

Refractive lens exchange—removal of the crystalline lens followed by IOL implantation—has the advantage of greatly expanding the range of refractive surgery beyond what can be achieved with other available methods. RLE also addresses all aspects of the dysfunctional lens syndrome, including presbyopia, early lens opacities, and lenticular higher-order aberrations (HOAs) associated with age. The procedure retains the normal contour of the cornea, which may enhance the quality of vision, and it can be used to treat presbyopia as well as refractive error through incorporation of multifocal, extended depth of focus (EDOF) and/or accommodating IOLs, maintaining stereopsis.

Disadvantages

The postoperative potential for positive dysphotopsias is an important consideration for diffractive, presbyopia-correcting IOL technology compared with other forms of vision correction. Patient expectations for excellent uncorrected vision may be higher for RLE than for cataract surgery, underscoring the need for thorough preoperative discussion, close attention to detail preoperatively and intraoperatively, and postoperative treatment of residual refractive error. Patients who can still accommodate may need enhanced preoperative counseling if accommodation will be lost through the procedure. The loss of accommodation can be demonstrated for the patient before surgery with the instillation of 1% cyclopentolate drops.

Patient Selection

Indications

The primary purpose of RLE is to correct refractive error. RLE may be considered for the correction of myopia, hyperopia, astigmatism, and presbyopia when alternative refractive procedures are not adequate to address the patient's refractive error. RLE is typically used for refractive correction of presbyopia or moderate to high hyperopia as well as in patients with lens opacity expected to progress quickly. It is generally not considered medically necessary and is usually not covered by the patient's insurance. All FDA-approved IOLs are approved specifically for implantation at the time of cataract surgery, and implantation for RLE is considered an off-label use in the United States.

Informed consent

Refractive lens exchange carries risks and complications identical to those for routine cataract extraction with IOL implantation. Potential candidates must be capable of understanding the short-term and long-term risks of the procedure. Patients should be informed that unless they are targeted for residual myopia with monofocal, toric, or accommodating IOLs, or have a multifocal IOL (MFIOL) implanted, they will not have functional near vision without correction. A consent form should be given to the patient before surgery to allow ample time for review and signature. A sample consent form for RLE for the correction of hyperopia and myopia is available from the Ophthalmic Mutual Insurance Company (OMIC) at www.omic.com.

Myopia

Refractive lens exchange can be considered in patients with myopia of any degree, although it is most commonly used in presbyopic patients with higher myopia, for whom corneal refractive procedures or PIOL implantation are not indicated. Myopia, however, is a significant risk factor for retinal detachment in the absence of lens surgery, and this risk rises with increased axial length. High myopia, defined as an axial length of 26 mm or greater, is an independent risk factor for subsequent retinal detachment after lens extraction. Thus, a thorough retinal examination, including peripheral retinal evaluation, is indicated in these eyes prior to consideration of RLE.

Alió JL, Grzybowski A, El Aswad A, Romaniuk D. Refractive lens exchange. *Surv Ophthalmol.* 2014;59(6):579–598.

American Academy of Ophthalmology Retina/Vitreous Panel. Preferred Practice Pattern Guidelines. *Posterior Vitreous Detachment, Retinal Breaks, and Lattice Degeneration.* American Academy of Ophthalmology; 2019. www.aao.org/ppp

Daien V, Le Pape A, Heve D, Carriere I, Villain M. Incidence, risk factors, and impact of age on retinal detachment after cataract surgery in France: a national population study. *Ophthalmology.* 2015;122(11):2179–2185.

Qureshi MH, Steel DHW. Retinal detachment following cataract phacoemulsification—a review of the literature. *Eye (Lond).* 2020;34(4):616–631. [Erratum appears in *Eye (Lond).* 2020. PMID: 31659283.]

Hyperopia

If the amount of hyperopia is beyond the range of alternative refractive procedures, RLE might be the only available surgical option, particularly in the United States. As with correction for myopia, the patient must be informed about the risks of intraocular surgery. A patient with a shallow anterior chamber from a thickened crystalline lens or small anterior segment would not be a candidate for a PIOL; RLE could be beneficial for such a patient both refractively and because of the reduced risk of angle-closure glaucoma postoperatively. In a highly hyperopic eye with an axial length less than 18 mm, nanophthalmos should be considered. Eyes with these characteristics have a higher risk of uveal effusion syndrome and postoperative choroidal detachment. (See BCSC Section 11, *Lens and Cataract,* for discussion of cataract surgery for a patient with high hyperopia and nanophthalmos.) Patients with hyperopia have a lower risk of retinal detachment than do patients with myopia.

Alió JL, Grzybowski A, Romaniuk D. Refractive lens exchange in modern practice: when and when not to do it? *Eye Vis (Lond).* 2014;1:10.

Astigmatism

With the advent of toric IOLs that cover an expanded range, patients with significant astigmatism are also candidates for RLE. In the United States, multifocal and EDOF toric IOLs, as well as a toric accommodating IOL, have been approved by the FDA. Thus, US patients planning to undergo implantation of toric IOLs have the option of monofocal outcomes as well as concurrent presbyopia correction.

Presbyopia

Discussion of the correction of presbyopia, in addition to that for correction of myopia, hyperopia, and/or astigmatism, should be a component of the preoperative discussion in applicable patients. RLE is often used primarily for the purpose of correcting presbyopia, with the implantation of multifocal, EDOF, or accommodating IOLs or the creation of monovision with lens implants. A patient selecting distance-focused toric or spherical IOLs in both eyes should be informed that reading glasses will be required for functional near vision.

Surgical Planning and Technique

Although RLE is similar to cataract surgery, there are some additional considerations for planning and performing the procedure, as the primary surgical goal is refractive rather than restoration of vision loss due to cataract. In contrast to keratorefractive procedures, which are usually performed bilaterally in the same surgical session, RLE is usually performed as sequential surgery on separate days to minimize the potential for bilateral endophthalmitis. However, practices continue to evolve, and some surgeons perform bilateral RLE in the same surgical session.

Preoperative corneal topography is essential to detect irregular astigmatism and to identify patients with corneal ectatic disorders such as keratoconus and pellucid marginal degeneration. Patients with these conditions may still have RLE performed; however, they must understand the limits of vision correction obtainable and that the quality of vision may still suffer postoperatively because of their irregular astigmatism. These patients must further understand that they are not good candidates for postoperative treatment with LASIK or photorefractive keratectomy to refine the refractive correction.

Surgeons need to identify the degree of corneal versus lenticular astigmatism present, as only the corneal astigmatism will remain postoperatively. The patient should be informed if substantial astigmatism is expected to remain after surgery and a plan devised to correct it in order to optimize the visual outcome.

Limbal relaxing incisions and arcuate keratotomies with either blade or femtosecond laser may be used to correct residual corneal astigmatism of less than 2.00 D (see Chapter 3). Supplemental surface ablation or LASIK could also be considered (see the section Bioptics). Although glasses or contact lenses are an alternative for managing residual astigmatism, refractive surgery patients frequently reject this option. Evaluation of posterior corneal astigmatism is important, for which against-the-rule astigmatism is treated more aggressively than with-the-rule astigmatism.

Some surgeons obtain preoperative retinal OCT to identify potential macular pathology. Careful attention should be paid to the peripheral retinal examination, especially in patients with higher myopia. If relevant pathology is discovered, appropriate treatment or referral to a retina specialist is warranted. In patients with high axial myopia, retrobulbar injections should be performed with caution because of the risk of perforating the globe. Peribulbar, sub-Tenon, topical, and intracameral anesthesia are alternative options.

Many surgeons believe that an IOL should be implanted after RLE in a patient with high myopia rather than leaving the patient with aphakia, even when little or no optical power correction is required. Plano IOLs are available if indicated. The IOL acts as a barrier to anterior prolapse of the vitreous, maintaining the integrity of the aqueous–vitreous barrier, in the event that Nd:YAG laser posterior capsulotomy is required. Some IOL models also reduce the rate of posterior capsule opacification.

Intraocular Lens Power Calculations in Refractive Lens Exchange

High patient expectations for excellent uncorrected vision after RLE make accurate IOL power determination crucial. However, IOL power formulas are less accurate at higher levels of myopia and hyperopia. In addition, in high myopia, a posterior staphyloma can make the axial length measurements less reliable. Careful fundus examination and B-scan ultrasound imaging can identify the position and extent of staphylomas. The subject of IOL power determination is covered in greater detail in BCSC Section 3, *Clinical Optics and Vision Rehabilitation,* and Section 11, *Lens and Cataract.*

In a patient with high hyperopia, biometry may suggest an IOL power beyond what is commercially available. The upper limit of commercially available IOL power is now +40.00 D. A special-order IOL of a higher power may be available or may be designed, but acquiring or designing such a lens usually requires the approval of the institutional review board at the hospital or surgical center, which delays the surgery.

Another option is to use a "piggyback" IOL system, in which 2 posterior chamber IOLs are inserted. One IOL is placed in the capsular bag, and the other is placed in the ciliary sulcus. When piggyback IOLs are used, the combined power may need to be increased +1.50 to +2.00 D to compensate for the posterior shift of the posterior IOL. One potential complication of piggyback IOLs is the development of an interlenticular opaque membrane. These membranes cannot be mechanically removed or cleared with the Nd:YAG laser; the IOLs must be explanted. Interlenticular membranes occur most commonly between 2 acrylic IOLs, especially when both IOLs are placed in the capsular bag. When used, piggyback lenses should be of different materials, ideally with one IOL placed in the bag and the other in the sulcus. Piggyback IOLs may also result in the shallowing of the anterior chamber and increase the risk of iris chafing, especially in smaller eyes.

Hill WE, Byrne SF. Complex axial length measurements and unusual IOL power calculations. *Focal Points: Clinical Modules for Ophthalmologists.* American Academy of Ophthalmology; 2004, module 9.

Shammas HJ. IOL power calculation in patients with prior corneal refractive surgery. *Focal Points: Clinical Modules for Ophthalmologists.* American Academy of Ophthalmology; 2013, module 6.

Complications

The intraoperative and postoperative complications for RLE are identical to those of cataract surgery. See BCSC Section 11, *Lens and Cataract,* for a comprehensive discussion of this topic.

Monofocal Intraocular Lenses

For some patients, the best IOL choice for implantation at the time of RLE is a monofocal IOL. A variety of IOL choices and styles is available, and all are utilized in routine cataract surgery as well (see BCSC Section 11, *Lens and Cataract,* for more detail). Patients without significant corneal astigmatism who desire best distance vision only, or individuals who have tolerated monovision well in the past and want it re-created after cataract surgery, are generally the best candidates for monofocal IOL implantation.

Toric Intraocular Lenses

Residual astigmatism after cataract surgery affects visual function and patient satisfaction. Large population analyses indicate that more than 50% of patients have 0.75 D or more corneal astigmatism at presentation for cataract surgery, and 15%–29% have 1.50 D or more corneal astigmatism. Thus, toric IOLs can address a major need for vision correction after crystalline lens removal. Current toric IOLs in the United States generally come in powers that can correct from 1.00 to 4.00 D of astigmatism at the spectacle plane, and wider power ranges are available outside the United States. These ranges are continually evolving.

Patient Selection

A toric IOL is appropriate for patients with regular corneal astigmatism, currently up to 4.00 D at the corneal plane (United States). Patients with astigmatism exceeding the upper correction limits require additional measures to obtain full correction. In addition to understanding the risks associated with intraocular surgery, patients must be capable of understanding the limitations of a toric IOL. Not all patients with toric IOL implantation achieve spectacle independence for distance vision. Further, patients should be informed that toric IOL implantation will not eliminate the need for reading glasses (unless monovision is planned). The patient also needs to be informed that the IOL may rotate in the capsular bag shortly after surgery and that an additional procedure may be required to reposition it. For patients with a significant potential risk of requiring silicone oil for retinal detachment repair in the future, nonsilicone IOLs are more appropriate choices than silicone toric IOLs. Also, surgeons may have a lower threshold to use a toric IOL for the treatment of against-the-rule astigmatism to account for posterior corneal astigmatism.

Planning and Surgical Technique

The amount, axis, and regularity of the astigmatism should be measured accurately. First, corneal topography is examined to determine the regularity and axis of astigmatism and identify eyes with irregular astigmatism or ectatic disease. Keratometry should be used to confirm the corneal power axis and provide the primary data for corneal astigmatic power. The axis of astigmatism from the refraction should not be the sole source for axis or power determination but rather should be considered in context with topographic and keratometric measurements.

Significant disagreement between measurements should prompt reexamination of the clinical data and may suggest the effect of lenticular astigmatism or posterior corneal astigmatism. Posterior corneal astigmatism may vary widely between patients, but may add 0.3–0.5 D of net against-the-rule astigmatic power in 80% of patients. Although technology to accurately measure the posterior corneal astigmatism is evolving, surgeons may use regression formulas, such as the Baylor nomogram (see Koch and colleagues reference), or theoretical formulas, such as the Barrett toric IOL formula (available at https://ascrs.org/tools/barrett-toric-calculator) to help compensate for the tendency of anterior corneal measurements to overestimate the with-the-rule corneal power and underestimate the against-the-rule corneal power. Intraoperative aberrometry may be useful in these cases.

The manufacturers of toric IOLs have online software available to aid in surgical planning. After the surgeon enters data such as keratometry measurements, axes, IOL spherical power generated by A-scan, average surgeon-induced astigmatism, and axis of astigmatism, these programs will generate the recommended power and model lens as well as orientation of the lens.

Many methods are available to mark the cornea prior to surgery. The surgeon establishes and marks the vertical and/or horizontal meridians with the patient in an upright position to avoid potential misalignment resulting from torsional globe rotation, which sometimes occurs in the supine position. Intraoperative alignment systems are available. Cataract surgery employing a wound that induces a predictable amount of astigmatism is necessary to achieve the intended benefit of a toric lens. All online toric IOL software requires input of the expected surgically induced astigmatism for lens power calculations.

After the IOL is injected into the capsular bag, the viscoelastic behind the IOL is aspirated and the IOL is rotated into position on the steep meridian. Some surgeons prefer to leave the toric IOL purposely underrotated by 10°–20° and then to rotate it into position after all viscoelastic substance has been removed. Others position the IOL in its planned orientation and then hold it in place with a variety of techniques while removing the viscoelastic material. If the IOL rotates beyond its appropriate position, it will need to be fully rotated around again, as the 1-piece IOLs tend not to rotate well against their haptics. This maneuver should be performed using irrigation or viscoelastic material to prevent capsule rupture during rotation.

Koch DD, Jenkins RB, Weikert MP, Yeu E, Wang L. Correcting astigmatism with toric intraocular lenses: effect of posterior corneal astigmatism. *J Cataract Refract Surg.* 2013;39(12):1803–1809.

Outcomes

In clinical trials of a 1-piece acrylic toric IOL, data provided by the FDA indicated uncorrected acuity of greater than 20/40 in 93.8% of 198 patients implanted with the IOL (all sizes combined). With the plate-haptic IOL, postoperative astigmatism was less than 0.50 D in 48% of patients and less than 1.00 D in 75%–81% of patients; results were 61.6% and 87.7%, respectively, for the 1-piece acrylic toric IOL.

For patients with corneal astigmatism greater than that correctable by toric IOLs, surgeons may opt to simultaneously or sequentially correct residual astigmatism using incisional or laser procedures.

Kessel L, Andresen J, Tendal B, Erngaard D, Flesner P, Hjortdal J. Toric intraocular lenses in the correction of astigmatism during cataract surgery: a systematic review and meta-analysis. *Ophthalmology.* 2016;123(2):275–286.

Complications Specific to Toric Intraocular Lenses

The primary complication of toric IOLs is the possibility of IOL rotation resulting in a misalignment of the astigmatic correction. Full correction is not achieved unless the IOL is properly aligned in the axis of astigmatism. Astigmatism calculations have shown that every 10° off-axis rotation of the lens reduces the correction by approximately one-third. Thus, at 30° the lens is functionally astigmatically neutral, and IOL misalignment greater than 30° can increase the cylindrical refractive error. In the FDA clinical trials for a plate-haptic toric IOL, 76% of lenses were within 10° of preoperative alignment, and 95% were within 30°. In the FDA clinical trials for the 1-piece acrylic toric IOL, the degree of postoperative rotation in 242 implanted eyes was 5° or less in 81.1% and 10° or less in 97.1%. None of the eyes exhibited postoperative rotation greater than 15°.

Typically, a misaligned IOL is recognized within days of the surgery; it should be repositioned before fibrosis occurs within the capsular bag. However, waiting 1 week for some capsule contraction to occur may ultimately help stabilize the IOL. An online calculator is available to help determine the exact amount of IOL rotation necessary to optimize visual outcome (www.astigmatismfix.com).

Visser N, Bauer NJ, Nuijts RM. Toric intraocular lenses: historical overview, patient selection, IOL calculation, surgical techniques, clinical outcomes, and complications. *J Cataract Refract Surg.* 2013;39(4):624–637.

Light-Adjustable Intraocular Lenses

The Light-Adjustable Lens (LAL; RxSight) is a 3-piece silicone-optic posterior chamber IOL that can be irradiated with UV light through a slit-lamp delivery system 2–3 weeks after implantation to induce a change in the shape, and thus the power, of the IOL (Fig 9-5). The lens received FDA approval in November 2017 and became commercially available in the United States in July 2019. Specific irradiation patterns can be applied to the lens to induce refractive shifts, treating −0.75 to −2.00 D of astigmatism and −2.00 to +2.00 D of manifest sphere. Several irradiation treatments are sometimes required, separated by 3 days, to achieve the intended effect. Once the goal refraction is obtained, a final irradiation is performed to "lock in" the prescription, after which no further adjustments can be made. At 6-month follow-up in an FDA trial of 600 patients, 70.1% of those receiving the LAL had uncorrected visual acuity of 20/20 or better compared with 36.3% of

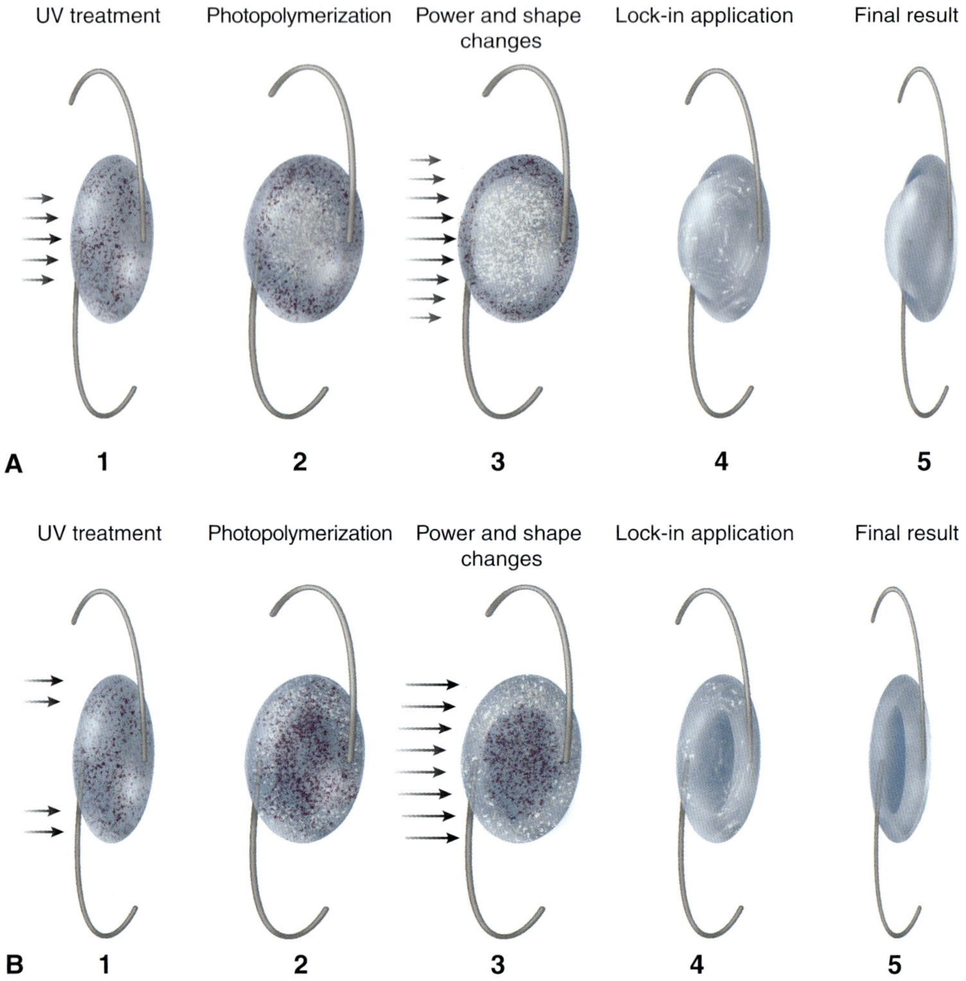

Figure 9-5 Schematic representation of the steps used in treating a Light-Adjustable Lens (RxSight). **Top row:** *1,* UV light is directed by the surgeon to the *center* of the lens. *2,* Photopolymerization occurs in the treated region. *3,* Unpolymerized macromers move to the light-exposed region (center), altering the lens shape and *increasing* the power. *4,* The entire lens is treated with UV light to polymerize and "lock in" all remaining macromers. *5,* The final lens power achieved after treatment matches the patient's individual prescription. **Bottom row:** *1,* UV light is directed to the lens *periphery*. *2,* Photopolymerization occurs in the treated region. *3,* Unpolymerized macromers move to the periphery, altering the lens shape and *decreasing* the power. *4,* The entire lens is treated with UV light to polymerize and "lock in" all remaining macromers. *5,* The final lens power achieved after treatment matches the patient's individual prescription. *(Illustration by Cyndie C. H. Wooley.)*

controls. At 6 months, 92% of LAL eyes were within 0.50 D of zero manifest refraction spherical equivalent (MRSE) and 83% within 0.50 D of cylinder target.

Prior to postoperative irradiation, the lens must be protected from sunlight exposure, which requires that patients wear full-time UV light–filtering sunglasses until the lock-in treatments are performed. The exposure to UV light during lock-in treatments results in transient erythropsia, in which objects appear tinged with red. Erythropsia occurred to some degree in 58% of FDA trial subjects, resolving in most patients over the first week after treatment but persisting in 2 subjects for longer than 6 months. Despite the refractive alterations available initially, after irradiation, the lens is functionally a monofocal IOL with all the limitations that come from that implantation strategy. See also Chapter 10.

US Food and Drug Administration. Light adjustable lens (LAL) and light delivery device (LDD). Medical devices website. PMA No. P160055. Accessed October 6, 2021. https://www.accessdata.fda.gov/scripts/cdrh/cfdocs/cfPMA/pma.cfm?id=P160055

Accommodating Intraocular Lenses

Accommodating lenses are another alternative for implantation during RLE. Currently, only 1 accommodating IOL and a similar accommodating toric IOL are FDA approved, although others are being investigated. Development is also currently under way for deformable IOLs. Additional investigational IOLs are discussed in Chapter 10.

Although the accommodating lens was designed to improve distance, intermediate, and near acuity through movement of its hinged haptics during the accommodative process, studies have found limited IOL movement and limited improvement in near acuity for most patients targeted for best distance acuity. Thus, many surgeons are utilizing a "mini-monovision" strategy when implanting the accommodating IOL, leaving the nondominant eye targeted for slight myopia (−0.50 to −0.75 D).

Gooi P, Ahmed IK. Review of presbyopic IOLs: multifocal and accommodating IOLs. *Int Ophthalmol Clin.* 2012;52(2):41–50.

Multifocal and Extended Depth of Focus Intraocular Lenses

Multifocal and EDOF IOLs have the ability to provide appropriate patients with functional vision at near, intermediate, and far distances in each eye. This ability stems from lens designs that split incoming light rays, creating different focal points or focal regions where objects will be clearest. However, all designs have potential trade-offs in vision quality and adverse effects, especially at night, and careful patient selection and counseling are necessary to achieve optimal outcomes. These types of lenses and their outcomes are discussed further in Chapter 10. Representative FDA-approved multifocal and EDOF IOLS are presented in Table 9-2.

Akella SS, Juthani VV. Extended depth of focus intraocular lenses for presbyopia. *Curr Opin Ophthalmol.* 2018;29(4):318–322.

Alió JL, Plaza-Puche AB, Férnandez-Buenaga R, Pikkel J, Maldonado M. Multifocal intraocular lenses: an overview. *Surv Ophthalmol.* 2017;62(5):611–634.

Patient Selection

Patients who are likely to be successful candidates for an MFIOL implant after lens surgery tend to be adaptable, to be less visually demanding, and to place a high value on reduced

Table 9-2 Representative Multifocal and Extended Depth of Focus (EDOF) Intraocular Lenses (IOLs) With FDA Approval

Focality	Model	Available Powers (D)	IOL Add Power (D)	Design	Manufacturer
Bifocal	Tecnis ZKB00	+5.00 to +34.00	+2.75	1-piece acrylic	Johnson & Johnson Vision
	Tecnis ZLB00	+5.00 to +34.00	+3.25	1-piece acrylic	Johnson & Johnson Vision
	Tecnis ZMB00	+5.00 to +34.00	+4.00	1-piece acrylic	Johnson & Johnson Vision
	Tecnis ZMA00	+5.00 to +34.00	+4.00	3-piece acrylic	Johnson & Johnson Vision
	Restor SV25T0	+6.00 to +34.00	+2.50	1-piece acrylic	Alcon
	Restor SN6AD1	+6.00 to +34.00	+3.00	1-piece acrylic	Alcon
	Restor SN6AD2	+6.00 to +34.00	+4.00	1-piece acrylic	Alcon
Trifocal	PanOptix TFAT00[a] TFAT30 TFAT40 TFAT50 TFAT60	+6.00 to +34.00 spherical, with 1.50 to 3.75 toric powers available in TFAT30 to 60 models	+3.25 near; +2.17, intermediate	1-piece acrylic	Alcon
EDOF	Symfony ZXR00 ZCU150[b] ZCU225 ZCU300 ZCU375 ZCU450 ZCU525 ZCU600	+5.00 to +34.00 spherical, with 1.50 to 6.00 toric powers available in ZCU150 to 600 models	+1.75[c]	1-piece acrylic	Johnson & Johnson Vision

D = diopters; FDA = Food and Drug Administration.

[a] Panoptix spherical and toric IOLs are also available in yellow chromophore, blue-light filtering TFNT00 series models.

[b] Initially released as ZXT Toric model, and subsequently replaced with ZCU Toric II model with squared and frosted edges to reduce edge glare and minimize rotation risk.

[c] Böhm M, Petermann K, Hemkeppler E, Kohnen T. Defocus curves of 4 presbyopia-correcting IOL designs: diffractive panfocal, diffractive trifocal, segmental refractive, and extended-depth-of-focus. *J Cataract Refract Surg.* 2019;45(11):1625–1636.

spectacle dependence at all distances. In addition, they should have good potential vision without significant pathology. Specific preoperative evaluation of macular function and anatomy may be warranted to exclude patients with macular degeneration, epiretinal membrane, or other conditions leading to suboptimal retinal function. Careful attention should be paid to evaluation of the corneal endothelium, as patients with Fuchs dystrophy may not be ideal candidates for MFIOLs. Significant anterior basement membrane dystrophy or tear film abnormality from dry eye syndrome or blepharitis may also adversely affect postoperative performance of these lenses. Multifocal IOLs are also more sensitive to residual ametropia than monofocal IOLs. Patients with more than 0.75 D residual astigmatism after MFIOL implantation frequently have suboptimal vision quality. As such, strategies to reduce postoperative spherical error and astigmatism, such as subsequent laser vision correction, may be needed more often in these patients than in patients receiving monofocal IOLs. Thus, these strategies should be evaluated and discussed before IOL implantation. Evidence has shown that patients generally have better visual outcomes if MFIOLs are implanted bilaterally, although mixing and matching with different multifocal, monofocal, and EDOF IOLs is sometimes used to meet the specific near, intermediate, and distance needs of individual patients.

Surgical Technique

The surgical technique for MFIOL insertion is the same as that used in standard small-incision cataract surgery with a foldable acrylic IOL. MFIOLs are much more sensitive than monofocal IOLs to minor optic decentration. If the posterior capsule is not intact, IOL decentration is more likely to occur, and adequate fixation for an MFIOL should be determined before implantation. Interoperative wavefront aberrometry and microscope-mounted, toric-IOL-alignment devices are available and may assist in the accuracy of intraoperative decisions on IOL power and alignment.

Patients are most likely to achieve independence from glasses after bilateral implantation of MFIOLs. Recent meta-analyses found bilateral MFIOL implantation associated with significant improvement in both distance and near visual acuity with each type of implant studied.

Rosen E, Alió JL, Dick HB, Dell S, Slade S. Efficacy and safety of multifocal intraocular lenses following cataract and refractive lens exchange: metaanalysis of peer-reviewed publications. *J Cataract Refract Surg.* 2016;42(2):310–328.

Adverse Effects, Complications, and Patient Dissatisfaction With Multifocal Intraocular Lenses

Patient concerns after MFIOL implantation can generally be divided into 2 categories: blurred vision and photic phenomena (glare, halos). Patients may experience both groups of symptoms. These symptoms can occur even after uneventful surgery with a well-centered MFIOL.

Patients with MFIOLs are more likely to have significant glare, halos, and ghosting than are patients with monofocal, toric, or accommodating IOLs. These issues stem from a variety of different sources, including residual refractive error, ocular surface disease, or intrinsic IOL problems. The reports of halos intrinsically related to the IOL tend to subside over several months, perhaps from the patient's neural adaptation, but they may be persistent. Because of a reduction in contrast sensitivity, the subjective quality of vision after MFIOL insertion may not be as good as after monofocal IOL implantation. The trade-off of decreased quality of vision in return for reduced dependence on glasses must be discussed fully with the patient preoperatively. With MFIOLs, intermediate vision may be less clear than distance or near acuity (see Chapter 10).

Some patients never adapt to MFIOLs and require IOL exchange to recover vision. All patients should be counseled as to this possibility before surgery. Patients with MFIOLs appear to be more sensitive to posterior capsule opacification (PCO) than individuals with monofocal IOLs. These patients benefit from Nd:YAG capsulotomy; however, tolerance of the MFIOL must be determined before undergoing the Nd:YAG capsulotomy, as an open posterior capsule significantly complicates IOL exchange. Intrinsic IOL symptoms usually appear very early if not immediately in the postoperative course and do not generally worsen over time. In contrast, symptoms from PCO are not present initially but gradually worsen over the first few weeks to months after the surgical procedure.

Braga-Mele R, Chang D, Dewey S, et al; ASCRS Cataract Clinical Committee. Multifocal intraocular lenses: relative indications and contraindications for implantation. *J Cataract Refract Surg.* 2014;40(2):313–322.

Hood CT, Sugar A. Subjective complaints after cataract surgery: common causes and management strategies. *Curr Opin Ophthalmol.* 2015;26(1):45–49.

Rosenfeld SI, O'Brien TP. The dissatisfied presbyopia-correcting IOL patient. *Focal Points: Clinical Modules for Ophthalmologists.* American Academy of Ophthalmology; 2011, module 8.

Bioptics

The term *bioptics* was suggested by Zaldivar in the late 1990s. It is used to describe the combination of 2 refractive procedures—1 intraocular and 1 corneal—to treat patients with refractive errors that are suboptimally treated with a single procedure. Examples include extreme myopia, high myopia or hyperopia with significant astigmatism, and MFIOL implantation in patients with significant astigmatism. In these cases, the intraocular procedure is performed first, with keratorefractive surgery performed after both anatomical and refractive stability are achieved, usually 1–3 months after the initial surgery. Ideally, a keratorefractive procedure is performed after YAG laser capsulotomy (if needed) to further stabilize effective lens position and manifest refraction prior to corneal treatment. Capsulotomy is typically not recommended prior to 3 months after IOL implantation.

Bioptics with LASIK or surface ablation are reasonable alternatives, depending on patient parameters. As new treatment options are developed, the possibilities for other combinations of refractive surgery will increase.

The ability to successfully combine refractive procedures further expands the limits of refractive surgery. The predictability, stability, and safety of LASIK increase when smaller refractive errors are treated. In addition, there is usually sufficient corneal tissue to maximize the treatment zone diameter without exceeding the limits of ablation depth. The LASIK procedure provides the feature of adjustability in the overall refractive operation. These benefits must be balanced against the combined risks of performing 2 surgical procedures rather than 1.

Trivizki O, Smadja D, Mimouni M, Levinger S, Levinger E. Bioptics for high hyperopia with combined multifocal intraocular lens implantation and excimer ablation in young patients. *Eur J Ophthalmol.* 2019;29(4):426–430.

Emerging Technologies

Because the creation of peripheral iridotomies before or during phakic IOL implantation may lead to complications such as iris bleeding or cataract, a posterior chamber PIOL with a central pore has been developed to allow the flow of aqueous through the center of the lens. This PIOL, which eliminates the need for additional iridotomies, is available outside the United States and is currently being evaluated by the FDA. In addition, several fluid-filled IOLs are under development and in early-stage clinical trials. These IOLs use the natural accommodative forces of the eye to shift internal fluid, changing the curvature of the IOL optic with resulting increased dioptric power and near focus. See Chapter 10 for further discussion.

CHAPTER 10

Accommodative and Nonaccommodative Treatment of Presbyopia

This chapter includes related videos. Go to www.aao.org/bcscvideo_section13 or scan the QR codes in the text to access this content.

Highlights

- Presbyopia, the loss of accommodation with age, affects approximately 100 million people in the United States.
- Strategies for correction of presbyopia include corneal, scleral, and lens-replacement surgery.
- New pharmacologic treatments and intraocular lens technologies in development appear to be especially promising.

Introduction

Presbyopia, the normal progressive loss of accommodation, affects all individuals beginning in middle age, regardless of any underlying refractive error. This relentless loss of near vision and dependency on glasses for near work may be particularly distressing for otherwise emmetropic individuals who previously enjoyed excellent uncorrected vision at all distances.

Interest in the surgical correction of presbyopia has resulted in several treatment options. These techniques include scleral modification, implantation of presbyopia-correcting intraocular lenses (IOLs), or creation of a multifocal cornea by use of lasers or alteration of the corneal stroma. More recently, the development of corneal inlays has introduced a new option for patients.

Overview of Strategies for Surgical Correction of Presbyopia

Scleral

- Incisional or laser modification: deep cuts or erbium:yttrium-aluminum-garnet (Er:YAG) laser treatment over the ciliary body area in an attempt to enhance accommodative effort and zonular function (see the section Scleral Surgery for potential complications)

Corneal

- Monovision: refractive target selected for near vision in nondominant eye treated with photorefractive keratectomy, laser in situ keratomileusis, or conductive keratoplasty
  - Modified monovision: manipulation of positive or negative spherical aberration to enhance uncorrected near vision
- Multifocal cornea: creation of multifocal zones with the excimer laser
- Corneal inlays: small-aperture or refractive implant in stroma of nondominant eye

Lens Based

- Monovision: selection of IOL for near vision in nondominant eye at the time of cataract surgery or refractive lens exchange
- Accommodating IOL: increase in IOL power during accommodative effort
- Multifocal or extended depth of focus IOL: use of concentric rings, zones, or diffractive optics to enhance near vision

Theories of Accommodation

The *Helmholtz hypothesis* or *capsular theory* of accommodation states that during distance vision, the ciliary muscle is relaxed and the zonular fibers that cross the circumlental space between the ciliary body and the lens equator are in a condition of "resting" tension. With accommodative effort, the ciliary muscle annular ring moves anteriorly and tension is released in the zonules, increasing the accommodative power of the lens. The reduced zonular tension allows the elastic capsule of the lens to contract, causing a decrease in equatorial lens diameter and an increase in the curvature of the anterior and posterior lens surfaces. This "rounding up" of the lens produces a corresponding increase in its dioptric power, enabling near vision (Fig 10-1). When the accommodative effort ceases, the ciliary muscle relaxes and the zonular tension on the lens equator increases to its resting state. This increased tension on the lens equator causes a flattening of the lens, a decrease in the curvature of the anterior and posterior lens surfaces, and a decrease in the dioptric power of the unaccommodated eye.

In the Helmholtz theory, the equatorial edge of the lens moves away from the sclera during accommodation and toward the sclera when accommodation ends. In this theory,

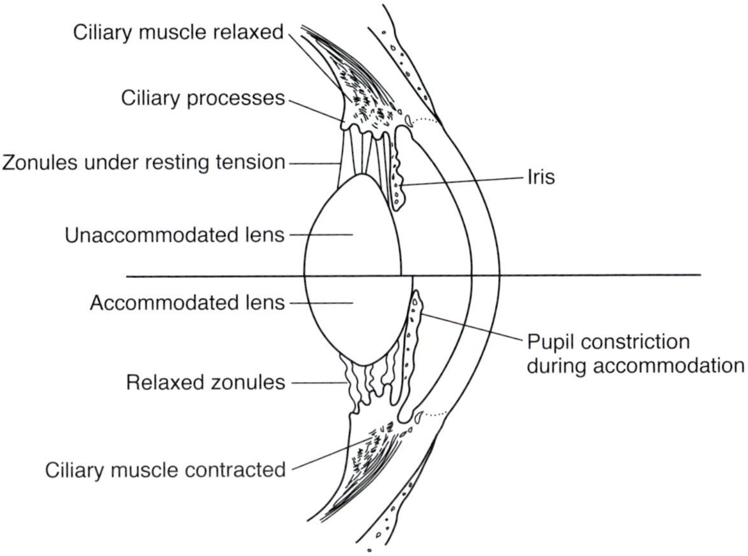

Figure 10-1 Schematic representation of the Helmholtz theory of accommodation, in which contraction of the ciliary muscle during accommodation *(bottom)* leads to relaxation of the zonular fibers. The reduced zonular tension allows the elastic capsule of the lens to contract, causing an increase in the curvature of the anterior and posterior lens. *(Illustration by Jeanne Koelling.)*

all zonular fibers are relaxed during accommodation and under tension when the accommodative effort ends. According to Helmholtz, presbyopia results from the loss of lens elasticity with age. When the zonules of an older lens are relaxed, the lens does not change its shape to the same degree as a younger lens does; therefore, presbyopia is an aging process that can be reversed only by changing the elasticity of the lens or its capsule.

Using model-based reasoning, Goldberg proposed another theory of accommodation with the help of a computer-animated 3-dimensional model of the eye and the accommodative system. Goldberg's *theory of reciprocal zonular action* describes 3 components of the zonules and posits that a synchronized movement by the ciliary body, zonules, and anterior hyaloid complex leads to a shift in the posterior lenticular curvature and refractive power (Video 10-1).

VIDEO 10-1 Computer model of accommodation.
Courtesy of Daniel B. Goldberg, MD.

Several other theories of accommodation have been proposed as well. Among them is the Schachar theory, but recent studies on humans and nonhuman primates do not support this mechanism of accommodation.

Glasser A, Kaufman PL. The mechanism of accommodation in primates. *Ophthalmology.* 1999;106(5):863–872.

Goldberg DB. Computer-animated model of accommodation and theory of reciprocal zonular action. *Clin Ophthalmol.* 2011;5:1559–1566.

Schachar RA. Cause and treatment of presbyopia with a method for increasing the amplitude of accommodation. *Ann Ophthalmol.* 1992;24(12):445–447, 452.

Strenk SA, Strenk LM, Koretz JF. The mechanism of presbyopia. *Prog Retin Eye Res.* 2005;24(3):379–393.

Accommodative Treatment of Presbyopia

Scleral Surgery

Several scleral surgical procedures have been evaluated for use in the reduction of presbyopia. Their objective was to increase zonular tension by weakening or altering the sclera over the ciliary body to allow for its passive expansion. Thornton first proposed weakening the sclera by making 8 or more scleral incisions over the ciliary body in a procedure called *anterior ciliary sclerotomy (ACS).* Results were mixed, and any positive effect appeared short-lived. A prospective study of ACS using a 4-incision technique was discontinued because of significant adverse events, including anterior segment ischemia. In 2001, the American Academy of Ophthalmology stated that ACS was ineffective and a potentially dangerous treatment for presbyopia. Use of scleral expansion bands placed directly over the ciliary body has had mixed results and has largely been abandoned.

However, one approach to scleral alteration is still under investigation. It involves use of an Er:YAG laser to create a series of micro-incisions or micropores in the sclera in an attempt to increase scleral plasticity over the ciliary body and thus improve the efficiency of accommodation.

Hipsley A, Hall B, Rocha KM. Long-term visual outcomes of laser anterior ciliary excision. *Am J Ophthalmol Case Rep.* 2018;10:38–47.

Hipsley A, Hall B, Rocha KM. Scleral surgery for the treatment of presbyopia: where are we today? *Eye Vis (Lond).* 2018;5:4.

Hipsley A, Ma DH, Sun CC, Jackson MA, Goldberg D, Hall B. Visual outcomes 24 months after LaserACE. *Eye Vis (Lond).* 2017;4:15.

Accommodating Intraocular Lenses

Accommodating IOLs attempt to restore a significant amount of true accommodation to patients with surgically induced pseudophakia. Accommodating IOLs were designed following the observation that some patients who received silicone plate-haptic IOLs reported better near vision than would be expected from their refractive result. Investigations revealed that during ciliary muscle contraction, forward displacement of the IOL led to an increase in the IOL's effective power and thus an improvement in near vision. However, some studies have questioned the amplitude of true accommodation that can be obtained solely on the basis of anterior displacement of the IOL optic. Other factors, such as pupil size, with-the-rule astigmatism, and mild myopia, may also contribute to unaided near visual acuity and increased depth of focus.

Some IOLs that use this accommodative approach are modified silicone plate-haptic lenses (Fig 10-2). These lenses may allow anterior movement of the lens during accommodation. Another possibility is that ciliary body contraction causes a steepening of the

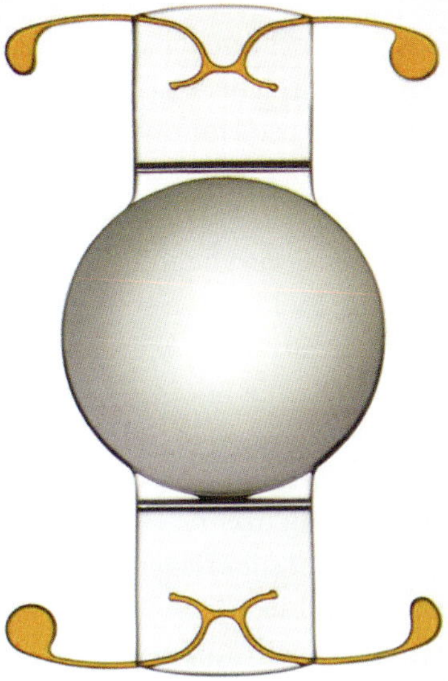

Figure 10-2 Accommodating intraocular lens with a flexible hinge in the haptic at the proximal end and a polyamide footplate at the distal end. The footplate functions to maximize contact with the capsule and ciliary body, and the hinge transfers the horizontal force into an anteroposterior movement of the optic. *(Courtesy of Carissa Hluchan and Michael Bono.)*

anterior optic surface, allowing for better near vision. Although the exact mechanism of the movement is unclear, it appears to be a combination of posterior chamber pressure on the back surface of the IOL and ciliary body pressure on the IOL that vaults the optic forward. The anterior displacement is postulated to result in an effective increase in optical power and near vision. The amount of power change is limited by the amount of movement (usually 1 mm or less) and is proportional to the base power of the IOL (anterior movement of a 15-D lens will result in a much smaller refractive change than a 30-D lens). As the posterior capsule contracts and stiffens over time, movement of the IOL may be limited. Newer accommodating IOL designs that employ different mechanisms of action are discussed later in this chapter in the Emerging Technologies section.

Pepose JS, Burke J, Qazi MA. Benefits and barriers of accommodating intraocular lenses. *Curr Opin Ophthalmol.* 2017;28(1):3–8.

Pepose JS, Burke J, Qazi MA. Accommodating intraocular lenses. *Asia Pac J Ophthalmol (Phila).* 2017;6(4):350–357.

Nonaccommodative Treatment of Presbyopia

Monovision

In the United States, monovision is the technique used most frequently for the nonspectacle correction of presbyopia. The term *monovision* typically refers to correcting 1 eye for distance (usually the dominant eye) and the other for near. Monovision can be achieved with contact lenses, laser in situ keratomileusis (LASIK), surface ablation (photorefractive keratectomy [PRK]), conductive keratoplasty (CK), or even lens-based surgery. A power difference of 1.25–2.50 D between the eyes is targeted on the basis of near-vision demands. Many refractive surgeons target mild myopia (–0.50 D to −1.50 D) for the near-vision eye in presbyopic and prepresbyopic patients. The term *mini-monovision* is used for myopia of –0.50 to –0.75 D; the term *blended vision* is used for myopia of −1.00 to −1.50 D. Mini-monovision is associated with only a mild decrease in distance vision, retention of good stereopsis, and a significant increase in the intermediate zone of functional vision. The intermediate zone is where many visual functions of daily life are performed (eg, looking at a computer screen or a car dashboard). For many patients, this compromise is an attractive alternative to constantly reaching for reading glasses. Selected patients who want better near vision may prefer a higher monovision correction (−1.50 D to –2.50 D) despite the accompanying decrease in distance vision and stereopsis. Leaving 1 eye nearsighted may lead to glare and halos from unfocused light when driving at night. This can be corrected with driving glasses.

The term *modified monovision* refers to the manipulation of spherical aberration (SA) to enhance near vision. Both negative and positive SA can aid near-vision performance; however, contrast sensitivity is compromised to some extent with this approach. Induction of SA to aid near vision has been described following laser vision correction and is the basis for the design of some IOLs.

Zheleznyak L, Sabesan R, Oh JS, MacRae S, Yoon G. Modified monovision with spherical aberration to improve presbyopic through-focus visual performance. *Invest Ophthalmol Vis Sci.* 2013;54(5):3157–3165.

Patient selection

Appropriate patient selection and education are fundamental to the success of monovision treatment. Although monovision can be demonstrated with trial lenses in the examination room, a contact lens trial period at home is often more useful to ascertain patient acceptance and the exact degree of near vision desired. For most patients, refractive surgeons routinely aim for mild myopia (–0.50 D to −1.50 D) in the nondominant eye.

The best candidates for monovision are individuals with myopia who are older than 40 years and who, because of their current refractive error, retain some useful uncorrected near vision. These patients have always experienced adequate near vision simply by removing their glasses and therefore understand the importance of near vision. Patients whose vision is neither presbyopic nor approaching presbyopia are typically not good candidates for monovision, as they are usually seeking optimal bilateral distance vision. However, those in their mid- to late 30s should be counseled about impending presbyopia and the option of monovision. Patients who do not have useful uncorrected near vision (ie, patients with myopia worse than –4.50 D or hyperopia) may be more accepting of the need for reading glasses after refractive surgery. A history of strabismus, phoria, or tropia warrants caution and a possible contact lens trial to avoid diplopia or other visual symptoms related to monovision.

Patients should understand that the loss of accommodation is progressive; thus, monovision may not be permanent and corrective glasses may eventually be required.

Monovision is also associated with a compromise in depth perception that may be bothersome to individuals who actively engage in sports such as tennis or skiing; patient counseling includes a discussion of these limitations. A difference of more than 2.00–3.00 D between the eyes can be difficult to tolerate because of the disparity in image size associated with anisometropia.

Reinstein DZ, Carp GI, Archer TJ, Gobbe M. LASIK for presbyopia correction in emmetropic patients using aspheric ablation profiles and a micro-monovision protocol with the Carl Zeiss Meditec MEL 80 and VisuMax. *J Refract Surg.* 2012;28(8):531–541.

Smith CE, Allison R, Wilkinson F, Wilcox LM. Monovision: consequences for depth perception from large disparities. *Exp Eye Res.* 2019;183:62–67.

Conductive Keratoplasty

In 2004, conductive keratoplasty (CK) received US Food and Drug Administration (FDA) approval for treatment of presbyopia in the nondominant eye of a patient with an endpoint of −1.00 D to −2.00 D (correction of hyperopia of 0.75 D to 3.00 D and up to 0.75 D of astigmatism). CK can be considered when other, more invasive procedures, such as LASIK or refractive lens exchange, may not be appropriate and is useful for the correction of low refractive error. The nonablative, collagen-shrinking effect of CK results from delivery of radiofrequency energy through a fine conducting tip that is inserted into the peripheral corneal stroma. As the current flows through the tissue surrounding the tip, resistance to the current creates localized heat. Collagen lamellae in the area shrink in a controlled fashion and form a column of denatured collagen. The shortening of the collagen fibrils creates a band of tightening and flattening in the periphery that increases the relative curvature of the central cornea (Fig 10-3).

For the treatment of hyperopia and presbyopia, the surgeon inserts the tip into the stroma in a ring pattern around the peripheral cornea. The number and location of spots determine the amount of refractive change, with an increasing number of spots and rings used for higher amounts of hyperopia. The CK procedure is performed under topical anesthesia and typically takes less than 5 minutes (Video 10-2). The collagen shrinkage leads to visible striae, which fade with time, between the treated spots. The treatment is not advisable for patients who have undergone radial keratotomy, and it is not FDA approved for such use.

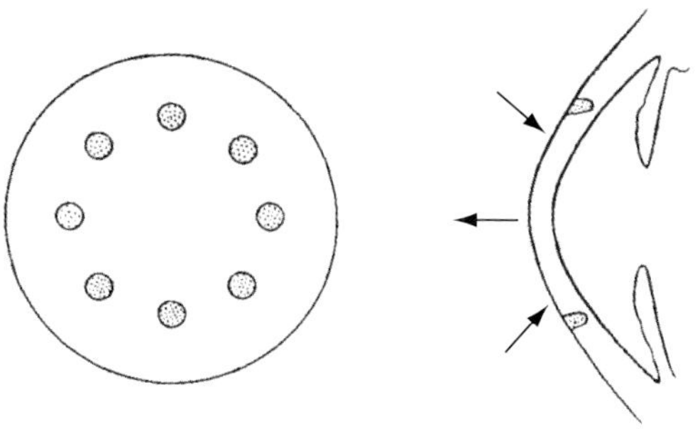

Figure 10-3 Schematic illustration of conductive keratoplasty. Note that uniform collagen shrinkage of the paracentral cornea results in steepening of the central corneal curvature.

VIDEO 10-2 Conductive keratoplasty.
Courtesy of Majid Moshirfar, MD, and Christopher Kurz, MD.

Despite initial reports of refractive stability, regression or lack of an adequate effect over time has been reported. In a long-term follow-up (mean, 73.1 months; range, 44–90 months) of patients enrolled in the phase 3 multicenter trial of CK, Ehrlich and Manche found nearly complete regression of treatment effect in the 16 eyes (of the original 25 eyes) available for follow-up.

Ehrlich JS, Manche EE. Regression of effect over long-term follow-up of conductive keratoplasty to correct mild to moderate hyperopia. *J Cataract Refract Surg.* 2009;35(9):1591–1596.

Other applications

Other potential off-label uses exist for CK. It can be used to correct hyperopia in cases of overcorrection of myopia after LASIK and PRK. In these procedures, CK obviates the need to lift or cut another flap.

CK may also be used to treat keratoconus and post-LASIK ectasia, although regression of effect may occur. Combination therapy with CK plus collagen crosslinking may be effective in achieving a change in corneal curvature that does not regress with time.

Chang JS, Lau SY. Conductive keratoplasty to treat hyperopic overcorrection after LASIK for myopia. *J Refract Surg.* 2011;27(1):49–55.

Kymionis GD, Kontadakis GA, Naoumidi TL, Kazakos DC, Giapitzakis I, Pallikaris IG. Conductive keratoplasty followed by collagen cross-linking with riboflavin–UV-A in patients with keratoconus. *Cornea.* 2010;29(2):239–243.

Multifocal and Extended Depth of Focus Intraocular Lenses

The number of IOL options for patients undergoing cataract surgery has increased in recent years. Patients may select a traditional monofocal IOL with a refractive target of emmetropia or monovision, or they may opt for a multifocal lens or accommodating IOL for greater range of focus. Table 10-1 provides an overview of presbyopia-correcting IOLs that are currently available or in development.

Several multifocal IOLs (MFIOLs) and extended depth of focus (EDOF) IOLs have been FDA approved in the United States. Since the first MFIOL was introduced, lens design has evolved. Diffractive lens designs employ a series of concentric rings to form a diffraction grating (see BCSC Section 3, *Clinical Optics and Vision Rehabilitation*), thus creating separate focal points for distance, intermediate, and near vision (Fig 10-4A). Multifocal lenses can be classified as either *bifocal,* if the lens provides focal points primarily for distance and near, or *trifocal,* if the lens supplies intermediate distance as well. Some diffractive lenses are *apodized,* meaning that the diffractive step heights are gradually tapered to yield a more even distribution of light, which theoretically allows a smoother transition between images from distant to near targets. In 2016, the FDA approved the first diffractive EDOF IOL (Fig 10-4B). This lens uses echelette diffractive optics to create an elongated focal zone, emphasizing intermediate to distance vision. The performance of MFIOLs and EDOF IOLs can be compared and contrasted with the aid of a defocus curve (Fig 10-5).

Table 10-1 **Intraocular Lenses for the Correction of Presbyopia**

Category	IOL Model (Manufacturer)	Design	FDA Approved	Comments
Accommodative	Crystalens (Bausch + Lomb)	1-piece plate haptic	Yes	See text
	TetraflexHD (Lenstec)	1-piece plate haptic	No	
	FluidVision (PowerVision)	1-piece fluid-filled lens	No	See text
	Juvene (LensGen)	2-piece design	No	See text and Video 10-2
	NuLens (NuLens Ltd)		No	See text
	Opira (ForSight Vision6)	2-piece modular design	No	See text
	Atia (Atia Vision)	2-piece modular design	No	Front optic can be exchanged
Multifocal	AcrySof IQ ReStor (Alcon)	Diffractive bifocal (apodized)	Yes	Available in 3 add powers and toric models
	Tecnis Multifocal (Johnson & Johnson Vision)	Diffractive bifocal (nonapodized)	Yes	Available in 3 add powers and toric models
	PanOptix (Alcon)	Diffractive trifocal (nonapodized)	Yes	Available in toric models
	M-flex (Rayner)	Zonal refractive bifocal	No	
	Lentis MPlus (Oculentis)	Zonal refractive bifocal	No	
Extended depth of focus	Tecnis Symfony (Johnson & Johnson Vision)	Echelette diffractive	Yes	Available in toric models
	IC-8 (AcuFocus)	Small-aperture technology	No	Optical principle similar to Kamra corneal inlay
	Mini Well (Sifi MedTech)	Central distance zone, surrounding distance zone with spherical aberration of the opposite sign, and a peripheral distance zone with monofocal characteristics	No	
	AcrySof IQ Vivity (Alcon)	Diffractive optics	Yes	Available in toric models
	IsoPure (PhysIOL)	Manipulates negative spherical aberration to achieve elongated focal zone	No	
Refractive index change	Sapphire (Elenza)	Electric current changes refractive index	No	
Other	Harmoni (Alcon)	2-piece modular design	No	Central optic can be changed from multifocal to monofocal (see text)
	Smart IOL (Medennium)	Acrylic gel injected into capsule after cataract removal	No	Gel takes the shape of capsule and crystalline lens (see text)

FDA = Food and Drug Administration; IOL = intraocular lens.

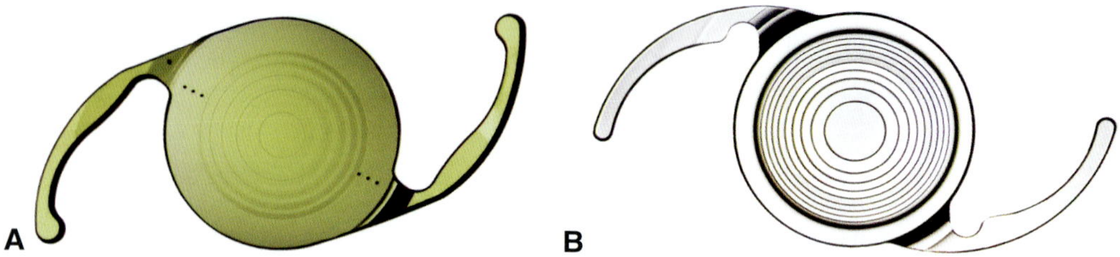

Figure 10-4 Examples of intraocular lenses (IOLs) that make use of diffractive optics. **A,** Trifocal IOL. **B,** Extended depth of focus IOL. *(Courtesy of Carissa Hluchan and Michael Bono.)*

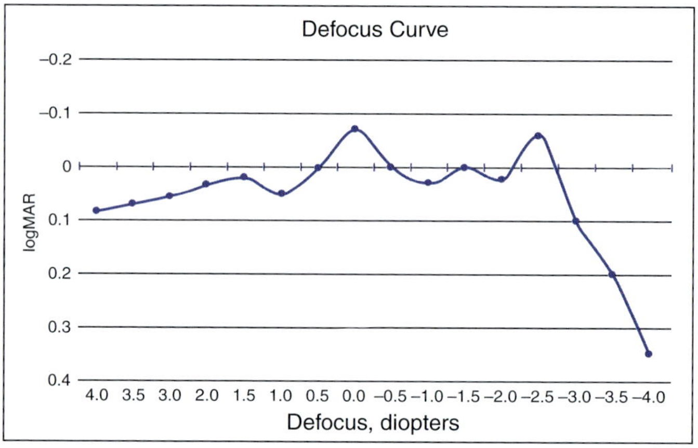

Figure 10-5 A defocus curve for a multifocal lens. Defocus curves are created by having the patient look through a series of positive and negative lenses (x-axis) and measuring the resulting binocular visual acuity (y-axis). This simulates what a patient will see at different distances. For example, a –2.00 D lens would simulate visual acuity at a distance of 50 cm (focal length [f] = 1/D). Pupil size, astigmatism, and spherical aberration can affect these measurements. The figure is designed to illustrate the concept of a defocus curve and is not representative of a particular lens. *(Courtesy of Michael Taravella, MD.)*

Zonal refractive lens design is another method of creating multifocality. Different zones of the lens have different refractive powers for distance and near. (See also BCSC Section 11, *Lens and Cataract,* Chapter 9, for further discussion and illustrations of MFIOLs.)

Böhm M, Petermann K, Hemkeppler E, Kohnen T. Defocus curves of 4 presbyopia-correcting IOL designs: diffractive panfocal, diffractive trifocal, segmental refractive, and extended-depth-of-focus. *J Cataract Refract Surg.* 2019;45(11):1625–1636.

de Medeiros AL, Jones Saraiva F, Iguma CI, et al. Comparison of visual outcomes after bilateral implantation of two intraocular lenses with distinct diffractive optics. *Clin Ophthalmol.* 2019;13:1657–1663.

US Food and Drug Administration. TECNIS Symfony Extended Range of Vision Intraocular Lens - P980040/S065. July 15, 2016. Accessed October 6, 2021. www.accessdata.fda.gov/cdrh_docs/pdf/P980040S065A.pdf

Patient selection

Patient counseling includes a discussion of the benefits and visual outcomes of MFIOLs and EDOF IOLs to ensure that the patient has realistic expectations. The preoperative examination is equally important; it is critical to rule out any macular or other ocular diseases, as MFIOLs are contraindicated in eyes with preexisting poor vision potential. Optical coherence tomography can be a useful adjunct for detecting significant macular pathology preoperatively. In addition, any ophthalmic abnormality that could increase ocular aberrations (eg, corneal scarring, irregular astigmatism, dry eye) can significantly decrease image quality with these lenses. The clinician should carefully consider the possibility of patient dissatisfaction with the quality of vision after MFIOL implantation. (See also Chapter 9.)

Complications

Patients who have suboptimal results or are dissatisfied with the quality of their vision with MFIOLs or EDOF IOLs should undergo a comprehensive evaluation from the ocular surface to the macula. The clinician should exclude possible causes of visual disturbance such as dry eye, residual refractive error, decentered lens or pupil, irregular astigmatism, vitreous opacities, cystoid macular edema, or epiretinal membrane. Posterior capsule opacification is of greater concern with multifocal than monofocal IOLs because minimal changes in the capsule can cause early deterioration in vision. To achieve optimal vision, patients with MFIOLs may require Nd:YAG laser capsulotomy earlier or more frequently than those with monofocal IOLs. However, if IOL exchange is being contemplated, Nd:YAG laser capsulotomy should be deferred. Other possible causes of visual disturbance should be excluded before an IOL exchange is considered.

MFIOLs and EDOF IOLs may cause glare and halos around lights at night, although newer MFIOLs incorporate technology that substantially reduces (but does not generally eliminate) these optical phenomena. Symptoms may be improved through the use of nighttime driving glasses or instillation of topical brimonidine drops to reduce mesopic pupil size. In addition, most of these symptoms will decrease over time through neuroadaptation. (See also Chapter 9.)

McMillin JC, Rocha KM, Barnwell EL, Haddad JS, Waring GO IV. Objective evaluation of vision quality in pseudophakic patients with posterior capsular opacification using double-pass retinal imaging. *Arq Bras Oftalmol.* 2019;82(3):189–194.

Shah VC, Russo C, Cannon R, Davidson R, Taravella MJ. Incidence of Nd:YAG capsulotomy after implantation of AcrySof multifocal and monofocal intraocular lenses: a case controlled study. *J Refract Surg.* 2010;26(8):565–568.

Multifocal Corneal Ablations

An excimer laser can be used to create a multifocal cornea. Prompted by the observation that the uncorrected near vision of many patients improved more than expected after

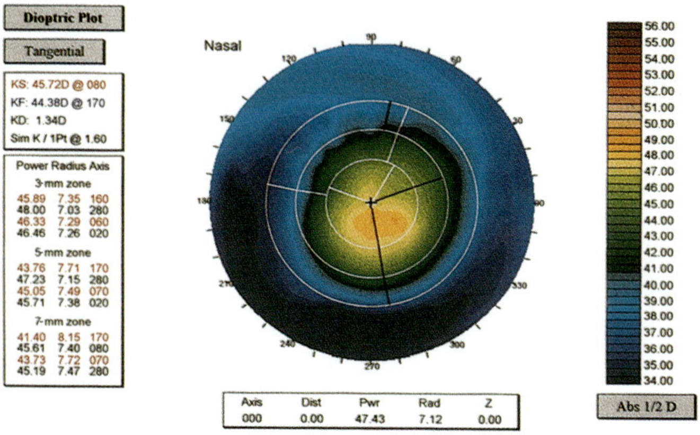

Figure 10-6 Multifocal ablation. Corneal topographic map showing a multifocal pattern after hyperopic laser in situ keratomileusis (LASIK) in a 62-year-old patient with preoperative hyperopia of +4.00 D. Postoperatively, the uncorrected distance visual acuity is $20/25^{-2}$ and at near is Jaeger score J1. Manifest refraction of −0.25 +0.75 D × 20 yields visual acuity of 20/20. Corneal topography demonstrates central hyperopic ablation *(green)* with relative steepening in the lower portion of the pupillary axis *(orange)*, which provides the near add for reading vision. *(Courtesy of Jayne S. Weiss, MD.)*

excimer ablation (Fig 10-6), ophthalmologists began to investigate the potential for improving near vision without significantly compromising distance vision. To this end, the following corneal ablation patterns have been employed:

- a small, central steep zone ablation, in which the central portion of the cornea is used for near vision and the midperiphery for distance vision
- an inferior near-zone ablation
- an inferiorly decentered hyperopic ablation
- a central distance ablation with an intermediate/near midperipheral ablation

Some of these patterns generate simultaneous near and distance images, whereas others rely on pupillary constriction (accommodative convergence) to concentrate light rays through the steeper central ablation. Although multifocal corneal ablation offers some potential advantages, the results of this technique are still under investigation.

Alarcón A, Anera RG, del Barco LJ, Jiménez JR. Designing multifocal corneal models to correct presbyopia by laser ablation. *J Biomed Opt.* 2012;17(1):018001.

Pallikaris IG, Panagopoulou SI. PresbyLASIK approach for the correction of presbyopia. *Curr Opin Ophthalmol.* 2015;26(4):265–272.

Stival LR, Figueiredo MN, Santhiago MR. Presbyopic excimer laser ablation: a review. *J Refract Surg.* 2018;34(10):698–710.

Corneal Inlays

Refractive errors, including presbyopia, may be treated by placing preformed tissue or synthetic material on or in the cornea. This approach alters the optical power of the cornea by changing the shape of the anterior corneal surface or by implanting a lens with a higher index of refraction than the corneal stroma. Intracorneal inlays with small apertures that use the pinhole effect to increase depth of focus have been developed. Corneal surface tissue addition procedures (ie, corneal onlays), such as *epikeratoplasty,* have fallen out of favor because of the poor predictability of the refractive and visual results, loss of corrected distance visual acuity (CDVA), and difficulty of obtaining donor tissue.

Homoplastic Corneal Inlays

Historically, a homoplastic inlay was created from a donor cornea by a lamellar keratectomy after removal of the epithelium and Bowman layer. The lenticule (fresh or frozen) was then shaped into a lens by means of an automated lathe and placed into a lamellar pocket or sutured onto the recipient corneal surface. This procedure, called *keratophakia,* has been used to correct aphakia and hyperopia of up to 20.00 D, but few studies of this procedure have been published. Early efforts, in which donor tissue was shaped by microkeratome before implantation, were hampered by low refractive predictability and complications including irregular lamellar resection, wound dehiscence, and postoperative corneal edema.

The procedure was originally intended to be used in conjunction with cataract extraction for the correction of aphakia, but its surgical complexity and unpredictable refractive results could not compete with aphakic contact lenses or the improved technology of IOL implantation. However, homoplastic keratophakia using excimer laser–shaped tissue obtained from small-incision stromal lenticule extraction (SMILE) procedures has been suggested for treating hyperopia, presbyopia, and ectatic corneal diseases. (See Chapter 6 for further information on SMILE.)

Ganesh S, Brar S, Rao PA. Cryopreservation of extracted corneal lenticules after small incision lenticule extraction for potential use in human subjects. *Cornea.* 2014;33(12): 1355–1362.

Riau AK, Liu YC, Yam GHF, Mehta JS. Stromal keratophakia: corneal inlay implantation. *Prog Retin Eye Res.* 2019;75:100780.

Sun L, Yao P, Li M, Shen Y, Zhao J, Zhou X. The safety and predictability of implanting autologous lenticule obtained by SMILE for hyperopia. *J Refract Surg.* 2015;31(6):374–379.

Alloplastic Corneal Inlays

Alloplastic inlays offer several potential advantages over homoplastic inlays, such as the ability to be accurately mass produced in a wide range of sizes and powers. Synthetic material may have optical properties that are superior to those of tissue lenses. Because of problems with re-epithelialization when synthetic material is placed on top of the cornea, such material generally has to be placed within the corneal stroma. For insertion of the inlay, a LASIK-type flap or a stromal pocket dissection can be performed; such procedures are technically easier than a complete lamellar keratectomy.

Experiments performed in the early 1980s using glass or plastic lenticules resulted in corneal opacities, nonhealing epithelial erosions, and diurnal fluctuation in vision because these materials blocked fluid and nutrients from reaching the anterior cornea. Previous-generation lenticule inlays were made of more permeable substances such as hydrogel, with or without microperforations, to increase the transmission of nutrients. Hydrogel inlays have an index of refraction similar to that of the corneal stroma, so these lenses have little intrinsic optical power when implanted. These hydrogel inlays were designed to change the curvature of the anterior cornea, inducing myopia or multifocality. Other mechanisms of action include inlays with refractive power and small-aperture inlays.

In 2015, the FDA approved a small-aperture corneal inlay (Kamra; CorneaGen) indicated for the improvement of near vision in presbyopic patients. This device is an ultrathin (5-μm), biocompatible polymer that is microperforated to allow improved nutrient flow. The inlay, which is usually implanted in the nondominant eye, is 3.8 mm in diameter, with a central aperture that is 1.6 mm in diameter. Although the inlay has no refractive power, the central aperture functions as a pinhole to increase depth of focus and improve near vision without changing distance vision (Fig 10-7). The surgeon inserts the device into an intrastromal pocket created by a femtosecond laser. The inlay is placed at a depth equal to or greater than 200 μm, centered on the patient-fixated, coaxially sighted corneal light reflex.

In the FDA study, an average gain of 3 lines of uncorrected near vision (UNVA) in the implanted eye was observed at 12 months. In addition, 95% of eyes achieved the primary efficacy endpoint of 20/40 or better UNVA and a primary safety endpoint of 0% eyes having greater than or equal to 2 lines of persistent loss of CDVA. Rare complications included refractive instability, decentration, and haze. In the FDA study, 2.9% of inlays were explanted, and all eyes from which the device was removed returned to their preoperative CDVA. Since then, deeper implantation (200–300 μm) has been found to decrease the risk of stromal haze and improve refractive stability. Laser vision correction is sometimes performed immediately before implantation of the inlay to bring the patient's refraction to an ideal preimplantation target of –0.50 D to –1.00 D.

Another inlay (Flexivue Microlens; Presbia) is a small, clear, hydrophilic acrylic inlay with an index of refraction different from that of the cornea. The inlay is placed in

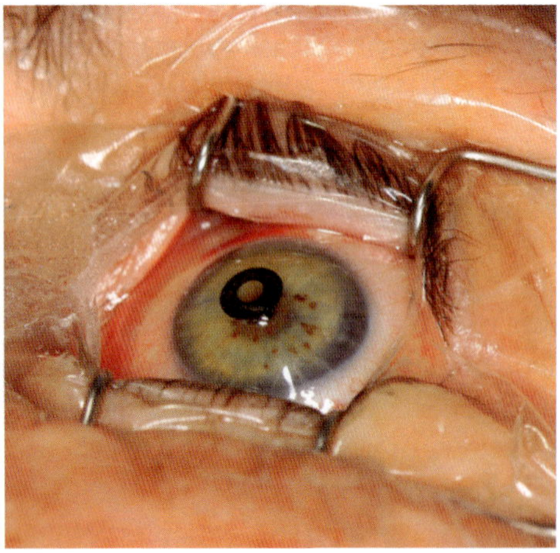

A

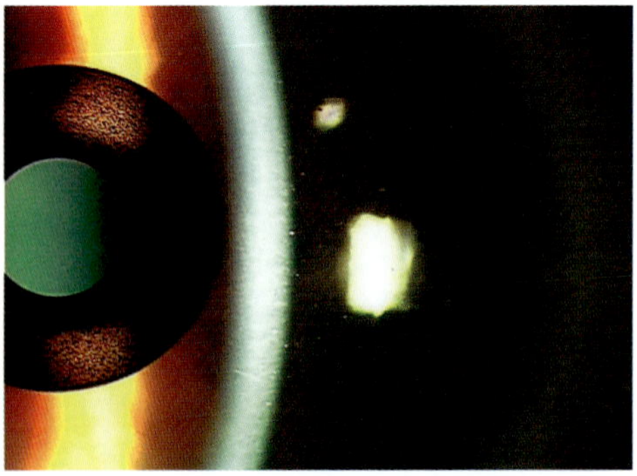

B

Figure 10-7 Small-aperture inlay. **A,** The device is placed in a deep lamellar pocket created by a femtosecond laser. **B,** Slit-lamp photograph of a small-aperture inlay in place. *(Courtesy of George O. Waring IV, MD.)*

a femtosecond-created corneal pocket 280–300 µm deep. A plano central zone is used for distance vision, while 1 or more concentric rings of varying additional power provide intermediate and near vision. The central zone is fenestrated to allow nutrient and oxygen diffusion across the cornea. In a study of 31 patients followed for 3 years after implantation in the nondominant eye, 76.9% of patients had UNVA of 20/25 (J1). Four devices were explanted: 3 for complaints of blurred vision at both distance and near in the implanted eye and 1 for a corneal ulcer. This inlay received the CE mark in 2009 but is not yet FDA approved.

Beer SMC, Werner L, Nakano EM, et al . A 3-year follow-up study of a new corneal inlay: clinical results and outcomes. *Br J Ophthalmol.* 2020;104(5):723–728.

Lindstrom RL, Macrae SM, Pepose JS, Hoopes PC Sr. Corneal inlays for presbyopia correction. *Curr Opin Ophthalmol.* 2013;24(4):281–287.

Tomita M, Kanamori T, Waring GO IV, et al. Simultaneous corneal inlay implantation and laser in situ keratomileusis for presbyopia in patients with hyperopia, myopia, or emmetropia: six-month results. *J Cataract Refract Surg.* 2012;38(3):495–506.

US Food and Drug Administration. Premarket Approval. KAMRA Inlay - P120023. April 17, 2015. Accessed October 6, 2021. www.accessdata.fda.gov/scripts/cdrh/cfdocs/cfpma/pma.cfm?ID=P120023

Vukich JA, Durrie DS, Pepose JS, Thompson V, van de Pol C, Lin L. Evaluation of the small-aperture intracorneal inlay: three-year results from the cohort of the U.S. Food and Drug Administration clinical trial. *J Cataract Refract Surg.* 2018;44(5):541–556.

Waring GO IV. Correction of presbyopia with a small aperture corneal inlay. *J Refract Surg.* 2011;27(11):842–845.

Emerging Technologies

Medical Treatment of Presbyopia

Pharmacologic therapy of presbyopia is based on 2 approaches. The first attempts to make the crystalline lens more pliable and flexible, reversing to some degree the natural age-related loss of elasticity. UNR844 chloride (UNR844-Cl; Novartis), also known as EV06, is a prodrug composed of lipoic acid choline ester 1.5%. As the drug penetrates into the eye, the lipoic acid converts to dihydolipoic acid, which breaks down disulfide bonds in the lens, softening the lens and improving its flexibility. This allows the crystalline lens to respond to accommodative effort. Preliminary results of a recent clinical trial have reported improvement in near function with the drug compared with placebo.

The second approach is to induce mild miosis, creating a pinhole effect and increasing the depth of field, ideally with minimal compromise in distance and night vision. Miotics currently in clinical trials include AGN-190584 (Allergan), aceclidine 2% (Presbyopia Therapies), and CSF-1 (Orasis).

Intraocular Lenses in Development

See Table 10-1, earlier in the chapter, which lists IOLs according to mechanism of action and FDA approval status. Some of the novel approaches to the correction of presbyopia are described in the following sections.

Accommodative mechanisms

Accommodating IOLs in use or development primarily employ 3 strategies to accomplish the necessary power change for near vision: a change in optic position, a change in the anterior curvature of the lens, or a change in refractive index.

As discussed earlier in the Accommodating Intraocular Lenses section, one approach is a single-optic IOL that makes use of anterior axial movement of the optic position to increase refractive power. The *Crystalens* (Bausch + Lomb; the only currently FDA-approved accommodating IOL) and *TetraflexHD* (Lenstec) employ this strategy.

Some IOLs in clinical trials or in development rely on a change in anterior curvature of the implanted lens; these lenses include FluidVision (Alcon) and Juvene (LensGen). The *FluidVision* IOL is completely hollow and filled with fluid. During accommodative effort, the capsular bag compresses and squeezes the lens. Fluid moves from the annular haptics into the body of the optic, increasing the anterior curvature and power of the lens. When the ciliary body relaxes again, the fluid moves from the optic back into the haptics, flattening the lens.

The *Juvene* IOL is a 2-piece device consisting of a larger base lens within a flexible outer silicone ring that is inserted into the capsular bag, followed by a smaller fluid-filled lens placed into the ring. Accommodative effort squeezes the silicone ring, which in turn compresses the fluid-filled lens, changing the anterior curvature of the lens and increasing its near power (Video 10-3).

VIDEO 10-3 Insertion of a Juvene intraocular lens.
Courtesy of Sumit (Sam) Garg, MD.

The *NuLens* (NuLens Ltd) relies on ciliary body contraction and relaxation to change power. The IOL consists of an anterior polymethyl methacrylate (PMMA) reference lens, a silicone gel–filled chamber, and a posterior piston. During accommodative effort, haptics placed in the sulcus generate a force that drives the piston forward; this in turn compresses the gel and pushes it through a small central aperture in the anterior PMMA portion of the lens. This changes the anterior curvature of the lens and provides near power.

The *Opira* (ForSight Vision6) and *Atia* (Atia Vision) IOLs are 2-piece modular systems that make use of ciliary body contraction to initiate power changes. The Opira is unique in that the anterior dynamic portion has haptics that straddle the edge of the capsulorrhexis (bag-in-the-lens concept), while the posterior portion provides optical power.

Other approaches

The *Sapphire* IOL (Elenza) uses an electric current to physically change the lens optics. A sensor built into the lens can detect pupil constriction as part of the accommodative reflex. An electric current is passed through the lens, altering the molecular configuration of the lens material and changing the power of the lens from distance to near. A small, wireless rechargeable battery powers the lens.

The *Harmoni* IOL (Alcon) is a modular system in which the central optic is detachable from the haptic base (Fig 10-8). Theoretically, this would allow for different types of

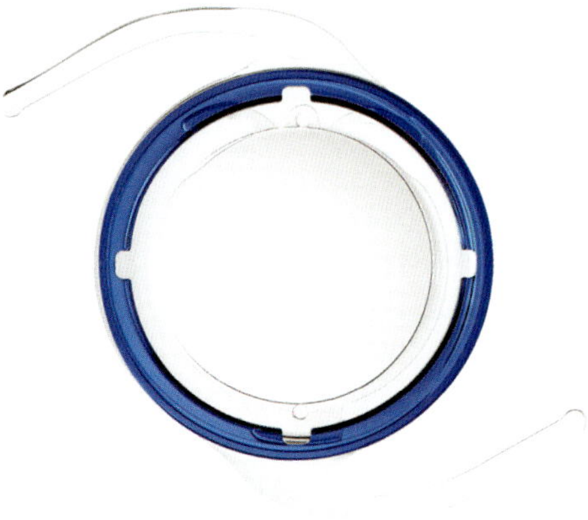

Figure 10-8 Example of a 2-piece modular lens (Harmoni). The central optic is detachable from the haptic base for ease of IOL exchange. *(Courtesy of Malik Kahook, MD.)*

optics to be used, including monofocal, multifocal, and toric lenses. The main advantage of this type of implant would be ease of exchange if a patient cannot tolerate a multifocal lens or if there is significant postoperative ametropia (ie, the refractive target was missed) in a monofocal lens.

Another type of lens, the *Smart IOL* (Medennium) is made from a thermoplastic acrylic gel. On insertion into the eye, the gel responds to body temperature and deforms to take the shape of the capsular bag. Theoretically, compression of this pliable lens by the capsular bag allows adjustment of its effective power in a manner analogous to the way the crystalline lens adjusts. Potential problems with this approach include difficulty in predicting the lens power that results from filling the capsular bag and uncertainty about management of posterior capsule opacification.

Alió JL, Ben-nun J, Rodríguez-Prats JL, Plaza AB. Visual and accommodative outcomes 1 year after implantation of an accommodating intraocular lens based on a new concept. *J Cataract Refract Surg.* 2009;35(10):1671–1678.

Saraiva J, Neatrour K, Waring GO IV. Emerging technology in refractive cataract surgery. *J Ophthalmol.* 2016;2016:7309283.

Additional Materials and Resources

Related Academy Materials

The American Academy of Ophthalmology is dedicated to providing a wealth of high-quality clinical education resources for ophthalmologists.

Print Publications and Electronic Products

For a complete listing of Academy clinical education products, visit our online store at:
https://store.aao.org/clinical-education.html

Or call Customer Service at 866.561.8558 (toll free, US only) or +1 415.561.8540, Monday through Friday, between 8:00 a.m. and 5:00 p.m. (PST).

Online Resources

Visit the Ophthalmic News and Education (ONE®) Network at https://www.aao.org/refractive-management-intervention to find relevant videos, online courses, journal articles, practice guidelines, self-assessment quizzes, images, and more. The ONE Network is a free Academy-member benefit.

Access free, trusted articles and content with the Academy's collaborative online encyclopedia, EyeWiki, at aao.org/eyewiki.

Get mobile access to the *Wills Eye Manual,* watch the latest 1-minute videos, and set up alerts for clinical updates relevant to you with the AAO Ophthalmic Education App. Download today: Search for "AAO Ophthalmic Education" in the Apple app store or in Google Play.

Basic Texts and Additional Resources

Azar DT, Gatinel D, eds. *Refractive Surgery.* 3rd ed. Elsevier; 2019.

Boyd BF, Agarwal S, Agarwal A, Agarwal A, eds. *LASIK and Beyond LASIK: Wavefront Analysis and Customized Ablations.* Slack; 2001.

Feder R. *The LASIK Handbook: A Case-Based Approach.* 2nd ed. Lippincott Williams & Wilkins; 2013.

Garg A, Rosen E, Lin JT, et al, eds. *Mastering the Techniques of Customized LASIK.* Jaypee Brothers; 2007.

Hardten DR, Lindstrom RL, Davis EA, eds. *Phakic Intraocular Lenses: Principles and Practice.* Slack; 2003.

Probst LE, ed. *LASIK: Advances, Controversies, and Custom.* Slack; 2003.

Troutman RC, Buzard KA. *Corneal Astigmatism: Etiology, Prevention, and Management.* Mosby; 1992.

Wang MX, ed. *Refractive Lens Exchange: A Surgical Treatment for Presbyopia.* Slack; 2015.

Waring GO IV, Rocha KM. *Femtosecond Lasers in Cornea and Lens Surgery.* Slack; 2020.

Requesting Continuing Medical Education Credit

The American Academy of Ophthalmology is accredited by the Accreditation Council for Continuing Medical Education (ACCME) to provide continuing medical education for physicians.

The American Academy of Ophthalmology designates this enduring material for a maximum of 10 *AMA PRA Category 1 Credits*™. Physicians should claim only the credit commensurate with the extent of their participation in the activity.

To claim *AMA PRA Category 1 Credits*™ upon completion of this activity, learners must demonstrate appropriate knowledge and participation in the activity by taking the posttest for Section 13 and achieving a score of 80% or higher.

This activity meets the Self-Assessment CME requirements defined by the American Board of Ophthalmology (ABO). Please be advised that the ABO is not an accrediting body for purposes of any CME program. ABO does not sponsor this or any outside activity, and ABO does not endorse any particular CME activity. Complete information regarding the ABO Self-Assessment CME Maintenance of Certification requirements is available at https://abop.org/maintain-certification/cme-self-assessment/.

To take the posttest and request CME credit online:

1. Go to www.aao.org/cme-central and log in.
2. Click on "Claim CME Credit and View My CME Transcript" and then "Report AAO Credits."
3. Select the appropriate media type and then the Academy activity. You will be directed to the posttest.
4. Once you have passed the test with a score of 80% or higher, you will be directed to your transcript. *If you are not an Academy member, you will be able to print out a certificate of participation once you have passed the test.*

CME expiration date: June 1, 2024. *AMA PRA Category 1 Credits*™ may be claimed only once between June 1, 2021, and the expiration date.

For assistance, contact the Academy's Customer Service department at 866.561.8558 (US only) or + 1 415.561.8540 between 8:00 a.m. and 5:00 p.m. (PST), Monday through Friday, or send an e-mail to customer_service@aao.org.

Study Questions

Please note that these questions are not part of your CME reporting process. They are provided here for your own educational use and for identification of any professional practice gaps. The required CME posttest is available online (see "Requesting Continuing Medical Education Credit"). Following the questions are answers with discussions. Although a concerted effort has been made to avoid ambiguity and redundancy in these questions, the authors recognize that differences of opinion may occur regarding the "best" answer. The discussions are provided to demonstrate the rationale used to derive the answer. They may also be helpful in confirming that your approach to the problem was correct or, if necessary, in fixing the principle in your memory. The Section 13 faculty thanks the Resident Self-Assessment Committee for drafting these self-assessment questions and the discussions that follow.

1. Which imaging technique for refractive surgery uses a low-intensity laser focused on the retina as a point source of light to assess the refractive state of the eye?
   a. Scheimpflug imaging
   b. thin-beam single-ray tracing
   c. spectral-domain optical coherence tomography
   d. Hartmann-Shack wavefront sensing

2. A patient with previous laser in situ keratomileusis (LASIK) and a refraction of −0.75 D undergoes surface ablation. What is the reason to use mitomycin C (MMC) in this case?
   a. In a patient with previous LASIK, MMC can prevent haze after surface ablation.
   b. MMC is approved by the US Food and Drug Administration (FDA) for the prevention of post–photorefractive keratectomy (PRK) haze.
   c. This small amount of treatment does not present a high risk of scarring, and MMC should be avoided because of potential toxicity.
   d. Irrigation of the cornea with MMC is performed to reduce pain and haze.

3. What is a disadvantage of small incision lenticule extraction (SMILE) compared with excimer-based refractive procedures?
   a. SMILE causes more disruption of anterior corneal innervation.
   b. SMILE results in less biomechanical stability.
   c. SMILE has more stringent specifications in terms of local environmental factors that can affect treatment predictability.
   d. SMILE has a more limited therapeutic range.

4. A 45-year-old patient with myopia desires monovision correction with LASIK. The nondominant right eye is chosen for near vision and has a refraction of −5.00 sphere. Assuming no nomogram adjustment is required, how many diopters of refractive treatment would be appropriate to program into the laser?
   a. −3.50 D
   b. −6.50 D
   c. −0.75 D
   d. −1.50 D

5. In refractive surgery, MMC is commonly employed in what concentration and for what duration?
   a. 0.002% for 2–4 minutes
   b. 0.02% for 12–120 seconds
   c. 0.2% for 12–120 seconds
   d. 2.0% for 10–30 seconds

6. Which organism is the most common pathogen in cases of infectious keratitis after LASIK?
   a. *Pseudomonas* spp
   b. *Staphylococcus* spp
   c. *Mycobacterium* spp
   d. *Nocardia* spp

7. Which refractive procedure is most likely to cause surgically induced ectasia?
   a. LASIK
   b. epikeratophakia
   c. PRK
   d. intrastromal corneal ring segment

8. Haze following PRK typically peaks approximately how long after surgery?
   a. 1–2 days
   b. 1–2 weeks
   c. 1–2 months
   d. 6–8 months

9. A patient with a refraction of plano +2.00 × 45 is scheduled for astigmatic keratotomy. Which operative plan is likely to achieve the best refractive result?
   a. paired arcuate incisions centered at 45° and 225° with an optical zone of 7 mm
   b. paired arcuate incisions centered at 135° and 315° with an optical zone of 4 mm
   c. paired arcuate incisions centered at 45° and 225° with an optical zone of 4 mm
   d. paired arcuate incisions centered at 135° and 315° with an optical zone of 7 mm

10. What is a risk factor for delayed epithelial healing after PRK?
    a. decentered ablation
    b. keratoconjunctivitis sicca
    c. hyperopia
    d. high myopia

11. Which wavelength of energy, when applied to the cornea, is characterized by high energy and precision, low penetration of tissue, and limited thermal spread?
    a. 193 nm
    b. 365 nm
    c. 1053 nm
    d. 2.13 μm

12. What is the most common risk factor for epithelial ingrowth following LASIK?
    a. epithelial defect near flap edge
    b. macrostriae
    c. Fuchs dystrophy
    d. high refractive error

13. Which refractive surgery places a patient at highest risk for a ruptured globe from blunt trauma?
    a. LASIK
    b. radial keratotomy (RK)
    c. refractive lens exchange with sclerocorneal incision
    d. refractive lens exchange with clear corneal incision

14. What is an appropriate initial option to improve myopic astigmatism caused by post-LASIK corneal ectasia?
    a. wavefront-guided enhancement
    b. refractive lens exchange
    c. radial and astigmatic keratotomy
    d. rigid gas-permeable contact lens

15. Why might increasing the optical zone in myopic LASIK or PRK limit the ability to treat patients with thinner corneas?
    a. It increases the risk of postoperative glare and halos.
    b. It increases the chance of regression.
    c. It decreases predictability of the refractive outcome.
    d. It increases the ablation depth.

16. A 26-year-old patient undergoes LASIK for the treatment of −9.00 D myopia. The ophthalmologist notes slightly decreased vision and glare symptoms 1 week postoperatively. The examination findings are normal with the exception of flap striae. What is the most likely cause of the striae?
   a. diffuse lamellar keratitis
   b. high myopic treatment
   c. ectasia
   d. epithelial ingrowth

17. A patient presents with nuclear cataracts in both eyes. He has a history of a bilateral 16-incision RK procedure with a 3-mm optical zone. His corrected distance vision is limited to 20/60 in both eyes related to the cataracts, and he undergoes cataract surgery and intraocular lens (IOL) implantation. At his 2-week postoperative visit, his vision is corrected to 20/25+ with a measured refractive error of +1.50 −0.50 × 120. He is very unhappy with his uncorrected vision, as he had hoped for either an emmetropic or a slight myopic outcome. What would be the best option at this point?
   a. Perform an IOL exchange, leaving him hyperopic.
   b. Plan a surface ablation to correct his hyperopic outcome.
   c. Inform him that this is a typical outcome in RK eyes and that glasses are the best option.
   d. Assure him that the hyperopia might lessen with resolution of corneal edema.

18. What is the best way to prevent post-LASIK macrostriae?
   a. meticulous flap realignment with minimal irrigation
   b. use of thin flaps
   c. use of sterile distilled water as the interface irrigating solution
   d. aggressive irrigation during flap repositioning to remove any debris

19. One month after a patient undergoes PRK, subepithelial haze develops. What is the preferred initial management?
   a. topical MMC
   b. oral prednisone
   c. observation
   d. phototherapeutic keratectomy

20. How does the Kamra corneal inlay correct presbyopia?
   a. It changes the refractive index of the cornea.
   b. It increases depth of field by using a small aperture.
   c. It steepens the cornea to induce myopia.
   d. It induces collagen shrinking to achieve myopia.

21. A 48-year-old woman has a persistent central corneal epithelial defect 2 weeks after PRK. She has a bandage soft contact lens in place and is using preservative-free artificial tears and topical nonsteroidal anti-inflammatory drugs (NSAIDs) every 2 hours. Her Schirmer test scores are normal. What is the best initial management option?
   a. Place a lower eyelid punctal plug.
   b. Discontinue topical NSAIDs.
   c. Add topical cyclosporine 0.05% eyedrops 2 times daily.
   d. Add topical prednisolone acetate 1% eyedrops 4 times daily.

22. In wavefront analysis, what type of optical aberration is coma?
   a. orthogonal astigmatism
   b. spherical aberration
   c. third-order aberration
   d. positive defocus

23. How are the incisions made for limbal relaxing incisions different from those made for arcuate keratotomy?
   a. more beveled
   b. more peripheral
   c. shorter
   d. shallower

24. What medical history finding in a 25-year-old man would be a relative contraindication for LASIK?
   a. asthma
   b. seropositivity for HIV
   c. depression
   d. multiple sclerosis

25. In LASIK, an RSB thickness of less than 250 μm is associated with which postoperative complication?
   a. haze
   b. ectasia
   c. epithelial ingrowth
   d. diffuse lamellar keratitis

26. A patient who presents 8 months after penetrating keratoplasty (PKP) with the concern of poor vision due to astigmatism is interested in laser refractive surgery. What is the appropriate recommendation for this patient?
   a. PRK is the best option because creation of a LASIK flap risks dehiscence of the graft.
   b. The patient should wait at least 1 year after PKP, and the refraction should be stable.
   c. LASIK is the best option to avoid postoperative haze induced by PRK.
   d. Because of the risk of graft dehiscence and the unpredictable nature of the results, laser refractive surgery should be avoided in patients who have undergone PKP.

27. How does laser refractive surgery affect the risk of retinal detachment in patients with myopia?
    a. The rapid increase and decrease in intraocular pressure during the procedure can stretch the vitreous base and lead to a posterior vitreous detachment (PVD), thereby increasing the risk of retinal detachment after refractive surgery.
    b. Acoustic shock waves from the laser could lead to the development of a PVD, thereby increasing the risk of retinal detachment after refractive surgery.
    c. Current data show that laser refractive surgery does not appear to increase or decrease the risk of retinal detachment.
    d. By eliminating myopia, refractive surgery reduces the risk of retinal detachment.

28. A patient experiences pain and light sensitivity 2 months after femtosecond laser–assisted LASIK. The eye appears white and quiet. What is the best initial treatment?
    a. flap lift with culture for suspected microbial keratitis
    b. intensive treatment with topical corticosteroids
    c. intensive treatment with topical antibiotics
    d. flap lift and irrigation of the lamellar space with sterile saline

29. Immediately after cataract surgery with a diffractive multifocal IOL, a patient reports visually disabling glare and halos that persist over the next several months. What is the best next step in management?
    a. IOL exchange with a refractive multifocal IOL
    b. IOL exchange with a monofocal IOL
    c. Nd:YAG capsulotomy; and, if that fails, an IOL exchange
    d. piggyback IOL

30. A 42-year-old man with adult-onset diabetes mellitus reports worsening vision at distance over the past 6 months. He has not worn eyeglasses or contact lenses but asks about the possibility of LASIK to correct his vision. He says that his blood glucose levels have ranged between 175 and 350 mg/dL (9.642–19.284 mmol/L) during the past 2 years, and his most recent HbA_{1c} was 8.5. Corrected distance visual acuity is 20/15 in each eye (right eye, 2.50 sphere; left eye, 2.00 sphere), and findings from the ophthalmologic evaluation are otherwise normal. What is the most appropriate initial management?
    a. contact lens fitting
    b. eyeglass correction
    c. improving glucose control prior to reevaluation
    d. LASIK surgery

31. Which condition might prevent a 25-year-old patient from being a good candidate for PRK?
    a. pregnancy
    b. posterior polymorphous corneal dystrophy
    c. high myopia
    d. asthma

32. How does a Placido disk–based corneal topography device determine elevation changes?
    a. scanning slit beam of light swept across the cornea
    b. laser reflected off the retina and captured by a lenslet array
    c. image of a series of concentric rings reflected off the cornea
    d. ultrasonic image of the corneal surface

33. In the creation of a lamellar flap for LASIK, what advantage does the femtosecond laser offer compared with a microkeratome?
    a. shorter procedure time
    b. lower total treatment cost
    c. more predictable flap thickness
    d. increased iris registration success

34. What characteristic would indicate that a patient is a poor candidate for LASIK?
    a. predicted postoperative keratometry of 52.00 D
    b. inability to make wavefront measure
    c. history of keloid formation
    d. RSB thickness of 300 µm

35. Why are accurate IOL calculations difficult in a patient who has had laser refractive surgery?
    a. Most traditional keratometers measure only the central corneal curvature.
    b. The axial length cannot be accurately measured.
    c. Tear film abnormalities make it difficult to obtain keratometry readings.
    d. The relationship between the anterior and posterior cornea has changed.

36. A visually significant interlenticular membrane develops in a patient with piggyback IOLs. What treatment is preferred for this patient?
    a. removal of the membrane(s)
    b. observation
    c. Nd:YAG capsulotomy membranolysis
    d. removal of the IOLs

37. How does conductive keratoplasty affect the cornea?
   a. It results in a permanent change in the shape of the cornea.
   b. It works by decreasing the curvature of the central cornea.
   c. It works by increasing the curvature of the central cornea.
   d. The effect is mediated by a holmium:YAG laser.

38. Which process is responsible for securing a LASIK flap immediately after surgery?
   a. endothelial pump activity
   b. corneal scarring
   c. corneal epithelialization and spreading
   d. flap position and shape

39. Binocular diplopia can occur in patients after LASIK as a result of which problem?
   a. decompensated phorias
   b. optic nerve ischemia
   c. corneal edema
   d. flap striae

40. What is the mechanism through which the femtosecond laser interacts with tissues?
   a. photocoagulation
   b. photoablation
   c. photodisruption
   d. photothermal effects

Answers

1. **d.** Wavefront aberrometry is used to assess the total refractive error of the eye, including both lower-order and higher-order aberrations. Of the 4 methods that are available clinically, Hartmann-Shack is the most common. In this technique, light from a low-power laser reflected off the retina is used as a point source of light. This light travels back through the optical system of the eye, then passes through an array of lenslets and focuses onto a detector. The divergence of the image from each lenslet from the expected focal point enables the reconstruction of the total wavefront. Thin-beam single-ray tracing, Tscherning, and optical path difference are other methods of aberrometry. Scheimpflug imaging is used in certain corneal topographers to determine the shape of the cornea. Spectral-domain optical coherence tomography is used in imaging but does not help to measure the refractive power of the eye.
2. **a.** Mitomycin C (MMC) is used off label to decrease the chance of corneal haze development after surface ablation in moderate to high treatments. It is also used even in small treatments in patients who previously had photorefractive keratectomy (PRK), laser in situ keratomileusis (LASIK), penetrating keratoplasty (PKP), or radial keratotomy (RK). MMC is not approved by the US Food and Drug Administration (FDA) for use in refractive surgery. The cornea is copiously irrigated with balanced salt solution (BSS) to remove MMC, and some surgeons apply chilled BSS after surface ablation in the belief that this reduces pain and haze formation.
3. **d.** The therapeutic range of small incision lenticule extraction (SMILE) is more limited than that of excimer treatments. The SMILE procedure (at the time of this publication) is approved for the treatment of myopia with or without astigmatism from −1.00 D to −10.00 D sphere, and from −0.75 D to −3.00 D cylinder with a manifest refraction spherical equivalent greater than −10.00 D. It is not approved for hyperopic treatments. However, SMILE is thought to be more stable biomechanically, less disruptive of anterior corneal innervation, and less affected by local environmental factors.
4. **a.** Monovision to modify presbyopia in phakic individuals can be an effective strategy for reducing dependence on spectacles. The process involves intentionally undercorrecting a myopic patient, overcorrecting a hyperopic patient, or inducing mild myopia in an emmetropic patient. Many refractive surgeons target mild myopia after treatment (−0.50 to −1.50 D) to achieve good uncorrected near- to intermediate-distance vision, making a treatment of −3.50 D (leaving a residual of −1.50 D) the correct answer choice. *Mini-monovision* would entail correction to achieve the lower end of myopia (−0.50 to −0.75 D) for the near-vision eye, resulting in only a mild decrease in distance vision, retention of good stereopsis, and a significant increase in intermediate-zone function. Blended vision would entail correction to achieve myopia in the range of −1.00 to −1.50 D.
5. **b.** MMC is commonly used off label to reduce the formation of haze after surface ablation procedures such as PRK or phototherapeutic keratectomy (PTK). Typical concentrations used are 0.01%–0.02%, applied for 10–120 seconds. Complications caused by dosage errors include corneal melting; other complications include infectious keratitis, delayed corneal healing, and corneal scarring.
6. **b.** Post-LASIK infectious keratitis typically begins 2–3 days after surgery and features a focal inflammatory reaction not necessarily confined to the flap interface. Often, there

is an inflammatory deep corneal and/or anterior chamber response. The pathogens that most commonly cause keratitis after laser ablation are the gram-positive bacteria *Staphylococcus* and *Streptococcus* spp. The next most common causative organisms are atypical *Mycobacterium* spp, *Nocardia asteroides*, and fungi. If infection is suspected, the flap should be lifted and the interface cultured and irrigated with antibiotics.

7. **a.** Ectasia is far more common after LASIK than after PRK. This is related to the residual stromal bed (RSB) thickness, which is far less after LASIK flap creation than after surface ablation. Intrastromal corneal ring segments (ICRS) can be used to reduce the irregular astigmatic error from ectasia but cannot prevent ectasia progression. Epikeratophakia, a largely obsolete procedure, featured the suturing of a donor lenticule on top of the Bowman layer of the host cornea.
8. **c.** Subepithelial corneal haze develops as a result of epithelial–stromal wound healing and appears several weeks after surface ablation, peaks in intensity at 1–2 months, and gradually diminishes or disappears over the following 6–12 months.
9. **a.** Arcuate, or astigmatic, keratotomy can be quite useful for the surgical management of astigmatism. The closer the incisions are to the center of the cornea, the more effect they have—and the greater their potential for inducing visually significant irregular astigmatism. An optical zone of 7–9 mm is typical, while a 4-mm optical zone is too narrow and would have a high incidence of irregular astigmatism. The incisions will flatten the cornea in the meridian of the incision and steepen the cornea 90° away when performed in an arcuate fashion, which is the most common pattern used for astigmatism. In this specific patient, incisions centered at 135° and 315° would increase the astigmatism and are in the wrong axis. It is critical to ensure that the incisions are performed in the correct axis for arcuate keratotomy.
10. **b.** Patients with ocular surface disease may have problems with epithelial healing. This is especially true in patients with large epithelial defects that occur after surface ablation procedures, such as PRK.
11. **a.** A variety of laser–tissue interactions are used in keratorefractive surgery. Argon-fluoride excimer laser generates a wavelength of 193 nm with high energy and precision but low tissue penetrance and little thermal spread, making this laser highly suitable for use on the ocular surface. Femtosecond laser generates a wavelength of 1053 nm that causes photodisruption, which transforms tissue into plasma with high pressure and temperature and leads to rapid tissue expansion. This forms microscopic cavities that are useful in the creation of stromal flaps and channels. Holmium:YAG laser generates a wavelength of 2.13 μm that has a photothermal effect. When applied to the anterior stroma, water in the cornea absorbs the energy and creates heat that shrinks surrounding collagen. This is useful in causing corneal steepening at the anterior surface, and this technique (laser thermokeratoplasty) is approved by the FDA for the treatment of low hyperopia. Collagen crosslinking devices produce a wavelength of 365 nm (ultraviolet A) that, while not used in refractive surgery, is used in the treatment of corneal ectasia.
12. **a.** Epithelial ingrowth is reported to occur in less than 3% of eyes undergoing LASIK. Epithelial defects along the flap edge are a major risk factor, as stromal edema can lead to poor flap adherence early after the surgery. This can allow epithelium to heal under the flap rather than over the top of the flap. Care should be taken to prevent epithelium from being caught under the flap at the time of LASIK. An additional risk factor is secondary flap lifts, such as those performed for an enhancement or surgical repositioning of flap striae. Although there can be a greater tendency for the flap to adhere poorly in the eyes

of patients with Fuchs dystrophy, this complication is unlikely to occur unless stromal edema is present. There does not appear to be any correlation with high refractive errors or flap striae.

13. **b.** Radial keratotomy (RK) incisions weaken the structure of the eye for years after the procedure. Traumatic injury can lead to rupture of RK incisions and has been reported up to 13 years after RK. Although refractive lens exchange with a sclerocorneal or clear corneal incision also creates a weak point, these incisions are not as susceptible to rupture as RK incisions. Full-thickness wounds are not created in LASIK, so there is less risk for a ruptured globe after LASIK than after RK.

14. **d.** Rigid gas-permeable (RGP) contact lenses are the gold standard for the correction of reduced vision due to ectasia. Surgical procedures that thin or destabilize the cornea (eg, LASIK, PRK, incisional procedures) might complicate the situation further. Ectasia can be progressive, so refractive lens exchange is also contraindicated. Because the contact lens fit and power can be modified as the ectasia progresses, RGP contact lenses are the most appropriate treatment. Corneal crosslinking is the first-line treatment to prevent further ectasia, but it does not improve vision as much as RGP contact lenses.

15. **d.** All photoablative procedures result in the removal of corneal tissue. The depth of myopic laser ablation by a broad-beam laser is estimated by the Munnerlyn formula:

$$\text{Ablation Depth } (\mu\text{m}) \approx \frac{\text{Degree of Myopia (D)} \times \text{Optical Zone Diameter [OZ (mm)]}^2}{3}$$

As the ablation diameter increases, the depth required for a given refractive correction increases by the optical zone squared. Thus, the increase in ablation depth is not linear and can rapidly exceed the structural capacity of the cornea to achieve the ablation depth and still maintain appropriate RSB thickness. However, complications of glare, halos, and regression increase when the optical zone decreases, and increasing the optical zone would actually improve these issues. For this reason, the optical zone should be 6 mm or larger.

16. **b.** When present, 95% of flap striae are noted by 1 week postoperatively. Risk factors include excessive irrigation under the flap at the time of surgery, thin flaps, or large ablations with subsequent mismatch of the flap to the underlying stroma. In this clinical situation, the striae are most likely due to the high myopic treatment. Diffuse lamellar keratitis (DLK) presents with haze near the edge of the flap to central diffuse haze. It can occur after a primary procedure or after flap lift or trauma. It is an inflammatory process that results in the accumulation of white blood cells in the interface. DLK does not present as flap striae. Ectasia does not occur at 1 week postoperatively and does not present as striae. Ingrowth is more likely to occur in patients with an epithelial defect at the time of surgery or after re-treatments.

17. **d.** After cataract surgery on eyes that had prior RK, short-term flattening of the cornea and hyperopic shift are frequently noted as a result of the corneal edema after surgery. Therefore, in the event of a refractive surprise, neither an intraocular lens (IOL) exchange nor PRK should be considered in post-RK eyes until the cornea and refraction stabilize, which can take several weeks to months.

18. **a.** The best way to prevent flap folds, or *macrostriae,* is meticulous flap realignment with minimal irrigation. Risk factors for the development of macrostriae include aggressive irrigation under the flap during LASIK flap repositioning (such as to remove debris), thin flaps, deep ablations with flap–bed mismatch, and postoperative flap slippage. In addition,

the use of hypotonic saline or sterile distilled water as the interface irrigating solution may cause flap swelling and reduce flap diameter, delay flap adhesion, and worsen striae after the flap dehydrates. When present, macrostriae almost always become apparent in the early postoperative period. It is important to recognize and address this complication early, as the success of interventions decreases greatly over time, and this problem can cause visually significant irregular astigmatism. The surgeon must examine the surgical eye(s) carefully to check for the presence of gross full-thickness folds (intraoperatively) or flap slippage (postoperatively).

19. **c.** Although subepithelial haze can occur early or late after PRK, the incidence peaks at 1 to 2 months and gradually diminishes over 1 year. Increased numbers and activity of stromal keratocytes may be the source of extracellular deposits. Haze is known to resolve spontaneously with normal wound remodeling; thus, observation is indicated soon after surgery. If clinically significant haze persists, superficial keratectomy or phototherapeutic keratectomy (PTK) may be performed but should be delayed for 6 to 12 months. Topical MMC may be used to prevent recurrence after superficial keratectomy or PTK. Steroids, typically applied topically, can be increased in patients with haze and in patients who are undercorrected to improve both haze and residual refractive error. Oral prednisone would not be indicated.

20. **b.** The Kamra inlay (CorneaGen) uses a 1.6-mm central aperture to produce a pinhole effect and increase depth of field in the nondominant eye, thus providing near vision. The Flexivue Microlens (Presbia; not FDA approved) is a hydrophilic acrylic clear inlay with a different index of refraction than the cornea and a central aperture for distance vision. A hydrogel inlay that steepened the central cornea to induce myopia (Raindrop Near Vision Inlay; Revision Optics) was formerly available but has been withdrawn. Conductive keratoplasty uses radiofrequency energy to shrink collagen and steepen the central cornea to achieve myopia.

21. **b.** Topical nonsteroidal anti-inflammatory drugs (NSAIDs) can be applied after surface ablation to reduce postoperative pain, but they can slow epithelialization and result in corneal melting, stromal scarring, and irregular astigmatism. Corneal epithelial defects after surface ablation typically heal in 3–4 days postoperatively. Topical NSAID drops should be discontinued for any patient who is not healing normally after refractive surgery. A frequent cause of delayed epithelialization is keratoconjunctivitis sicca, which can be treated with increased lubrication, topical cyclosporine, and/or temporary punctal occlusion; however, this patient has normal Schirmer test scores and is already receiving frequent preservative-free artificial tears, so these measures are not indicated as first-line treatments. Topical steroidal anti-inflammatory drops such as prednisolone acetate will not likely improve epithelialization in this case.

22. **c.** Optical aberrations measured by wavefront analyzers, such as the Hartmann-Shack wavefront sensor, can be described by an infinite number of systems. Zernike polynomials, one set of wavefront descriptors, are the mathematical formulas used to describe surfaces. The most important Zernike coefficients affecting visual quality are coma, trefoil, and spherical aberration. Coma and trefoil are third-order aberrations. With coma, light rays at one edge of the pupil come into focus before rays at the opposite edge; the effective image resembles a comet, having vertical and horizontal components. Coma is common in patients with decentered corneal grafts, keratoconus, and decentered laser ablations. Lower-order (second-order) aberrations include myopia, hyperopia, and regular astigma-

tism. Myopia produces positive defocus, hyperopia produces negative defocus, and regular (cylindrical) astigmatism produces a wavefront aberration that has orthogonal and oblique components. Spherical aberration, a fourth-order aberration, is the most clinically significant higher-order aberration. It increases depth of field, but decreases contrast sensitivity, causes night myopia, results in halos around point images, and is commonly increased after myopic LASIK and surface ablation.

23. **b.** The closer an incision is to the center of the visual axis, the greater the effect on the refractive error of the eye. Arcuate keratotomy (AK) incisions have been made at various optical zones. Limbal relaxing incisions (LRIs) are placed closer to the limbus than AK incisions. In general, to achieve a similar effect, LRIs should be longer than AK incisions, although this is not specific to the definition. In addition, the cornea is thicker in the periphery; therefore, LRIs should generally be deeper than AK incisions for the equivalent refractive result. The degree of beveling is not specifically different for most surgeons' technique for astigmatic incisions.

24. **b.** Immunocompromised status, including HIV infection or AIDS, represents a relative contraindication to refractive surgery because of the potential for increased risk of infectious complications. The FDA recommends that patients with an immunodeficiency disease not undergo LASIK because the risk outweighs the benefits. Although the other responses do not represent contraindicated states per se, it is important to assess for conditions associated with each of them: atopy in the case of asthma, optic neuritis in the case of multiple sclerosis, and dry eye disease due to antidepressant use in the case of depression.

25. **b.** While exact mechanisms of postrefractive corneal ectasia are not fully known, an RSB thickness of less than 250 μm is a recognized risk factor for this postoperative complication. Flap creation thicker than anticipated, preoperative forme fruste keratoconus, higher myopic correction, thin corneas, and multiple laser ablations are also risk factors. However, no single risk factor is an absolute predictor of ectasia after LASIK. In order to reduce the risk of this complication, surgeons should review topography and perform pachymetry prior to surgery. In addition, the RSB thickness should be calculated. It can be estimated preoperatively by subtracting the anticipated flap thickness plus ablation depth from the central corneal thickness; however, intraoperative pachymetry is the most accurate way to measure flap thickness and calculate the RSB thickness to confirm whether it is safe to proceed with ablation. Although the other 3 answer choices are complications of LASIK, they are not related to the RSB and can occur at any RSB thickness.

26. **b.** Laser refractive surgery is an option for improving ametropia after PKP. Most surgeons advocate waiting at least 1 year after transplant and an additional 4 months after sutures are removed. Moreover, refraction and corneal topography should be stable, as measured on 2 consecutive visits at least 1 month apart. Both LASIK and PRK are options for patients who have had PKP. To avoid postoperative haze associated with PRK, MMC should be used. LASIK after PKP is subject to the same patient evaluation constraints as conventional LASIK. There is a small but significant risk of wound dehiscence during both LASIK and PRK; therefore, the graft–host interface must be carefully inspected for areas of variable coaptation. Although the results of laser refractive surgery in post-PKP eyes are less accurate and predictable than in eyes with naturally occurring refractive errors, the surgery can still significantly reduce refractive error and improve the visual outcome when combined with glasses or contact lenses.

27. **c.** Patients with high myopia are at a higher risk of retinal detachment, but LASIK and PRK do not appear to increase the risk for these patients compared with patients in similar populations who have not had laser refractive surgery. While it has been proposed that intraocular pressure changes or acoustic shock waves from the laser can induce a posterior vitreous detachment, studies do not show an increased retinal detachment risk in patients after laser refractive surgery. Although laser refractive surgery eliminates the refractive component of myopia, the natural history of the highly myopic eye is unchanged. Therefore, the elevated retinal detachment risk of a myopic eye remains.
28. **b.** Postoperative photophobia with good acuity is a rare entity that can occur weeks to months after femtosecond laser–assisted LASIK. Patients develop acute onset of pain and photophobia in a white and quiet eye in which both the cornea and the flap interface appear normal. The treatment consists of frequent application of topical corticosteroids and cyclosporine. The flap does not have to be touched.
29. **b.** All multifocal lenses have the potential to cause halos. Many patients experience a decrease in halos over several months, possibly from neuroadaptation. However, if the halos are persistent and disabling, an IOL exchange with a monofocal IOL may be the only option. A piggyback IOL would not address the halos. Although patients with multifocal IOLs may be more sensitive to the visual effects of posterior capsule opacification (PCO), symptoms from PCO are typically not present initially but gradually develop over the first few weeks to months after surgery. In contrast, intrinsic IOL symptoms appear early, if not immediately, in the postoperative course and stay consistent over time. Moreover, performing an Nd:YAG capsulotomy would make future lens exchanges more difficult.
30. **c.** Refractive error can fluctuate with changes in the blood glucose level, so the blood sugar of a patient with diabetes must be well controlled at the time of evaluation to ensure an accurate refraction. For this reason, diabetic patients with labile blood glucose should be carefully counseled if eyeglasses or contact lenses are to be prescribed. Elective ocular surgery should not be performed in a diabetic patient with poor or erratic blood glucose control.
31. **a.** Pregnancy and breastfeeding can cause a temporary change in refraction, which makes refractive surgery potentially less accurate. Many surgeons recommend waiting at least 3 months after delivery and cessation of breastfeeding before performing the refractive surgery evaluation and procedure. High myopia, posterior polymorphous corneal dystrophy, and asthma are not contraindications for PRK.
32. **c.** A Placido disk–based corneal topography instrument captures and analyzes the image of a series of concentric rings reflected off the corneal surface. The computer measures the distance from the edge of each ring to the next ring along multiple semi-meridians and generates a map of the corneal surface that would be required to produce the captured image. These data are frequently expressed in pseudocolor maps. The system can present the pseudocolor maps in several ways, including axial curvature, tangential curvature, and best-fit sphere; it can also show an image of the rings themselves as seen by the computer.
33. **c.** Several studies have compared the benefits of the mechanical microkeratome with those of femtosecond lasers in creating flaps. Minimal differences between the techniques have been found for most patients. However, the flap thickness achieved with the femtosecond laser is generally more predictable, with less variability than flaps created with a mechanical microkeratome. See Chapter 4, Table 4-1, which summarizes the advantages and disadvantages of the femtosecond laser.

34. **a.** There seems to be an increase in spherical aberration in patients with a postoperative keratometry of greater than 50.00 D. For this reason, such patients are usually not good refractive surgery candidates. The current guidelines recommend a minimum RSB thickness of 250 μm, although this is not based on any controlled prospective studies. A history of keloid formation is not a contraindication to LASIK. If a reliable wavefront measurement cannot be obtained, then conventional LASIK can be performed.

35. **d.** Numerous formulas have been developed to help with IOL selection after refractive surgery, but there is no infallible way, at present, to calculate IOL power because of the nature of the postrefractive cornea. Standard IOL calculations make certain assumptions about the relationship between the anterior and posterior curvatures of the cornea, which is altered by photoablation. In addition, the effective central optical zone after refractive surgery is typically small, and most keratometers measure corneal curvature several millimeters away from the center of the cornea, resulting in inaccurate estimation of the true central corneal power. Because the eye's axial length does not change after laser refractive surgery, axial measurements should remain accurate. Some formulas rely on keratometry to estimate the effective lens position, which may be inaccurately estimated, resulting in errors, depending on which IOL formula is used. Tear film abnormalities may make it difficult to obtain keratometry readings; however, this effect, if properly treated, does not contribute errors to the IOL calculations.

36. **d.** Piggyback lenses may be used in patients who require more correction than a single IOL can provide or in patients who have a refractive surprise after cataract surgery. The conventional implantation technique involves placing one IOL in the capsular bag and a second IOL with its haptics in the ciliary sulcus. Interlenticular membranes have been reported to occur between 2 acrylic IOLs, especially when both lenses are implanted in the capsular bag. The preferred treatment is to remove the IOLs. Observation alone will result in progressive visual deterioration and delay and potentially complicate definitive intervention. Nd:YAG capsulotomy and intraocular removal of the membrane do not prevent progression.

37. **c.** Conductive keratoplasty (CK) works by radiofrequency shrinkage of collagen lamellae in the cornea. It is approved by the FDA for the treatment of hyperopia and presbyopia. The CK probe is applied at various intervals in the periphery of the cornea. A small corneal scar is initially seen, which fades over time. The peripheral shrinking of the corneal collagen results in an increase in the curvature of the central cornea. The holmium:YAG laser has been used in laser thermokeratoplasty, which CK has replaced. One disadvantage of CK is that the effects are often temporary.

38. **a.** Immediately after LASIK, corneal suction pressure from dehydration by the endothelium provides adhesion to secure the flap. Corneal scarring has a role in the late postoperative phase, but not immediately after surgery. Healing of the corneal epithelium does not play a significant role in flap adherence. The flap position and shape do not provide any adhesive effect.

39. **a.** Rare complications of LASIK include optic nerve ischemia, premacular subhyaloid hemorrhage, and macular hemorrhage from prior lacquer cracks or choroidal neovascularization. Diplopia can occur in patients who have iatrogenic monovision or problems of accommodation when they have had prior strabismus. Decompensated phorias can also manifest after LASIK. Typically, flap striae would cause monocular diplopia or multiple images, rather than binocular symptoms. Screening for decompensated phorias with a contact lens trial might be useful.

40. **c.** The femtosecond laser is used to create flaps for LASIK, channels for stromal inlays, and keratoplasty incisions, as well as in femtosecond laser–assisted cataract surgery. It works by a mechanism called *photodisruption.* This process occurs when tissue is changed into plasma that leads to the formation of stromal microscopic cavities. Contiguous photodisruption allows for creation of the corneal flap, channel, or incision. *Photothermal* laser effects cause tissue modification as illustrated by use of a holmium:YAG laser, which generates heat that results in collagen shrinkage. An example of *photoablation* is the excimer laser used in LASIK and PRK. This process breaks chemical bonds within tissue. *Photocoagulation* is primarily used in retinal lasers and results in a thermal burn to tissue.

Index

(*f* = figure; *t* = table)